HOW TO PREPARE FOR THE DENTAL ADMISSION TEST (DAT)

Richard A. Lehman

CONTRIBUTING AUTHORS

Suzanne L. Khalil, M.F.A.
Ph.D. Candidate
Department of Psychology
Arizona State University

A. W. Whitehead,
D.M.D., M.Ed., M.B.A.
Director, Student Affairs
University of Pittsburgh
School of Dental Medicine

Sharon Joyce, M.Ed.
Former Director of Admissions
University of Pittsburgh
School of Dental Medicine

Jason L. Burak
D.M.D. Candidate
University of Pennsylvania
School of Dental Medicine

Scott M. Blyer
D.D.S. Candidate
SUNY-Stony Brook
School of Dental Medicine

Assaf T. Gordon
M.D. Candidate
University of Pittsburgh
School of Medicine

Brian Stern
D.M.D. Candidate
University of Pittsburgh
School of Dental Medicine

Thomas J. Meals
D.M.D. Candidate
University of Pittsburgh
School of Dental Medicine

BARRON'S

CS ChemDraw™ by CambridgeSoft Corporation was the chemical structure drawing program used to illustrate the chemical structures.

Reading Comprehension Test (excerpts in Model Examinations A and B): Reprinted with permission from *The Compendium of Continuing Education in Dentistry* 18(10): 1002, 1006–1010, 1997.

Reading Comprehension Test (excerpts in Model Examinations A and B): from *Clinical Periodontology*, 8th edition by Fermin A. Carranza, Jr., et al. Copyright © 1995, pp. 17–21, 36–39. Reprinted with permission from W. B. Saunders Company, Philadelphia, Pennsylvania.

© Copyright 1999 by Richard A. Lehman

All inquiries should be addressed to:
Barron's Educational Series, Inc.
250 Wireless Boulevard
Hauppauge, NY 11788
http://www.barronseduc.com

Library of Congress Catalog Card No. 98-33115

International Standard Book No. 0-7641-0577-9

Library of Congress Cataloging-in-Publication Data
Lehman, Richard A.
   How to prepare for the dental admission test, DAT / Richard A. Lehman.
      p.   cm.
   Includes bibliographical references.
   ISBN 0-7641-0577-9
   1. Dental schools—United States—Entrance examinations—Study guides.   2. Dentistry—Ability testing.   3. Dentistry—Examinations, questions, etc.   I. Title.
   (DNLM: 1. Dentistry examination questions. 2. Aptitude Tests.
3. Educational Measurement.   WU 18.2 L523h 1999)
RK76.L44   1999
617.6′0076—dc21
DNLM/DLC
for Library of Congress   98-33115
                                                                                   CIP

Printed in the United States of America
9 8 7 6 5

CONTENTS

PREFACE

ACKNOWLEDGMENTS

This test preparation guide is the result of the cooperative work of many individuals. I would like to thank the faculty, staff, and administration at the University of Pittsburgh School of Dental Medicine for unanimously supporting my efforts in writing and editing this book. I am indebted to Grace Freedson and Lynne Vessie, as well as many others at Barron's Educational Series, Inc., for their assistance during the working stages of the manuscript. I also must acknowledge that this massive project originated in the mind of Scott Blyer; I merely acted on his idea.

I would also like to express my gratitude to a few contributors who unselfishly devoted their time and energy: David Dorenfeld for preliminary work on the Perceptual Ability Test; Jay Haraphongse for putting together information on the Canadian DAT; Yulia Mayzenberg, Lavinia Wu, Andrew Cheifetz, Robert Laughlin, Andrew Diamond, and Christine Wankiiri for permission to reprint their AADSAS personal statements; Steven Marsh, D.D.S., Ben Williamowski, D.D.S., and Janet Century, D.M.D., for their insights regarding the profession of dentistry. I would like to thank Edward Thibodeau, D.M.D., Ph.D., for his review and analysis of the entire manuscript; R. Mundell, Ph.D., and N. Long, D.D.S., for their constructive criticism of the manuscript; Dev Chandra for his work on the organic chemistry questions; Thomas Meals for his continued help with illustrations and for his assistance in the last-minute crunch; Corinne Caccas for her efforts in reviewing and selecting the reprinted Personal Statements; Brian Stern for the Reading Comprehension Test review; Scott Blyer for the general chemistry review; Assaf Gordon for the biology review; Suzanne Khalil for the Perceptual Ability Test review; Jason Burak for the Quantitative Reasoning Test review; Sharon Joyce and A. W. Whitehead, D.M.D., for insights into the application process; Cassandra Allen for reviewing the general chemistry and organic chemistry sections for errors and omissions. I am grateful for the continued guidance and encouragement that I have received from my friend and dental confidant, Noushin Azizi.

I am eternally indebted to Suzie and James Fourtier, Jonathan Bassman, and Julie Du for their assistance in putting the final work together.

To Suzie, James, Jon, Julie, Ne, and Papa—thank you for your unwavering love and support. Thanks Dad and Liz for encouraging me to write the original proposal for this book. And finally, thanks Mom for encouraging me to pursue dentistry in the first place. You knew all along that the biological sciences coupled with the hands-on, intricate work specific to dentistry would be a perfect compliment to my interests and abilities. I love you all.

A NOTE TO THE APPLICANT

Dear Future Colleague,

You have purchased the only comprehensive DAT review written specifically for the dental school applicant. The review chapters are tailored to the scope of examination established by the ADA Department of Testing Services. Much effort has gone toward including only the most relevant material, that which has the highest probability of appearing on the exam.

You will find that some other concerns and questions of many applicants are addressed in the chapter titled Dental Education and Practice. Information about the American Association of Dental Schools Application Service (AADSAS), letters of recommendation, the Personal Statement, and interviews, as well as some material on career options and dental organizations, is included in this chapter.

Some available DAT review guides rename chapters adapted from MCAT preparation materials, whereas other guides provide no review of the subject matter. Also, because Barron's Educational Series, Inc., a proprietary corporation not affiliated with the American Dental Association or the American Association of Dental Schools, publishes this book, the contents are not "sugar-coated"; you are getting a realistic picture of what to expect on the DAT, in dental school, and in a career in dentistry.

The DAT, and therefore this book, should be treated with much seriousness as your future may be determined by your performance on this exam. While an excellent score on the DAT *does not* ensure that you will be accepted into a dental school, a low score does ensure that you will *not* be accepted. The DAT will most likely be the most important examination you will ever take: it will affect not only your admission to a *university*, but also your admission to a *career*. In a real way, your future as an aspiring dentist is riding on this test.

Believe it or not, admissions officers want to accept you into their dental schools. The two numbers that are used to screen applicants initially are the GPA and DAT scores. Make sure your scores on the DAT are competitive. Do not give the admissions officers a reason to reject you!

Hopefully, this book will serve as a valuable study aid and as a resource to assist in your preparation for the DAT and for the application procedure that will soon ensue.

I wish you the best of luck on the DAT and in your dental career.

Sincerely,

Richard

Richard A. Lehman

ABOUT THE AUTHOR

Frustrated by the lack of test preparation material available during his review for the DAT, Richard A. Lehman assembled a team of professors, dentists, dental students, and other individuals to write the first complete test preparation book specifically for the DAT. As contributing editor of the official *ASDA Handbook: A Resource Guide for Predental Students*, he has considerable insight into the concerns of the dental school applicant.

A graduate of Pennsylvania State University, Richard is currently studying at the University of Pittsburgh School of Dental Medicine and School of Public Health in the D.M.D. and M.P.H. degree programs, respectively. He is the president of his dental school class and holds a national ASDA leadership position on the Editorial Board. Richard is actively involved in the pursuit of knowledge through research. He is a member of the Author's Guild, National Institute of Dental and Craniofacial Research (NIDCR), Alpha Omega Dental Fraternity, and the American Student Dental Association (ASDA).

In his free time he enjoys skiing, cycling, and running. As for his ambition in life, he says he would like to become a dentist when he grows up.

This book is dedicated to the applicant who seeks a career in dentistry because of three motivational factors: an intellectual curiosity in the sciences, a true love for intricate artistic work, and a humanistic instinct to provide care to others.

It is this individual who will find the greatest satisfaction and reward through the practice of dentistry.

INTRODUCTION

ABOUT THE DAT

The American Dental Association Department of Testing Services annually reports on the *appropriateness* of the DAT. It has been proved through statistical analysis that the test battery is a significant indicator of success in dental school as well as a valuable indicator of performance on Part I of the National Board Dental Examinations. The DAT is also used as a method of standardizing and quantifying the undergraduate preparation received at various academic institutions.

The Dental Admission Testing Program is administered by the ADA Department of Testing Services. It consists of *four timed sections*:

- **Survey of the Natural Sciences (SNS)**
- **Perceptual Ability Test (PAT)**
- **Reading Comprehension Test (RCT)**
- **Quantitative Reasoning Test (QRT)**

Although there are only four timed sections, there are six scored sections. Notice in the list below that the Survey of the Natural Sciences has three scored sections that are administered in one timed section. *You will receive the following* ***eight*** *score reports*:

- **Biology** (Questions 1–40 of the Survey of the Natural Sciences)
- **General Chemistry** (Questions 41–70 of the Survey of the Natural Sciences)
- **Organic Chemistry** (Questions 71–100 of the Survey of the Natural Sciences)
- **Quantitative Reasoning**
- **Reading Comprehension**
- **Total Science** (a combination of the biology, general chemistry, and organic chemistry raw scores)
- **Academic Average** (a composite score that is an average of the quantitative reasoning, reading comprehension, biology, general chemistry, and organic chemistry scores)
- **Perceptual Ability** (a score that is not incorporated in the other composite/combination score reports; it is always reported separately)

The specifics regarding the number of questions and the time allotted for each section are as follows for the Dental Admission Testing Program:

SECTION	QUESTIONS	TIME AVERAGE	AVERAGE TIME PER ITEM
Survey of the Natural Sciences	100 questions; (40 Biology, 30 General Chemistry, 30 Organic Chemistry)	90 minutes	54 seconds/question

(continued)

SECTION	QUESTIONS	TIME AVERAGE	AVERAGE TIME PER ITEM
Perceptual Ability Test	90 questions (composed of 6 different sections)	60 minutes	40 seconds/question (see section for specifics on timing)
BREAK		15 minutes	
Reading Comprehension Test	50 questions (three passages with 16–17 questions following each passage)	60 minutes	20 minutes/passage
Quantitative Reasoning Test	40 questions	45 minutes	1 minute 7 seconds/question
TOTAL	280 questions	4 hours 30 minutes (start to finish)	

SCORING

The DAT is scored on a 30-point scale with 30 being the highest mark and 1 being the lowest. *There is no penalty for wrong answers.* The total number of correct answers on each section is the raw score. The score on each section that is reported to you and to the dental schools you select is your *standard score*. It is the standard score that is used to compare one administration of the exam to another. The actual derivation of the standard score is quite complex: it utilizes a log ability scale based on the Rasch psychometric model. What you need to know is that a score of 16 is about the national average on most sections of the DAT. You should aim to get above this national average on all sections. A composite score of 17–18 is currently the average of enrollees in the first-year classes. *Therefore, a score of 17–18 should be your goal.* A standard score of 17–18 converts roughly to a raw score of 65–75% of questions answered correctly, so of 40 biology questions, for example, you should be able to answer approximately 28–30 correctly.

The average standard score report from the 1997 computerized DAT (N = 1,719) was 16.60 with an average standard deviation of 2.93. This means that approximately 65% of test takers received a standard score between 13.67 and 19.54. Approximately 92% scored between 10.73 and 22.47 (*Note*: standard score reports are given in whole numbers; fractional numbers are used for statistical analysis only). The average scores over the past years show an upward trend, as the applicant pool becomes more and more competitive.

HISTORY OF THE DAT

The Dental Admission Testing Program began in 1945 with a test battery that included sections on mathematics, verbal reasoning, reading comprehension, science, and object visualization/chalk carving. In 1972, organic chemistry was added to the test battery and the chalk carving was replaced with a perceptual-motor ability test. In 1981, the format was changed again to include a Reading Comprehension Test, Quantitative Ability Test, Perceptual Ability Test, and Survey of the Natural Sciences. In 1993, a paper-folding section was added to the DAT.

In 1996, a computerized version of the test was piloted. After statistical information from the computer-based examination was collected and analyzed, the

Council on Dental Education and Licensure voted to discontinue the administration of the written DAT as of the October 1998 examination. Ten minutes have been added to the Reading Comprehension Test. Students may take the current computer-based examination almost any day of the year through Sylvan Learning and Technology Centers.

A NOTE TO CANADIAN STUDENTS

There are some distinct differences between the American Dental Admission Test (DAT) and the Canadian Dental Aptitude Test (DAT). The following major differences should be noted:

- **The Canadian DAT is administered in the written format, as opposed to the computerized American DAT.**
- **The Canadian DAT includes a *Carving Dexterity* Test; the American DAT does not.**
- **The Canadian DAT does not include *organic chemistry* in the Survey of the National Sciences Test, nor does it have a *Quantitative Reasoning Test*. The American DAT has both.**

The Canadian Dental Association (CDA) and the ADA sample exams included in the test preparation materials of these two bodies are *identical*, word for word, for the following sections: perceptual ability, biology, general (inorganic) chemistry, and reading comprehension. Therefore, this book is well suited for review of the sections tested on the Canadian DAT battery with the exception of the Carving Dexterity Test. A lengthy explanation, including helpful hints, of exactly what is tested in the soap-carving section is included in *Preparation Manual: Dental Aptitude Test*, published by the CDA.

Practice for this section of the Canadian DAT is essential, and you can purchase practice materials directly from the CDA at the following address:

The Dental Aptitude Test Program
c/o Canadian Dental Association
1815 Alta Vista Drive
Ottawa, Ontario K1G 3Y6
phone: 613-523-1770

Specific information regarding the administration of the CDA can readily be obtained from the Ottawa office of the DAT program or from faculty of the 10 Canadian dental schools. Contact information for these schools is included in WWW Addresses in the appendix of this book.

Other publications, all free, offered by the CDA include *Dentistry: Is It for You?*, *Accredited Dental Education Programs*, and *Dental Practice in Canada*.

THE ART OF TEST TAKING

In order to take the Dental Admissions Test (DAT), you need only to pay the required fee, register, show up at the testing site, and spend several hours answering the battery of test questions. Alternatively, you have chosen to do more than just take the test. By purchasing this book, you have begun a commitment to something much greater. Your decision to engage in test preparation is a sign that you seek to take control of the test and that you believe that performance is largely a result of preparation. Hopefully, the following comments regarding test preparation for the DAT will prove useful.

Studying and Preparation Strategies

Study What You *DON'T* Know

After a few weeks of studying for this exam, you will find that much of the material looks familiar. Concentrate on acquiring the information you don't have rather than continuously reviewing the information that you've read before. This tip seems obvious, but failure to follow it is the downfall of many test takers.

Utilize All Your Senses

Read the material, write the material, and speak the material to maximize the experience of learning. If you enhance the learning experience, you will enhance your ability to recall that experience.

Use Repetition

Read, write, and speak the information for 6 weeks, and you will be able to recall important facts with greater ease.

Don't Study Just the Sciences

Any single low score on any section could be reason to *not* accept you, whereas a single high score will *not* greatly help your application. High scores across *all* sections are what is desired.

For the SNS, Create Mnemonics

For an easier way to remember unfamiliar or unrelated science information, make up mnemonics. Major corporations that rely on phone orders usually spell out a familiar word to make it easier for their customers to remember their phone number (1-800-GO FEDEX is a lot easier to recall than 1-800-463-3339). Make up phrases and words that stand for difficult to remember items of information in biology, chemistry, and organic chemistry.

Allow Sufficient Time

Do not schedule your examination before you can realistically be prepared to take it. Only you will know how much time you will need to spend reviewing. Use the model exams in this book to gauge your proficiency with the subject matter. Schedule a date that will permit you to critically and thoroughly review all the material for the exam. Usually 6 weeks is sufficient for the average student; but, depending on how much time you will dedicate to studying each day, you may require only 4 weeks, or as many as 8, to fully cover all the material.

Be Disciplined

This is the common strategy of all test takers who score in the top few percentiles. It is through hard work that high marks are achieved. Discipline yourself to a regimented schedule of studying for the DAT. Do not let anything come between you and the scores you desire. Between now and your test date, many things will try to distract your attention from your studies, but *be disciplined*!

Test-Taking Strategies

Answer EVERY Question

On the DAT, unlike the SAT, you are *not* penalized for wrong guesses. You will have a 20% chance of guessing the correct answer if you respond randomly.

Beware of *All* and *None*

The ADA Department of Testing Services does not want to have to rescore examinations and answer inquiries regarding ambiguous questions. Therefore, "gentle" words, such as *usually*, *often*, and *rarely*, are preferred in answer choices. "Harsh" words—*always*, *never*, all, *none*—can prove disastrous if any one exception can be argued. If you are really baffled on a question, steer clear of choosing an answer containing a "harsh" word.

Be Knowledgeable About Distracters

The wrong answer choices to a question are termed distracters because their purpose is to distract the test taker from the obvious correct answer. The ADA Department of Testing Services does not really want to confuse you; rather, it wants the correct answer to blend in with the wrong answers. The distracters lure the test taker from the correct answer by presenting possible answers that may be partially correct. On any given question, the distracters will be similar in their "degree of distraction." The following example will illustrate how to identify and eliminate distracters.

1. What is the first day of the week?
   A. January
   B. Monday
   C. Saturday
   D. 1st
   E. Sunday

It is obvious that Sunday, answer E, is correct. However, this simple example clearly shows how difficult science answers will be structured. Answers A and D test to see whether you can identify the days of the week. January is the first month of the year, and the 1st is the first day of the month. If you did not know the days of the week but you knew the months of the year, you might be distracted because January is the first month of the year. Answer C not only is a day of the week, but also starts with the same letter as the correct answer. This could distract the test taker who could identify the days of the week and who may have read once that Sunday is the first day of the week. The last distracter, answer B, Monday, is the type that you will find on the most difficult questions. Even if you know the days of the week and their sequence, you may still accidentally choose this distracter if little thought is put into selecting the answer. While Monday is the first day of the work week, it is not the first day of the calendar week.

Supplemental information must be used to eliminate the wrong answers. Do not get caught in the trap of choosing the most familiar and comfortable answer. On a difficult organic chemistry question involving an obscure reaction that you are not familiar with, undoubtedly at least two familiar reactions will appear in the answer choices as distracters. You will want to choose one of these as the correct response because we all like to feel comfortable with our answers. Use any knowledge you possess about any answer choices to identify distracters and thus eliminate them.

Draw It

You will almost always be able to more clearly understand what is being asked if you can sketch a chart, a figure, or some other graphical representation of the question you are asked. You will be given an unlimited amount of paper at the Sylvan Learning Center; use it to your advantage.

Know the PAT Directions

Before the test date, be sure that you know exactly what you will be asked to do in each section of the Perceptual Ability Test. For the other tests, the directions are rather straightforward; for the PAT, however, they are not as clear-cut. A sufficient review of the material presented in this book should clear up any confusion as to what will be required of you on the PAT's six sections.

Be Sensible About Sleep, Eating, and Exercise

To give a peak performance on the day of the test, you will need to take care of yourself in the days prior. Eat right, get plenty of sleep, and exercise the week before the test. Getting adequate sleep the night before will not compensate for a series of late nights. Also, it is generally difficult to sleep the night before the test.

Get Ready the Night Before

The night before the test, you should have everything accounted for so that no last-minute stresses will distract you on test day. Be sure that everything you need is in order and that plans are set for your timely arrival at the test site. Again, your focus on the test is reinforced by a general sense of control over the situation. Have clear plans for the test day that include what you will eat, wear, and take to the center.

Be Prepared to Succeed

At the test site, remain calm. Don't be concerned about sweaty palms or a slightly racing heart. You know that you are prepared, and your body is reflecting the excitement that you feel—you are ready to peak!

About Anxiety

By viewing your future goals as intimately connected to your actions in the present, you will undoubtedly acknowledge the value of engaging in preparative measures to ensure future success. You will possess a sense of control over your performance. Control will help you to stay focused, to remain in the present, and to use the mental tools that you have worked hard to refine. When you possess a high level of self-control, anxiety can serve you positively in two ways: It can help to keep you motivated as you actively prepare and it can even help boost performance on the day of the test.

It is normal to be anxious about the DAT. In fact, it would probably be a sign of concern if you had no qualms about the test. The fact that you possess a degree of anxiety suggests that you respect the difficulty of the test, the importance of peaking on test day, and the value of a high score. Anxiety will be your mentor, reminding you to actively prepare for this test. Anxiety will help to ensure that you have taken care of important details, such as verifying that you have the proper identification and familiarizing yourself with the best way to get to the test site. On the day of the test, if you maintain a sense of being in control of your own destiny, as discussed above, you will walk into the testing center confident that your hours of preparation will pay off. During the test, your slightly rapid heart rate will serve to keep you working at a productive pace. You will remain alert, and you will perform to your best ability.

Become Comfortable with the Computerized Format

Because the test will be administered on computer, you should be certain to clear up any concerns about the computer format prior to your test date. It is strongly suggested that you order the computer tutorial from the ADA Department of Testing Services. This will help you to know what the test will look like on the computer screen and how you can register your answers appropriately. You should also consider ahead of time how you will use your scratch paper. Although you will be given an unlimited supply, you must become comfortable with using it instead of marking directly on the test. There are suggestions for how to make the best use of scratch paper throughout this review guide.

DENTAL EDUCATION AND PRACTICE

THE APPLICATION PROCESS

Timeline of Events

Understanding the sequence of events in the application process should reduce the confusion and alleviate some stress. However, it should be noted that there is no correct sequence. You should use this timeline as a suggestion; then create your own timeline tailored to your individual situation.

When should you take the DAT? With the computerized format, you are now able to take the test at your convenience, so, the best answer is as soon as you are adequately prepared. Schedule time to review for the DAT, and then arrange an appropriate date with your local Sylvan Technology and Learning Center. You should try to take the DAT before the fall semester of your senior year (or the fall of the year prior to matriculation if you are not currently enrolled).

Note: You do not have to take the DAT before applying through the American Association of Dental Schools Application Service (AADSAS). Filling out and submitting your application early is imperative to maximizing your chances for acceptance. When you take the DAT, your scores will be sent directly to the dental schools to which you are applying through AADSAS.

The following timeline is a suggestion of when events should occur for the typical undergraduate who is seeking admission to dental school. Some extra suggestions have been included; however, they are not essential and are indicated with an asterisk (*).

Junior Year—Fall

- Start saving money for AADSAS fees and interviews.*
- Informally visit and tour the dental schools you have an interest in attending.*
- Keep your grades up.
- Intern with a dentist.*

Junior Year—Spring

- Register for the DAT (or summer between junior/senior year). First, send appropriate application materials to the ADA. You will receive a card instructing you to register with Sylvan. The 800 number will be indicated. Schedule your test date with the National Registration Center.
- Schedule a meeting with the Pre-Health Professions Advisor in your college or with faculty members to lay the groundwork for your letters of recommendation.
- Practice a mock dental school interview with your Pre-Health Professions Advisor, a faculty member, or a dentist.

- Start drafting your Personal Statement and have it reviewed by an on-campus writing specialist.
- Complete the Personal Statement.

Junior/Senior Summer

- Apply through AADSAS.
- Make sure you have appropriate clothes for an interview.
- Ask yourself these questions: Have you paid all necessary secondary processing fees to the schools to which you have applied? Have you submitted any additional information that was requested?

Senior Year—Fall

- Check your application status at the schools to which you have applied. A school will notify you if you are invited for an interview. Not all candidates are interviewed; only those who pass the first round of reviews from the Admissions Committee are invited to the school. It can't hurt, though, to inquire about your application status; and if your application is missing anything, the director of admissions will let you know.
- After an interview, send a follow-up thank you note to your interviewer.
- Keep in mind that the agreed national notification date for the AADS is December 1.
- If (When) you are accepted, remit a deposit to the school of your choice and withdraw your application from the others.
- Complete all necessary paperwork.
- Notify your Pre-Health Professions Officer of your decision, and thank him or her for help. Or, if you used individual faculty members and health practitioners, let them know of your decision and express your appreciation.
- If you plan to apply for financial aid, file your taxes as soon after January 1 as possible, as this will facilitate the process of awarding financial aid.

Senior Year—Spring

- Receive and complete financial aid paperwork provided by your school's Financial Aid Office.
- Complete orientation forms, and take care of predental school tasks, such as collecting teeth and getting your hepatitis shots.*

Senior Year—Summer

- Find housing accommodations.
- Try to network with current dental students, who can give you advice regarding books to buy, the best place to set up your bank account, and other details to make your transition to dental school as easy as possible.

American Association of Dental Schools Application Service (AADSAS)

In order to apply to most dental schools (50 out of 54 U.S. schools and all 10 Canadian schools), you must use a universal application that is offered through the American Association of Dental Schools Application Service (AADSAS). The AADSAS application enables a student to apply to several schools with greater ease and has helped Admissions Committees to efficiently process and review applications.

AADSAS serves merely as a clearinghouse for applications; this service plays no role in the evaluative aspect of the admissions process. Students who apply through AADSAS submit transcripts, a Personal Statement, a list of intended future coursework, information regarding participation in activities, financial aid requests, and letters of recommendation. For a fee, AADSAS processes all of this information and then disseminates it in a profile folder and on diskette to each school that the candidate has indicated an interest in attending. Thus, with one AADSAS application, a student can apply to several schools.

After all required documents and fees have been submitted to AADSAS, the service generally takes from 3 to 6 weeks to process an application and send it to all of the candidate's requested schools. Upon receipt of your official AADSAS identification number, you can be confident that your materials are on the way to the schools you indicated.

Once the AADSAS profile folders and diskettes are received by a dental school, the Admissions Committee reviews them and then selects candidates for interviews. The main items of information from the AADSAS application that the Admissions Committee will weigh are your grades (science and nonscience), Personal Statement, letters of recommendation, and DAT scores.

It should be mentioned that, although most schools rely solely on the information provided by the AADSAS application, some schools also have secondary applications. It is important, therefore, that you find out exactly what is required in the application process for each individual school.

Common mistakes to avoid in filling out the application include not following the specific directions provided by AADSAS and leaving blanks. If you are not sure how to answer something on the AADSAS application, call the service directly or call a dental school admissions officer for advice. Mistakes made on the AADSAS application can hold up your application for weeks. As time is of the essence, avoid submitting an AADSAS application with errors.

In the event that you become aware of an error made on an application that has been submitted to AADSAS and disseminated to the schools you indicated, you must request AADSAS to complete the paperwork needed to issue a revised application to each school to which you are applying.

Although not required, it is suggested that you submit an AADSAS application prior to your senior year. In the event that you do apply earlier, however, you will need to update your application with current grades (up to and including fall grades from your senior year) and note any other additions or changes by using the revised application form provided by AADSAS.

AADSAS applications are usually made available in the middle of the summer. To request an application, or to receive more information, you can contact the service directly at 800-353-2237 or 202-667-1887 or at the following address:

1625 Massachusetts Avenue, NW
Suite 600
Washington, D.C. 20036-2212

The service can also be reached by e-mail: aadsas.appl@aads.jhu.edu or on the web: http://www.aads.jhu.edu.

In addition to providing the application service, the American Association of Dental Schools provides a useful guide that is recommended for review by prospective dental students. Published yearly, *Admission Requirements: United States and Canadian Dental Schools* ($25) includes each school's most recent incoming class profile (average DAT scores, GPAs, etc.). Additionally, information is given about the program offered by each dental school, and the composition of the student body is described. For more information about this and other resources, refer to the Appendix section titled Other Publications and Resources (page 427).

Letters of Recommendation

Letters of recommendation play a key role in Admissions Committees' decision-making process. They serve as an analysis and critique of your abilities and true desire to attend a school of dental medicine. Most dental schools require a minimum of three letters of recommendation for your file to be considered complete. These letters should come from faculty members, preferably in the sciences, of your college.

Admissions Committees prefer to review letters that not only comment on your intellectual abilities but also address your personal demeanor. Because you are attempting to enter a profession that requires patient interaction, your communicative skills and compassion should be critically assessed. Furthermore, as the competitiveness for positions in dental schools escalates, Admissions Committees are adamant about selecting students who have experience in dental medicine, whether this be observational or hands-on. Recommendations can serve to address any experience you have had in the field of dentistry.

Generally speaking, if you and another applicant appear similarly qualified on paper—same grades, DAT scores, and the like—your letters of recommendation could be the deciding factor between your admittance and the other candidate's.

If you are serious about attending dental school, it is suggested that you start finding possible recommenders during your undergraduate studies. This means that you should attend classes, be prepared, sit in the front row, ask questions, and approach faculty members early on to disclose your desire to study dentistry. Although you will not formally need to secure your letters until your junior year, if you identify yourself—favorably, of course—early, you will be remembered later.

The type of institution you attend may dictate the type of recommendation letter dossier you will compile. Some colleges have Pre-Health Profession Committees. If you attend a large university, more than likely there is an on-campus Pre-Health Professions Office. This office is specifically designed to advise and assist students whose goal is to attend a graduate health professions school, whether it be medical, dental, physical therapy, or other. (Some smaller colleges also have these resources.)

Undergraduate students are often unaware that a Pre-Health Professions Office exists at their college or university, or they assume that this office is only for students preparing to gain admittance to medical school. If you are unsure as to whether your undergraduate college or university has a Pre-Health Professions Office, check with your academic advisor.

The Pre-Health Professions Office is responsible for compiling and mailing out your letters of recommendation, thereby helping to ensure their confidentiality. Whether or not you make use of a Pre-Health Professions Office, you will be asked to sign a statement that you waive the right to read your letters of recommendation. Although you have the option to retain this right, the norm is to waive it. The person you ask to write a letter for you may not give an entirely reflective and honest account of your abilities if you have access to his or her statement.

Some colleges have the Pre-Health Profession Committee write a profile on you that is mailed to the schools you wish to attend. If your school adheres to this practice, you probably will need to make a formal appointment for an interview with the Pre-Health Profession Committee. You should take this interview very seriously; it will be similar to any formal interview you will have at a dental school. The individuals who comprise the Pre-Health Profession Committee are professionals who either have been selected or have volunteered to serve as reviewers of the potential pre-health professions candidates at their particular college or university. There will be faculty from the sciences, student service personnel, and the chair of the Pre-Health Professions Office, who may be either a faculty member or a student service professional.

Appearing before the Pre-Health Profession Committee is a rigorous process. Prior to your interview, the members will often request to review a Personal Statement (this can be the same statement that you submit to AADSAS) and your official college transcripts. During your scheduled formal interview, they will review your grades and ask you about your desire to attend dental school, your exposure to dental medicine, and your hobbies and activities (see "The Interview," page 17). After you meet with the Pre-Health Profession Committee, the members will review your candidacy, draft a comprehensive letter, or complete a Likert scale form that assesses your abilities. The committee then assigns a recommendation rank. Usually the rank represents some variation of "Highly Recommend;" "Recommend;" "Recommend with Reservation;" or "Do Not Recommend."

Given that this can be an arduous process, why would a student choose to go through the Pre-Health Profession Committee? *A letter of recommendation from the Pre-Health Profession Committee is preferred over individual letters from faculty.* This is not to say that you will be penalized if your school does not have a Pre-Health Profession Committee. However, Admissions Committees are aware that the Pre-Health Profession Committee is an assemblage of persons who possess the knowledge base and skills to accurately assess future health care practitioners.

While some Pre-Health Professions Offices actually issue the recommendations, others make it the student's responsibility to approach faculty recommenders for the written assessment. The faculty submit their recommendations directly to a Pre-Health Professions Office, which, in turn, will compile the letters and mail them out at the student's request.

It is obviously in your best interest to approach professors with whom you have had some interaction, even if limited, or for whom you performed well in their course(s). Ideally, your recommenders are professors who know you well and have seen your potential. After selecting these professors, you should arrange individual meetings with them to discuss your goals and reasons for selecting the dental schools you have chosen.

If your hands-on or observational experience in dentistry has been only with family members, it is suggested that these persons not write recommendations. Given the familial connection, such endorsements are not appropriate and will not be given serious consideration.

Regardless of whether you are using a Pre-Health Profession Committee or an assemblage of faculty recommenders, you should provide these persons with your personal statement, resume, and transcript. The more documentation you provide, the easier it will be for them to write strong letters.

When you meet with the Pre-Health Profession Committee or with your faculty recommenders to discuss your goals and reasons for applying to dental school, you should also address your strengths and weaknesses. Be honest about any shortcomings in your academic record. Nobody but you can provide the personal insight that is often needed to humanize data and to account for any blemishes that appear in your file. It is important that you state what you have done to overcome setbacks or how you have dealt with adversity.

Once you have completed the appropriate meetings, be sure that the committee or individual faculty members have all they need to complete the recommendation. Find out when your committee letter or individual faculty letters will be complete. If you are not making use of a Pre-Health Profession Committee, and individual faculty members are writing the recommendations, it is suggested that you collect and mail them. These recommendations *must* be sealed and bear the instructors' signatures across the seal of the envelopes.

Lastly, acknowledge the time and effort that went into writing the recommendations by sending thank you letters to the committee or your individual faculty recommenders. Also, once a decision has been made concerning your dental schooling, you should notify those who offered you their support.

Supplemental Letters of Support

In some circumstances it is appropriate to submit more than the required number of letters of recommendation. If you have spent time observing or assisting in a dental office or have performed some type of noteworthy community service, you may also submit supplementary letters of recommendation. Although most schools request only three letters of recommendation, *it is acceptable to go over this limit* within reason. If you are going through the committee process and its members are writing your formal letter, you may ask to have a supplemental letter or supplemental letters added. Generally, the committee will readily comply with this request.

A Special Note to Nontraditional Students

If you have made the decision to attend dental school after being in the work force for a number of years, you may also submit supplemental letters from your employer(s). However, it is still advisable to follow the protocol of submitting letters from faculty members, preferably in the sciences. If your alma mater has a Pre-Health Professions Office, you should still, as an alumnus/alumna, have access to its services. Otherwise, you should follow the recommendations for traditional students in this situation.

Personal Statement

Your essay is the first form of personal contact that the Admissions Committee has with you. It is of utmost importance, therefore, that you write an essay that is truly reflective of your motivation to attend dental school. This essay serves as a unique personal window that only you can open for your readers.

In all strong essays, candidates use this opportunity not only as a means of introduction, but also as a way to highlight personal strengths and, where applicable, address any weaknesses that may have a bearing on their candidacy.

The Personal Statement is an appropriate vehicle to describe any honors you may have been awarded, whether academic or civic, and to tell why you were so recognized. Furthermore, any experiences you have had in the field of dentistry, such as an internship with a general practitioner, should be highlighted and explained in the Personal Statement. It is not enough to write that you have had "hands-on" experience. What did you do? What did you learn? Why did this experience or these experiences solidify your decision to attend dental school?

Also, you may describe any leadership positions you held during your undergraduate tenure, write about clubs you have been involved with, and/or discuss practical work experiences you have had. The point of providing this information is to demonstrate to the Admissions Committee that you are a well-rounded individual.

Address the depth of your experiences. For example, how did being a class officer help you to learn to work with others? Has your involvement in civic organizations heightened your compassion for others? Give concrete evidence as to why these activities have been meaningful to you, and also explain how they have contributed to your candidacy for dental school.

If you are applying to dental school after being out of college for a number of years, you should focus on your life experiences after earning your undergraduate degree. This out-of-school time will not be seen as a weakness in your essay if you compose a thoughtful statement integrating your recent activities with your aspirations. What wisdom and insight have you gained since leaving school? More importantly, why have you decided to pursue dental medicine; what has made you decide to change your career track? Or, if you are already working in the field of dentistry, as a hygienist, for example, why is it now important for you to further your education?

In addition to writing about your strengths, you may also wish to address any weaknesses in your overall application. For example, if your grades suffered during a particular semester, explain why. Perhaps a parent died or you were ill. In addressing your weaknesses, you should not elaborate in great detail; the gravity of a situation such as the death of a parent is well understood. Nor should weaknesses be the focus of your Personal Statement. You have only one page in which to clearly and concisely present yourself, so strategically compose your essay with an emphasis on the positive.

Because the Personal Statement serves as the Admissions Committee's first assessment of you as an individual, it is important to attract their attention at the outset. An opening paragraph that begins "Ever since I was a young child I have wanted to attend dental school" is trite and probably untrue. Approach this component of your application as an opportunity to be creative.

Brainstorm some experiences that you have had within the field of dentistry. Think of quotations to incorporate that summarize you as a person, embody your ethics, or have been of particular inspiration to you. Have a theme to your essay. Use humor with care—don't become too comedic, and be sure to avoid sarcasm. Most important, what have you accomplished in your life that sets you apart from the other 1,000 candidates applying to dental school? Don't trivialize your successes; be proud of your achievements while maintaining a sense of humility.

As the Personal Statement is part of your application to graduate school, it should be flawless and presented in a professional manner. Essays that are handwritten or contain many errors in spelling or grammar are unacceptable. Before submitting your final draft, proofread it several times. Also, find someone in your school's writing center who will critique and, where necessary, correct your Personal Statement. You might ask the faculty members writing your letters of recommendation or perhaps someone in a Pre-Health Professions Office to give you feedback on your essay.

It is expected that the Personal Statement be formally presented in a black, easy-to-read font. Before you print out your statement on the official form provided by AADSAS, make duplicates of the form and test-run your final essay through the computer's printer. You may discover that you need to adjust your margins to fit within the AADSAS format.

However you choose to approach the writing of your Personal Statement, try to readily embrace the task, rather than viewing it as an arduous chore. Remember that the words you write serve as a precursor to any interviews you wish to secure. A well-written, well-executed Personal Statement should pique the Admissions Committees' curiosity about you as a candidate and make them want to learn more during an interview.

Three Personal Statements from successful applicants are reprinted here to provide you with examples of well-written essays. Proper names have been omitted, but the essays are otherwise reprinted as they appeared on the AADSAS form. Examine how each statement contains details that shed light on the uniqueness of the applicant.

Personal Statement 1

Science and artistry, two seemingly unrelated terms, share a harmonious relationship with each other. I believe that dentistry reveals this intrinsic and unconstrained association, allowing the two terms to be juxtaposed in a natural way. I have devoted 16 years to the piano and 12 years to the flute; the two instruments have become prominent defining factors in my life. With the many required hours of practice each day and with the number of different performances, I have acquired a deep happiness and satisfaction in producing the art forms with my hands and fingers. Because of the emphasis I have placed on the development of manual dexterity, I feel that the career that I choose should in some way incorporate my hands to a large degree. I am a steadfast believer that the hands have an amazing power to heal.

I liken the practice of dentistry to the learning of a new musical piece: both facilitate the satisfaction of beginning a project and having a final product to show at the end. In dentistry, a problem is recognized; then certain skills are employed to remedy it. Whether it be filling a cavity or replacing a crown, the acquired techniques and skills are utilized and directed toward the specific situation. With the piano and flute, I slowly work each key, measure by measure, from the beginning, until the time tuning of the piece is accomplished. Both dentistry and the playing of an instrument require the mechanical skill that develops through years of training. The idea of focusing my mind on something specific and then applying a certain technique to achieve the desired goal appeals greatly to me.

Many people question health practitioners about the reasons they choose their certain profession. The answer "I want to help people" has been stated so frequently that it almost seems cliched; however, I truly believe that the words warrant greater respect. When I was seven, a tragic accident ended my brother's life. From that episode of my life, a seed was implanted within my mind to one day serve others and help them in some way, whether by performing music, saving lives, aiding in the betterment of health, or by other means. With involvement in activities that serve the community—soup kitchens, ministry within the church, performances at hospitals and geriatric homes, volunteering at the local hospitals, and charity concerts—I have realized that I ultimately want a profession that enables me to serve others. Because of my combined need to help people and love for science, I have found that dentistry has the special characteristics that many other occupations do not afford.

I hope that one day, as a practicing dentist, I will be able to help people feel better about themselves. I want to help people attain a beautiful smile and increase their level of self-esteem and confidence. Having grown up in Taiwan in the 1930's and 40's, my parents were not so fortunate as to have had the dental treatment that the present generations receive. I see how, in every photo, there is always embarrassment at being unable to show a nice smile because they are so ashamed of their teeth. I see the suffering and the pain that they go through, having received numerous crowns, bridges, and root canals. It is important to inform people that maintaining personal health and caring for one's teeth and gums are vital to everyday life. I want to show people that they can exercise control over their own health. Dentistry undoubtedly allows the possibility of achieving this goal.

Personal Statement 2

At the age of eleven, I possessed the facial structure of the nation's favorite TV horse, Mr. Ed. People were forced to duck whenever they came face to face with my teeth. Fortunately, my parents eagerly placed me in the hands of my would be hero, Dr. [omitted], who gave me not only a smile to be proud of but also the self-confidence and courage to venture into the most terrifying stage of life: adolescence. Amazing! The truth is, dentistry had fascinated me long before my braces came into existence. My lifelong exposure to the health care field, my innate interest in dentistry accompanied by the hands on experience I have gained in the profession throughout the years, and finally my desire to dedicate my life to the service of others are some of the reasons I have decided to pursue a career as a dentist.

As the daughter of a physician, the hard work, sacrifice, and devotion involved in the delivery of quality health care are well known to me. I was first exposed to patient care and interaction at the age of fifteen when my father asked me to work for him as an office clerk, and a short time later as a medical assistant. After seeing my father skillfully and confidently helping other human beings,

I knew my future work would be in the health care field. Although many of my summers were spent working as a medical assistant, never did I stray from my lifelong desire to become a dentist. Given my profound interest in dentistry, I contacted my regular dentist, Dr. [omitted], in [omitted], Georgia, and asked for the opportunity to observe him at work. My fascination lead me to advance from the status of "tourist," to volunteer worker, and finally to part-time employee during the summers of '91, '93, and '96. Currently I am volunteering six to eight hours a week at his office while I also work part-time as a medical assistant at my father's surgical practice. Not only does a career in dentistry give me the ability and freedom to establish my professional independence, but also the ongoing scientific and technical advancements in the field ensure continuous challenges and motivation, while allowing me the opportunity to enrich my life through humanitarian service to my community. I anticipate with much excitement the intellectual and personal challenges the dental field will provide throughout my years of practice.

At this time my primary interest lies in the field of pediatric dentistry. Because of the absence of a pediatric dentist in [omitted], I have had the delight of working with the many children who come into Dr. [omitted] office. For me, children are magical. I vowed to dedicate my future work to children in the summer of 1994 when I volunteered at the [omitted] Oncology Clinic for Children in [omitted], Georgia. Here I devoted my time to the entertainment and supervision of the children (patients and siblings) in the playroom. This experience reinforced the profound and innate joy the ability to help others as well as working with children gives me.

The highlight of my undergraduate studies at [omitted] University occurred during my senior year when I was granted the privilege to do research in the field of reproductive biology at the [omitted] Primate Research Center of [omitted] University. During the course of the year I studied the effects of certain cryoprotective additives on the biological and biophysical parameters of human embryos, and cow and rhesus monkey oocytes. Dissecting cow and rhesus monkey ovaries and extracting and recovering oocytes, along with their subsequent handling through the use of special pipettes, not only sharpened my mechanical abilities but also showed me how much I enjoyed the mechanical challenge of precision work. Thus, while patient care is to be my primary focus as a dentist, I nonetheless intend to actively engage in research while in dental school. Having lived in a rural area for almost ten years now, I know from firsthand experience the lack of and need for qualified and specialized health care professionals. I enjoy the life-style small towns have to offer, and as a result I plan to settle down in a rural area following my dental education. My ultimate goal is to better serve the more underprivileged communities with little or no access to dental care.

I would like to give back to dentistry what it has given to me: dedication, excellence, and compassion. There are currently five physicians, three physical therapists, three nurses, one speech therapist, and one optometrist in my family. I have had sufficient exposure to every single one of these areas, and not one of them has been able to captivate my interest as has dentistry. The beauty of dentistry lies within its power to coalesce the sciences, arts, and humanities to make it the unique vocation that it is. I desire more than anything the opportunity to be part of a field that allows me to help my fellow human beings while offering me the challenge and satisfaction necessary to lead a fulfilled and productive life.

Personal Statement 3

From my first retainer, to braces, to oral surgery, my teeth and I have experienced many of the services of the dental profession. No matter how physically uncomfortable a procedure, the dentists always treated me and their other patients with a compassion and devotion that instilled a certain resolve in me to pursue the field of dentistry.

My exposure to the dental profession has mostly been from the chair, and it was not until about a year ago that I came to the realization that dentistry was the perfect career for me. Past experiences and current visits to my own dentist to view the inner workings of the field have encouraged my desire, and everything about my decision began to fall into place. My attraction to dentistry began about seventeen years ago with my PlayDoh Dental Set. I spent many fun-filled hours making teeth, drilling, and pulling. At age five I remember discussing setting up a dental office with my friend. Of course, then it would have been a "you hold them down and I'll yank" type of practice. Luckily, I've become more sensitive since then! I know that my quest to become a dentist is real. I am adamant about committing to this intense, yet rewarding path.

To make sure that my choice was the right one, I spent a number of days in my dentist's office. The doctors there amazed me, not only by the technology used, but also by giving me a glimpse into the doctors' rapport with their patients. I was fascinated that children who are normally apprehensive about spending time in a dentist's chair could leave the office with a shine on their teeth and a smile on their faces. I spoke to a number of people in the field, and they were all dedicated, sincere professionals who left me feeling confident about my decision to attend dental school.

Apart from the actual dental work, I know that the doctor must have a trusting, caring relationship with each patient. This interaction is not something that can be obtained from books. My experience with community service both in high school and at [omitted] University has helped me to develop a greater understanding of people.

As a college freshman, I began with a volunteer organization and tutored a high school senior who read at a first grade level. While pleased with his progress, I realized that he needed more structured assistance than I could offer. I expressed my concerns to his guidance counselor and teacher, and succeeded in getting him into the school's special program. I was instrumental in starting an after school study program at an area high school. During my sophomore year, I assisted a graduate by teaching high school ESL students. This class was very rewarding. I taught half the students by myself, which gave me greater confidence speaking in front of people and articulating my ideas. For the past three years, my roommate and I have been a part of Project [omitted]. We pick up perishables from local businesses and deliver them to various shelters in the area to aid the homeless.

My greatest achievement as a volunteer has been working for "[omitted]." I have contributed a lot of time and effort to this program, ultimately serving as president for the past two years. "[omitted]" distributes donated furniture to those in the greater Providence area who cannot afford to buy their own. When out on a shift, I meet many people who directly benefit from "[omitted]." I have had many memorable experiences as a member of this organization.

In addition to these volunteer organizations, other extracurricular activities include intramural soccer and ice-skating. I played hockey for many years and take advantage of the time I can spend in an ice rink. From a teaching assistant in immunology, to an ice-skating instructor, to president of "[omitted]," my extracurricular activities have broadened my perspective and enriched me as a person. I especially enjoy interacting with children and had a job as a camp counselor for the past three summers.

This summer I am involved in research at [omitted] Cancer Center. Interning in the Human Immunogenetics Laboratory affords me the opportunity for intellectual growth and increased technical aptitudes. Not only am I gaining a great deal of knowledge from assisting in the lab on a groundbreaking study, but also the molecular biological protocol involves manipulating DNA and bacteria, which requires a delicate, exacting hand—excellent practice for dentistry.

I am excited at the prospect of embarking on a career in dentistry. I hope to incorporate my desire to work with children, and participate in current research along with my dental education and career. I look forward to it with great anticipation.

The Interview

Much preparation is required for an interview. The 20 to 30 minutes you spend in an interview may be the final contributing factor determining your acceptance to dental school. Interviewers are continually amazed at the number of applicants who drift into admissions interviews without any apparent preparation and only the vaguest idea of what they are going to say. Since the interview plays such a critical role in the selection process, you should prepare for it as you would for any other examination on which you would be evaluated.

In preparation for an interview, research the dental school that you will be visiting. Then prepare a short personal history that will help you focus on the important aspects that you would like to convey during the interview. Review the highlights of your undergraduate experience, summer jobs, research, volunteer work, and experience with dentistry. It is important to be able to relate some personal experiences and history in the interview in order to establish a rapport with the interviewer. The picture you provide to the interviewer must convince him or her that you are the best candidate for admission. Be ready to state why you chose the field of dental medicine and what unique perspectives you can bring to that particular school. Having a strong sense of oneself and taking adequate time to prepare will help the dynamics of the interview.

Applicants who have thoroughly prepared will enter into the interview process with focus and confidence. Be aware that the interview will start the moment you walk into the room. Your posture and manner will create a first impression. For this reason you should practice how to enter a room, sit, and stand. Maintain eye contact and a pleasant look. Positive facial expressions and body language set the mood for a constructive interview and can help conversation flow. You will want to manage the interview through posture, voice, and manner and to engage the interviewer by conveying thoughts and feelings with enthusiasm throughout the interview.

Listed below are some questions that interviewers frequently ask. Practicing your responses to these questions out loud will help you to become a more articulate and polished speaker.

- Why do you want to be a dentist?
- What originally stimulated your interest in dental medicine?
- What steps have you taken to acquaint yourself with what a dentist does?
- What do you do in your spare time?
- With so many well-qualified candidates, why should we invite you to enroll at our school of dental medicine?
- As an interviewer, what should I look for in a candidate?
- What prompted you to apply to our school?
- How would your plans differ if we were now under socialized medicine?
- What do you think is the most pressing issue in dental medicine today?
- What was the last book that you have read? Or favorite book?
- Have you previously applied to other educational programs (i.e., medicine, public health, or M.S. program)?
- How has your undergraduate major prepared you for dental school and a career in dentistry?
- What are your biggest fears?
- What are your strengths? Weaknesses?
- Is there anything else you would like us to know that hasn't yet been conveyed in your application?

Throughout the entire interview process, speak about those areas that you know best or feel passionately about. Your enthusiasm and interest, shown in your voice and accompanying facial expressions, will engage the interviewer. With proper preparation and confidence, you will have a successful interview.

Most interviews will have a traditional one-on-one format. Some schools, however, use a committee interview, which can be a bit more daunting than just meeting with one faculty member or dental school administrator. Prior to your interview, contact the Admissions Office and ask which format that particular school uses. If the answer is a committee format, you may want to practice before a simulated committee of friends or family. Generally speaking, the questions will be the same as in a one-on-one interview, but being questioned by more than one person can be a nerve-wracking experience. If you prepare for a committee interview, it will pose no greater challenge than the one-on-one format. Try to remember to address all interviewers rather than focusing on the person who asked you a particular question. If you stumble over a question, ask whether you can come back to it later; the interviewers know that you are human and it's normal to be a bit nervous.

An interview is your opportunity to view the school as a prospective applicant who may become an enrolled student. Not only are you being interviewed; this is your turn to interview the school. Therefore, be prepared to ask some questions of the interviewer regarding the dental school or even the dental profession. This will convey the message that you have a serious interest in the particular school or the future of dentistry.

Listed below are some commonly asked questions from prospective students:

- What is the faculty/student ratio? What percentage of the faculty is full-time? Part-time?
- What is the male/female ratio of the dental student body? Minority student enrollment? In state/out-of-state enrollment?
- What were last year's statistics for your incoming class? GPAs? DATs?
- How many of your graduates specialize in ortho, perio, endo, oral surgery, etc.?
- How many attended GPRs or AEGDs? How many went into the military?
- How much is tuition? How much are instruments, supplies, and other expenses? Is financial aid available? Are scholarships, grants, and fellowships available?
- What is the average student indebtedness at graduation?
- Are there opportunities for research?
- Can I pursue any other degrees, such as an M.P.H. or M.B.A., while I am a dental student here?
- How did your students perform on the National Boards last year?
- What can you tell me about the patient pool and how patients are assigned?
- Where do most of the dental students live? What is an average figure for the cost of living?
- Is the school located in a safe area?
- How are curriculum problems addressed and are there any?
- Do the students have any participation in the decision-making process for the school?
- What clubs, student dental organizations, and fraternities exist?
- With all of the school requirements, is it difficult to participate in extracurricular activities?

Most interviews are scheduled so that you will have the opportunity to meet current dental students, admissions staff, financial aid officers, and, of course, faculty members. You should also be provided with a tour of the facilities so that you can view the clinics and preclinics, library space, computer facilities, and the like. While you are visiting the dental schools where you have been invited to interview, ask questions! In particular, take time to speak frankly with one or more dental students. It is through your communication with the student body that you will gain the most insight into the real inside workings of the school. For example, a stressed and tired dental student will not hold back on revealing what he or she perceives as inadequacies in the system. Listen closely, and note the school's weaknesses as well as its strengths.

Remember: The purpose of an interview is not to line you up in front of a firing squad. Rather, the goal should be a positive exchange of information between you and the interviewer(s). Ultimately you are looking for a good fit between your expectations of a dental program and the reality of what that particular school offers. The Admissions Committee is likewise looking for confirmation that you would be successful at this institution and that it would benefit by having you as a member of their next incoming class.

Financial Aid—A Brief Overview

There are two major types of financial aid, *gift aid*, which refers to scholarships and grants, and *nongift aid*, which refers to loans. Unfortunately, at the graduate school level, there are no grants similar to what you may have had as an undergraduate student, such as the federal Pell Grant, or a state-sponsored grant. Scholarships are available: some are merit based; others are not. More than likely, the dental school you attend will award merit-based scholarships once you have matriculated and are a dental student. These merit-based awards will be disbursed based on grades and class rank, so be sure to work hard in dental school. Other scholarships may be based on involvement in research, clubs, and other activities, or on other criteria, such as representation of a minority group in the field of dentistry.

The first step in applying for financial aid, if you intend to take out student loans, is to file a Free Application for Federal Student Aid (FAFSA). Anyone who plans to apply for student loans *must* have this application on file with the federal government. In order to file the FAFSA, if you worked you should complete your federal income tax return as soon after January 1 as possible. This is also the date when the FAFSA forms for the upcoming school year become available.

Keep in mind that, by virtue of the fact that you will be a graduate student, you are now independent for financial aid purposes. *Do not* report parental/guardian information on the FAFSA unless otherwise requested by your dental school's financial aid office. We suggest that you submit your completed FAFSA to your financial aid office so that a professional financial aid officer can check for errors; corrections can take up to 6 weeks.

The FAFSA is a tool used by the federal government to calculate students' Expected Family Contribution (EFC). This is not as intimidating as it sounds; rather, it is a number used in calculating your need for financial aid.

After the FAFSA has been filed, within 4 to 6 weeks, you will receive a Student Aid Report (SAR) in the mail. It is always printed on colored paper and is typically five pages long. The SAR is simply a printed-out report of all the information you provided on the FAFSA. The second step in applying for financial aid is to submit your SAR to the dental school you will be attending. The financial aid office needs the SAR to obtain your EFC.

The third step in applying for financial aid (if you plan to borrow funds) is to obtain and complete a Stafford Loan application. After the federal government has processed your FAFSA, you will receive a Stafford Loan application in the mail. By then, you should also receive from your dental school financial aid office an award letter that will notify you of how much, if any, funds you will need to borrow for school. Your award letter is a simple equation:

Budget Amount – EFC = Need

After you have received your award letter and have completed your Stafford Loan application, return the loan application(s) to your financial aid office to double-check the material for accuracy. Your financial aid office also has a responsibility to "certify" all loans, that is, approve you for the funds requested on your loan application(s).

Once the loan application process has been completed, you have finished—for one financial aid cycle. You will have to complete all necessary paperwork on a yearly basis, however, while enrolled in school. Keep in mind, too, that if you need to defer payment on student loans obtained when you were an undergraduate, you will need to do that every semester while in dental school. Your financial aid office should have all the appropriate deferment forms.

The Stafford Loan Program is the most comprehensive and accessible loan to dental students who are U.S. citizens or permanent residents. Listed below is a description of the federally regulated Stafford Loan Program (students may be eligible for these amounts depending on the dental school).

LOAN NAME	MAXIMUM AMOUNT	GRACE PERIOD	INTEREST RATE
Stafford (subsidized)	$8,500	6 months	Caps @ 8.25%
Stafford (unsubsidized)	$30,000	6 months	Caps @ 8.25%

However, even with the maximum total award of $38,500 through the Stafford Loan Program, some dental students find that they are still short of funds for school. Most of those students, will apply for a DEAL Loan, which has rates similar to those of the Stafford Loan while the student is enrolled; however, the interest rates fluctuate while the borrower is in repayment. Finally, another loan is the Health Professions Loan (HPL), which is subsidized while the dental student is in school and carries a 5% interest rate; but the amounts awarded are usually low compared to the amounts available through the Stafford or DEAL Program. Also, even though a student is independent for financial aid purposes, for the HPL parents must submit a signed tax return and complete a school-specific supplemental application.

For more in-depth information pertaining to financial aid for dental school, you should refer to the *Admission Requirements: United States and Canadian Dental Schools*, published yearly by the American Association of Dental Schools. You may order this publication from the AADS.

A Note to Foreign Dental School Applicants

A major problem for foreign applicants is that the formula AADSAS uses for calculating grades is not always comparable to a foreign scale. If you have determined that AADSAS calculated your foreign transcripts incorrectly, you will want to approach the individual dental schools to rectify the problem. One possibility is to provide each dental school you wish to attend with a notarized copy of your transcript. The school, in turn, can have the transcript evaluated by the on-campus office that works specifically with international students. Instead, you can expedite the process by having your foreign transcripts evaluated by an outside agency, such as Educational Credentials Evaluators, Inc. [P.O. Box 92970, Milwaukee, WI 53202-0970; (414) 289-3400] and then provide that evaluation not only to AADSAS but also to the schools you would like to attend. Even with this preliminary evaluation done, keep in mind that, if you are accepted to dental school, the individual schools will eventually need proof of your original foreign credentials.

One of the most serious problems associated with foreign students who choose to pursue an education in the United States is the lack of financial aid that is available to them. Generally speaking, unless a student holds a green card/is a permanent resident, he or she is ineligible for financial aid programs such as the Stafford loan. Also, in order to apply for studies in the United States, students have to provide proof of sponsorship. There are a few sources of loans to foreign students, the largest being the International Education Finance Corporation [424 Adams Street, Milton, MA 02186; (617) 696-7840]. This company has a loan program specifically for Canadian students as well as one for other international students who are pursuing a graduate degree. Another lender, Nellie Mae [Grad Excel Program, 50 Braintree Hill Park, Suite 300, Braintree, MA 02184-8753; (800) 634-9308] offers some loans to nonresidents. However, the guidelines for eligibility for the loan programs offered by these two companies are strict; credit history is weighed strongly, and in most cases nonresidents who apply for these loans must have a cosigner who is a U.S. citizen or a permanent resident.

If English is your second language, some dental schools may require that you take the TOEFL (Test Of English as a Foreign Language) test. This varies from school to school: some schools use the DAT reading comprehension score to ascertain language ability, others do not. Therefore, check with the dental schools to which you are applying to see what their policies are toward non-native language speakers.

Most dental schools with English prerequisites do accept Grade 13 English and the Canadian DAT. However, to be sure, you should call all the dental schools in the United States that you are interested in attending to check their individual requirements.

DENTAL SCHOOL

In almost all dental schools, the first 2 years are primarily devoted to courses in the basic sciences and preclinic dental sciences. Most courses have both a didactic (lecture format) and laboratory component. All schools teach the following courses within the first 2 years as they are tested subjects on Part I of the National Board Dental Examinations:

- Anatomic Sciences
- Biochemistry
- Physiology
- Microbiology
- Pathology
- Dental Anatomy and Occlusion

Although pharmacology is not tested on Part I, it is often taught in the second year so that the students may begin practice in the clinic by their third year.

The third and fourth years are taught mostly in the clinic. The emphasis is on radiology, operative dentistry, anesthesia, and the clinical specialties of periodontics, endodontics, prosthodontics, pedodontics, orthodontics, and oral surgery.

Some schools have unique programs integrating the science disciplines, whereas others teach via a "problem-based learning" format or a "case-based learning" format. Some schools have condensed the basic science curriculum into 14–18 months. Some of these alternative curricula are very interesting and should be fully investigated if you are considering a school that provides such an education.

The following is a sample schedule similar to most dental school curricula:

First Year

General Histology

Embryology

Oral Histology

Biochemistry

Dental Materials

Dental Anatomy

Amalgam Restoration

Functional Waxing

Gross Anatomy

Neuroanatomy

Head and Neck Anatomy

Preventative Dentistry

Occlusion

Composite Restoration

Physiology

Cast Restorations

Second Year

Pathology

Oral Radiology

Anesthesia

Microbiology

Pharmacology

Pediatric Dentistry

Removable Partial Dentures

Periodontology

Occlusion

Behavioral Science

Nutrition

Radiology

Oral Surgery

Orthodontics

Endodontics

Dental Materials

Complete Dentures

Fixed Partial Dentures

Third Year

Oral Pathology

Oral Medicine

Anesthesia

Oral Surgery

Prosthodontics

Orthodontics

Endodontics

Periodontics

Pediatric Dentistry

Radiology

Abnormal Psychology

Radiology

Anesthesia

Geriatrics

Esthetic Dentistry

TMD Management

Electives

Fourth Year

Ethics

Practice Management

Dental Public Health

Oral Medicine

Emergency Care Clinic

Implantology

Diagnosis and Treatment Planning

Maxillofacial Prosthodontics

Oral Surgery

Pediatric Dentistry

Prosthodontics

Restorative Dentistry

Periodontology

Orthodontics

Electives

THE PROFESSION OF DENTISTRY

Dentistry is the branch of the healing arts devoted to maintaining and treating the oral cavity and maxillofacial complex. A dentist is a scientist dedicated to providing a high quality of health care through prevention, diagnosis, and treatment of oral diseases. The dentist contributes enormously to the state of a person's health and quality of life. Through prevention of decay, periodontal disease, malocclusion, and oral-facial anomalies, dentistry provides an invaluable service to the public.

The opportunities and responsibilities of the dental profession in today's society are dynamic and make the field one of the most exciting, challenging, and rewarding professions. The dental profession includes involvement in research, public health, and patient care. Each discipline contributes to the overall general welfare of the public.

Dentistry offers many challenges and rewards. The profession is one of autonomy; becoming a dentist allows you the freedom to be your own boss. Today's private-practice dentist is more than a clinician. Dentists also must be business-people and managers. As a manager, you must constantly be aware of the consumer, the government, and third-party representatives. Your knowledge and ability as a businessperson is as important as your clinical skills.

Dentists need a thorough understanding of how to manage themselves, their staff, and their patients. Strong communication skills are essential in this management process. Communication skills include interpersonal skills, listening skills, speaking skills, and nonverbal skills. No matter how good a dentist's clinical skills may be, the quality of his or her communication skills will greatly impact the dental practice. The ability to provide dental services depends on the ability to inform patients about their dental needs. Uninformed patients will not perceive the importance of good dental health. Excellent patient relationships help ensure the best treatment for the patient and also will benefit the dental practice, leading to increased patient referrals and recommendations. Strong interpersonal communicative skills promote the sort of caring, friendly atmosphere vital to a successful practice.

Dentistry is both an art and a science. The outstanding dentist possesses both superior manual dexterity and technical expertise. A dentist restores a patient's dentition to be both functional and aesthetically pleasing. Restoring teeth, especially cosmetic dentistry, improves the self-esteem of patients. For most dentists, the greatest satisfaction is derived from improving patients' self-esteem through restoring their smiles.

Dentistry offers various opportunities from which an individual can choose based on his or her personality and career objectives. The following are some of the options that should be anticipated and considered:

- Solo practice
- Associateship
- Academics
- Dental research
- Service in the federal government
- Public health care

Because of the dynamic state of U.S. health care, new career options are being developed every year. New opportunities for dental health care providers are being created in private practice, industry, government, dental societies, national scientific organizations, and educational institutions.

A basic question that a recent graduate must ask him- or herself is whether to pursue a solo or an associate practice. Historically, one of the factors in selecting dentistry as a career has been the opportunity to be one's own boss. Approximately 150,000 dentists are practicing in the United States. Most dentists have been trained as general dentists. General dentists may choose a solo or an associate (group) practice.

The solo practitioner is independent and has complete autonomy in making decisions and in setting practice policy. He or she can make choices that influence the day-to-day operations of the practice and the potential for financial reward. The dentist is responsible solely for all decisions and takes a greater financial risk. A solo practitioner must be a self-starter. The daunting tasks of selecting a community, deciding on a location, securing a lease, designing an office, selecting equipment and supplies, hiring and training staff—thousands of important and minute details are all part of starting a practice.

An associateship position gives the recent graduate an opportunity to gain more knowledge in all aspects of dental practice. An associate agrees to work in a practice for a certain period of time as either an independent contractor or as an employee. The vast majority of new graduates who go directly into private practice are doing so as associates. This is also true for dentists completing residency or graduate programs. The high financial investment and uncertainty involved in starting a solo practice are the main reasons for recent graduates to choose an associateship. Rising educational debt may also preclude the graduate from starting a solo practice. Moreover, an associateship position helps to facilitate the transition from the academic environment to clinical practice, increases clinical knowledge and speed, and, in some cases, allows the associate to buy into a practice. Being an associate requires flexibility in treatment planning and the ability to practice in someone else's office. The associate has less discretion and decision-making authority than solo private practice affords. Associateship agreements are varied and should be structured to fit the needs of all parties. Some associateships are based on the current owner's retiring and phasing out of the practice; some are simply an employer-employee situation; and in some a new practitioner is considered an independent contractor.

A dental general practice residency (GPR) is an excellent opportunity to gain additional knowledge beyond dental school. The challenges of providing quality dental care to the medically compromised, the mentally and physically handicapped, and the dental phobic attract many graduates to apply for a GPR. A GPR may offer training in anesthesiology, medicine, and emergency and trauma cases and is usually a one-year residency program that offers a stipend or small salary. This valuable experience provides the student with additional knowledge and skills that may motivate a decision to specialize in some area of the dental profession.

In addition to general practice, there are eight recognized specialties: dental public health, endodontics, oral and maxillofacial pathology, oral and maxillofacial surgery, orthodontics and dentofacial orthopedics, pediatric dentistry, periodontics, and prosthodontics. Specialties require additional training after receiving a dental degree and are very competitive. The cost and the number of years required for a particular program vary from institution to institution. Specialty programs enable an individual to concentrate in one field of dentistry and to perfect his or her clinical skills in that area. Generally, a specialist's services are more costly; therefore, these practitioners have higher incomes than general dentists.

Following are brief descriptions of the procedures dentists perform in each specialty field, the additional education required beyond dental school, the length of the program, and the number of programs available:

- **Dental public health:** Individuals who enter the dental public health field are involved in developing policies and programs that affect the community at large. The individual may earn a certificate or a master's or doctoral degree. Most of the programs are between 12 and 24 months long, and there are currently 22 programs.
- **Endodontics:** Endodontists diagnose and treat diseases and injuries specific to the dental nerves, pulp, and tissues that affect the vitality of the tooth. Programs offer certificates or master's degrees. The lengths of the program vary but are usually 24 months, and there are currently 47 programs.
- **Oral and maxillofacial pathology:** Oral pathologists are dental scientists who study and research the causes, processes, and effects of diseases with oral manifestations. These diseases may be confined to the mouth and oral cavity. Oral pathologists do not deal with patients directly. They provide critical diagnostic and consultative biopsy services to dentists and physicians in

the treatment of their patients. Programs offer certificates or master's and/or doctoral degrees. The length of the program is usually 36 months, and there are currently 15 programs.

- **Oral and maxillofacial surgery:** Oral surgeons provide a broad range of diagnostic services and treatments for diseases, injuries, and defects of the neck, head, jaw and associated structures. Programs offer certificates or master's and/or doctoral degrees and most are at least 48 months long. Currently, there are 109 programs.
- **Orthodontics and dentofacial orthopedics:** Orthodontists treat problems related to irregular dental development, missing teeth, and other abnormalities. Orthodontists establish normal functioning and appearance for their patients. Some programs offer certificates; others, master's degrees. Most of the programs are 24 to 36 months in length, and there are 53 programs.
- **Pediatric dentistry:** This field specializes in treating children from birth to adolescence. Also, practitioners may treat disabled patients beyond the age of adolescence. The programs may offer certificates or master's and/or doctoral degrees. Most of the programs are 24 to 36 months in length. There are currently 57 programs.
- **Periodontics:** Periodontists diagnose and treat diseases of the gingival tissue and supporting bone of the teeth. Some programs offer certificates; others, master's or doctoral degrees. Most programs are 36 months in length, and there are 52 programs.
- **Prosthodontics:** Prosthodontists replace missing teeth with fixed or removable substitutes. Again, some programs offer certificates; others, master's or doctoral degrees. Training may be from 12 to 36 months, and there are currently 70 programs.

The decision as to what to do after receiving a dental degree takes as much thought as making the initial decision to enter the dental profession. Recent graduates must take into consideration their financial situations upon graduation and their personal and career goals.

There was a time when almost any professional could walk into a bank, spend less than a half-hour with a loan representative, and be approved for a large loan. This situation came to an abrupt halt in the 1980s. Although it is not impossible to obtain a loan, approval is far from automatic. Factors such as credit rating, positive cash flow, net asset value, and other criteria are considered. Although professionals, dentists no longer are treated any differently than small business owners when applying for a loan. With the exception of service in the federal government and an associateship, however, applying for a bank loan is usually inevitable.

The level of prior indebtedness plays a major role in the path that the recent graduate follows. Whether right out of school or after completing a general residency program, most recent graduates become associates or buy existing practices. Starting a solo practice from scratch is very risky and entails a large financial burden that few students can afford.

To enjoy dentistry, one must be happy with his or her personal and professional choices. An imbalance leads to unhappiness and stress. Since the dentist wears many hats, dentistry can be a very stressful profession. Mitigating the burden involved in fulfilling the many obligations of dentistry must be a general sense of contentment and well-being that comes from satisfaction with the profession.

The future of dentistry is bright. The professional rewards of being a dentist are numerous. Dentists obtain personal satisfaction from helping others and are highly regarded by the community. In addition, dentists are well paid. The average income for a dentist is in the upper 8 percent of family incomes in the United States. The increasing public awareness of the importance of oral health has resulted in a greater demand for dental insurance. The number of persons who have dental insurance has grown from fewer than 5 million to more than 100 million. Increases in preventive, geriatric, and cosmetic dental care also have contributed to growth in the demand for dental services.

We are in the age of high technology, and the dental profession is continually changing with new advances. The CAD/CAM, computer-generated radiographs, improved restorative materials, and new antiplaque agents and vaccines are only a few of the recent advances in dentistry. A dentist's education is not completed after earning a dental degree, which is only the beginning. With the advances in technology, a dentist must continually enroll in continuing education classes, review dental journals, and participate in the local dental society. The opportunities for continuing education are numerous; courses are offered in everything from practice management seminars to dental materials and are available from universities, private industry, and national and local dental societies.

Dentistry is an exciting and rewarding profession. As a healing art, the profession continues to advance at a rapid pace, changing the day-to-day operations of the dental practice. Thanks to modern miracles, people are living longer and the need for continued preventive and restorative dentistry will continue to rise.

Paradoxically, as the demand for dental services has increased, over the last decade or more, there has been a steady decrease in the number of dentists graduating in the United States. This has led to a decrease in the ratio of dentists to patients in the population. The American Dental Association has predicted that by the year 2010 the patient/dentist ratio will be approximately 1,800/1.

The dental profession has been fortunate that managed care has not affected dentistry as much as medicine. It is true that dentists are now working harder for the same income, but they still enjoy a very comfortable life. The average net income of solo dentists working 32 hours or more a week is $125,730. It is predicted that, with the shortage of dentists after the year 2000, the average income will greatly increase and that the impact of managed care and third parties will be minimal. In summary, dentistry provides many opportunities for an individual and can be very fulfilling professionally and personally.

Interviews

Three transcribed interviews with practicing dentists follow. Each interviewee offers a different perspective on the field of dentistry. These interviews are included, not to provide a comprehensive picture of the entire profession, but rather to inspire you to call your local practitioners and interview them. Tailor your interviews to your own needs by asking questions relevant to your interests in dentistry. Almost all practitioners respond well to aspiring dentists; let them relate their success stories to you. They will be able to convey the real-life struggles and triumphs of dentistry better than any text.

Dr. Roberta Doyle

Q. *How long have you been in practice?*

A. About 16 years.

Q. *Do you own your practice?*

A. Yes.

Q. *What factors made you want to pursue dentistry as a career?*

A. My parents wanted me to be a physician, but that wasn't exactly what I wanted. I'm artistic, and dentistry is a good combination of medicine and art.

Q. *Please describe your practice (location, staff, hours, etc.).*

A. My practice is in downtown suburbia. I have 12 employees. My regular hours are 7:45 A.M.–5:15 P.M. Monday through Friday, with lunch hours available.

Q. *What have been the most rewarding aspects of dentistry for you?*

A. I like to see my patients walk out feeling good—I like to change their perspectives.

Q. *What have been the biggest challenges in your practice?*

A. Owning my own business and being the one to take care of people, I'm running the show.

Q. *Were you given training for the business aspect of your work?*

A. No, but I knew a lot about it.

Q. *What have been the most significant changes in dentistry that you have seen?*

A. The big changes have been in bonding.

Q. *What about the social changes you've seen?*

A. Better dental health.

Q. *Would you do it all over again?*

A. Yes, definitely.

Q. *What qualities do you think make an excellent dentist?*

A. You need ethics and good communication skills, and you must be good at working with people. It's really a people-oriented job.

Q. *What advice would you convey to dental school applicants?*

A. It's a lot of hard work, so be prepared. You have to also be willing to do a lot of different things; you won't just come out of dental school and be a hit.

Q. *How has being a woman influenced your career?*

A. In school, it was harder to be a woman, but once I got out I found it to my advantage. I'm a general dentist, so I go directly to the public. People perceive that I am more gentle, so they come and seek treatment more readily. I don't know how I would feel if I were a specialist because then I'd be relying on men for referrals.

***

Dr. Ben Williamowsky

Q. *Where did you go to dental school?*

A. University of Maryland–Baltimore.

Q. *When did you graduate?*

A. 1948.

Q. *Did you do a postdoctoral program? GPR, AEGD, Specialty?*

A. No, I was a general dentist.

Q. *How long were you in practice?*

A. I was in practice for 48 years, but I have been retired for 2 years.

Q. *What factors made you want to pursue dentistry as a career?*

A. If there was anything definitive, I would say it was that my cousin was a dental student. He took me to NYU and showed me around. I was 13 or 14 years old at the time, and I thought I wanted to be a physician. When I saw what my cousin Sam was doing, I wanted to be like him.

Q. *Please describe your practice (location, staff, hours, etc.).*

A. There were many changes during my 48 years. In the last 25 years of practice, at first I had one partner. We were multidisciplined—we did some of everything other than orthodontic care. We did some surgery, some periodontal work, and general dental work. No HMOs. The staff consisted of nine full-time and a few part-time employees besides the dentists. Later there were two partners, and then a third a couple of years prior to my retirement. There were eight operators.

Q. *What have been the most rewarding aspects of dentistry for you?*

A. The relations with people. I really miss that.

Q. *What have been the biggest challenges in your practice?*

A. Keeping up with all of the new things.

Q. *What have been the most significant changes in dentistry that you have seen?*

A. The sophistication of dental practices, I would say. It used to be "Fill 'em and drill 'em," but now there's reconstruction and implants. In the last 10–15 years of my practice, I didn't do more than a couple per year of denture sets on new patients.

Q. *What changes do you anticipate? Where is dentistry headed in your opinion?*

A. Well, the biggest problem on the horizon is insurance—HMOs. In the ending years of my practice, I was discouraged by the need to focus on how to deal with insurance, rather than concentrating on actual dentistry. Maybe that's just a phase, though, I don't know.

Q. *What qualities do you think make an excellent dentist?*

A. A good dentist relates well to people and has artistic or visual-conceptual abilities. Also, a good dentist, when faced with disease and pain, sees it as a challenge to heal the ailment.

Q. *What advice would you like to convey to dental school applicants?*

A. A lot of dental schools have changed in that they realize their job is to help the students graduate, not challenge them to fail. If there is a choice of schools, go to them and talk with some students and see how their professors treat them. Also, everyone seems to think that it's 4 years and then, BOOM!—you're a dentist. Plan to spend at least one year in residency.

***

Dr. Steven Marsh

Q. *What have been the most significant changes in dentistry that you have seen?*

A. The dental materials have changed greatly. I don't use amalgam or silver in my practice anymore. We not only restore teeth and make them stronger, but they look a lot better. There is much more emphasis on cosmetic dentistry now.

Q. *What changes do you anticipate? Where is dentistry headed in your opinion?*

A. I anticipate an even greater emphasis on cosmetic dentistry.

Q. *Would you do it all over again?*

A. Absolutely. It's been a wonderful experience.

Q. *What qualities do you think make an excellent dentist?*

A. You have to have what we call a "good eye" for aesthetics, you must be terrific with your hands, and probably the #1 quality is the ability to have good relations with people, be it with patients or staff.

Q. *What advice would you like to convey to dental school applicants?*

A. You can control your own destiny with this career. It's one of the few fields left where you assume all of the responsibility. You can practice and market yourself however you desire. It's the kind of career where you can support your family, and you won't be traveling all over the country like some salespeople.

References

American Association of Dental Schools, *Admission Requirements: United States and Canadian Dental Schools 1999–2000*, 36th Edition. Washington, DC: 1998.

American Association of Dental Schools, *Applicant Analysis, 1996 Entering Class*. Washington, DC: 1998.

American Association of Dental Schools, *Opportunities for Minority Students in the United States Dental Schools: 1997–1999*, 2nd Edition. Washington, DC: 1997.

American College of Dentists, *Dentistry: A Health Profession, A Guide to Professional Conduct*. Gaithersburg, MD: 1997.

American Dental Association, *ASDA Handbook: A Resource Guide for Dental Students*. ASDA Publishing Company. Chicago, IL: 1996.

American Dental Association, *Dental Admission Testing Program User's Manual, 1997–1998 Report 3*. ADA Publishing Company. Chicago, IL: 1998.

American Dental Association, *Dental Admission Testing Program Validity Study, 1992–1993 Report*. ADA Publishing Company. Chicago, IL: 1994.

American Dental Association, *1996/97 Survey of Predoctoral Dental Educational Institutions: Academic Programs, Enrollment, and Graduates,* Volume 1. ADA Publishing Company. Chicago, IL: 1997.

Department of University Relations, *Bulletin: University of Pittsburgh School of Dental Medicine, 1996–1998*. Pittsburgh, PA: 1996.

SURVEY OF THE NATURAL SCIENCES REVIEW

The following chart shows the expected number of questions, by major subject area, in each of the three parts of the Survey of the Natural Sciences section of the Dental Admission Test. For a detailed listing of content in each subject area, see the outline at the beginning of each review section. Remember that this review is not intended to be a substitute for a comprehensive 1-year course in each of these subjects.

CONTENT SPECIFICATIONS FOR BIOLOGY, GENERAL CHEMISTRY, AND ORGANIC CHEMISTRY

1. BIOLOGY (40 QUESTIONS)

SUBJECT AREA	EXPECTED NUMBER OF QUESTIONS
Origins of Life, Cell Metabolism, Thermodynamics, Enzymology, Organelle Structure and Design	13
Biological Organization and Relationship of Major Taxa	4
Structure and Function of Vertebrate Systems	8
Descriptive Embryology and Developmental Mechanics	4
Mendelian Inheritance, Chromosomal Genetics, Meiosis, Molecular/Human Genetics	7
Natural Selection, Population Genetics, Populations and Community Ecology, Animal Behavior	4

2. GENERAL CHEMISTRY (30 QUESTIONS)

SUBJECT AREA	EXPECTED NUMBER OF QUESTIONS
Atomic and Molecular Structures	3
Periodic Properties	2
Stoichiometry	4
Gases	3
Liquids and Solid	1
Solutions	3
Acids and Bases	3
Chemical Equilibrium	3
Oxidation Reduction Reactions	3
Thermodynamics and Thermochemistry	2
Chemical Kinetics	2
Nuclear Reactions	1

(continued)

3. ORGANIC CHEMISTRY (30 QUESTIONS)

SUBJECT AREA	EXPECTED NUMBER OF QUESTIONS
Bonding, Aromaticity	3
Nomenclature	2
Stereochemistry	3
Chemical and Physical Properties of Molecules, Organic Analysis	3
Acid-Base Chemistry	3
Mechanisms (Energetics, Structure, Stability)	6
Reactions of the Major Functional Groups, Synthesis	10

BIOLOGY REVIEW OUTLINE (SNS Q1–Q40)

    I. OVERVIEW

    II. ORIGINS OF LIFE

        A. First Living Cells
        B. Theories

            Spontaneous Generation
            Amino Acid Stew

    III. CELL METABOLISM

        A. Chemical Pathways

            Anabolic Reactions
            Catabolic Reactions

        B. Cellular Respiration

            Anaerobic versus Aerobic Respiration
            Glycolysis
            Krebs Cycle
            The Electron Transfer Chain

                The Role of Oxygen
                Oxidation-Reduction Reactions

            Fermentation

        C. Photosynthesis

            Autotroph versus Heterotroph
            Light Reactions—Chlorophyll
            Dark Reactions

                Carbon Fixation
                Calvin-Benson Cycle
                C_4 Photosynthesis

    IV. THERMODYNAMICS

        A. Kinetic and Potential Energy
        B. First and Second Laws of Thermodynamics

V. ENZYMOLOGY

    A. Chemical Reaction

        Exergonic versus Endergonic Reactions
        Activation Energy and Catalysts

    B. The Lock and Key Model

        Active Site and Induced Fit
        Cofactors and Coenzymes
        Competitive and Noncompetitive Inhibition
        Enzyme Regulation

            Feedback Inhibition
            Allosteric Regulation

VI. ORGANELLE STRUCTURE AND FUNCTION

    A. Prokaryotic Cells—Bacteria
    B. Eukaryotic Cells

        Cytoplasm
        Nucleus
        Ribosomes
        Endoplasmic Reticulum
        Golgi Apparatus
        Secretory Vesicles and Exocytosis
        Lysosomes and Endocytosis
        Vacuoles
        Mitochondria
        Choloroplasts
        Cytoskeleton and Microfibers

    C. Cell Membranes

        Lipid Bilayer

            Phospholipids
            Membrane Proteins

        Fluid Mosaic Model
        Movement Through Membranes

            Diffusion
            Osmosis
            Hypotonic and Hypertonic Solutions
            Facilitated Diffusion and Active Transport

        Osmoregulation

    D. Cellular Reproduction

        Cell Cycle
        Interphase—S, G_1, and G_2 Phases
        Mitosis

            Prophase
            Metaphase
            Anaphase
            Telophase

Cytokinesis

Control of Cell Division

Meiosis and Gametes

VII. BIOLOGICAL ORGANIZATION AND RELATIONSHIP OF MAJOR TAXA

A. Binomial Nomenclature

B. Taxa

C. Five Kingdom Classification

Monera

Protista

Fungi

Plantae

Animalia

D. Phylum Tree of Animalia

Lower Invertebrates

Porifera

Cnidarians

Platyhelminthes

Nematoda

Higher Invertebrates

Mollusca

Annelidae

Arthropoda

Lophophorates

Echinodermata

Chordata

E. Taxonomy

Phenetic Classification

Cladistic Classification

VIII. STRUCTURE AND FUNCTION OF VERTEBRATE SYSTEMS

A. Integumentary System

Anatomy of Skin

Epidermis

Dermis

Functions of the Skin

Thermoregulation

Protection

B. Skeletal System

Types of Bone

Long Bone

Flat Bone

Short Bone

Irregular Bone

Bone Tissue

Haversian Systems
Spongy Bone
Bone Marrow

Connective Tissues

Cartilage
Tendons
Ligaments

Skeletal Structure

Axial Skeleton
Appendicular Skeleton
Joints

C. Muscular System

Types of Muscle

Smooth Muscle
Cardiac Muscle
Skeletal Muscle

Structure of Skeletal Muscle

Muscle Fibers
Thick and Thin Filaments
Sarcoplasmic Reticulum and T-Tubules
Z-Lines

Sliding Filament Model
Fatigue

D. Circulatory and Lymphatic Systems

Blood

Plasma
Red Blood Cells
Hemoglobin
White Blood Cells
Lymphocytes
Blood Clotting

Arteries and Veins—Systolic and Diastolic Blood Pressure
The Heart—Events of a Heartbeat
The Lymphatic System

Interstitial Fluid Buildup
Lymph Vessels
Role in Immune System

E. Immune System

Pathogens

Bacteria
Protozoans
Viruses
Viral Attack

Humoral versus Cell-mediated Response
Cells of the Immune System

Macrophages
Antibodies

Efferent

Transmission of Information

Resting Potential
Action Potential
Propagation of the Impulse
Transmission between Cells
Processing Information

Central and Peripheral Nervous Systems

Sensory Organs
Autonomic and Somatic NS
Sympathetic and Parasympathetic NS

J. Endocrine System

Hormones

Steroid Hormones
Polypeptide Hormones
Amino Acid Hormones

Secondary Messengers and the Cascading
Effect

K. Reproductive System

Gamete Production

Male—Spermatogenesis
Female—Oogenesis

Hormones and the Reproductive Pattern

Androgens
FSH and LH Hormones
Estrogen
Menstrual Cycle
Conception

IX. DESCRIPTIVE EMBRYOLOGY AND DEVELOPMENTAL MECHANICS

A. Cleavage

Determinate Cleavage
Indeterminate Cleavage

B. From Morula to Gastrula

Blastulation—Blastoceal
Gastrulation—Gastrula layers
Neurulation

C. Development of the Fetus

Placenta
Umbilical Cord

X. MENDELIAN INHERITANCE

A. Genes

Principle of Segregation—Alleles
Principle of Dominance—Dominant and Recessive Expression
Genotype versus Phenotype

XV. POPULATION GENETICS

   A. Hardy-Weinberg Equilibrium

   B. Mutations or Random Events

      Genetic Drift
      Founder Effect

   C. Reproductive Isolation

      Allopatric Speciation
      Parapatric Speciation
      Sympatric Speciation

XVI. COMMUNITY ECOLOGY AND POPULATION ECOLOGY

   A. Communities

      Succession
      Niche

         Competitive Exclusion Principle
         Fundamental versus Realized Niche

   B. Community Interactions

      Competition—Intraspecific versus Interspecific Competition
      Predation—Predator/Prey Oscillations
      Mimicry

         Batesian Mimicry
         Mullerian Mimicry

      Symbiosis

         Parasitism
         Mutualism
         Commensalism

   C. Ecosystems

      Trophic Levels
      Producers
      Consumers
      Decomposers
      Food Webs

   D. Populations

      Carrying Capacity (K)
      K-Selected Species
      r-Selected Species

XVII. ANIMAL BEHAVIOR

   A. Nature versus Nurture

      Nature—Fixed Action Patterns
      Nurture

         Habituation
         Imprinting
         Classical Conditioning
         Operant Conditioning

   B. Social Behavior and Kin Selection

I. OVERVIEW

The biology section is the first of the three science sections that comprise the Survey of the Natural Sciences; it is followed by the chemistry section and then the organic chemistry section. There are 40 biology questions, whereas the chemistry sections each have 30 questions. Even though there is no division between the three science sections on the actual examination battery, you will receive three separate scores.

Biology can be an overwhelming subject. There are many levels to life, including cell structure, cell metabolism, animal functioning, and community processes. Before you begin reading the text that follows, carefully examine biology questions from past examinations. Get a feeling for what information you will need to recall and to what degree of detail. For instance, you will not be asked how the theory of evolution was developed historically, but you may be tested on the definition of natural selection. In other words, focus on what the test wants you to know, then acquire that knowledge through this chapter on biology.

Your time will be best spent in learning the major biological concepts first, and then filling in detailed information. The questions on the biology section are mostly conceptual, testing your understanding of processes, functions, and organization of biological systems. An example of this type of learning would be to first review the major topics covered in the discussion of the circulatory system and then learn the divisions of the heart. Finish your review of the heart with an understanding that the sinoatrial node is the pacemaker because it has the fastest depolarization rate. At this level of understanding you should begin to piece the big picture together.

Regarding the types of questions on the biology section, you need to realize what types of information are more likely to be tested. Given the topic of the histologic layers of arteries and veins, you *may* be asked on the DAT what layers (or tunics) are adjacent to Auerbauch's plexus in arteries. But you are far more *likely* to be asked *why* arteries have a thicker layer of musculature than do veins. The answer to the latter question incorporates more information. Again, focus your review on learning the concepts; they are the subject matter of the questions most frequently asked. Then fill in the details.

This chapter reviews the life sciences as outlined in the DAT Scope of Examination. The figures that accompany the text are an important part of the review process. The level of understanding and the concepts covered are directed toward achieving success on the biology questions of the DAT. By the end of this chapter, you should possess a working knowledge of most of the terms and ideas included in the DAT. The following is the Scope of Examination as described by the ADA Department of Testing Services:

- Origins of Life
- Cell Metabolism (including Photosynthesis)
- Thermodynamics
- Enzymology
- Organelle Structure and Function
- Biological Organization and Relationship of Major Taxa (using the Five Kingdom system)
- Structure and Function of Vertebrate Systems (Integumentary, Skeletal, Muscular, Circulatory, Immunological, Digestive, Respiratory, Urinary, Nervous, Endocrine, Reproductive)
- Descriptive Embryology and Developmental Mechanics
- Mendelian Inheritance
- Chromosomal Genetics
- Meiosis
- Molecular and Human Genetics

Kaplan

- Natural Selection
- Population Genetics
- Community Ecology and Population Ecology
- Animal Behavior (including Social Behavior)

As you will notice, the two chemistry chapters that follow (pages 106–188) are written in outline format, whereas the biology section is not. *To maximize readability, the biology subtitles within the major topics have been omitted.*

Our discussion of biology begins with the building blocks of life. Living things are made up mostly of carbon-based compounds. Carbon has the unique chemistry to form the large, complex, and diverse macromolecules of life. In fact, carbon compounds are studied in their own special field—organic chemistry. The macromolecules that play key roles in biological functioning are lipids, carbohydrates, nucleic acids, and proteins. Lipids are a diverse group of molecules that are insoluble in water. Many lipids are made up of fatty acids, or long hydrocarbon chains each with a carboxyl group at one end. Lipids have a variety of uses: fats store energy, phospholipids are the principal components in cell membranes, and steroids, such as cholesterol, play key roles in hormonal regulation.

Carbohydrates, commonly called sugars, are carbon compounds that fit the formula ratio of 1:2:1 for carbon, hydrogen, and oxygen. An individual sugar molecule, such as glucose, is called a simple sugar. A molecule formed from two joined sugars is a disaccharide, a group that includes the ordinary table sugar sucrose. Complex carbohydrates, or polysaccharides, are compounds with varying numbers of covalently bonded sugars. This group includes such compounds as starch (acts as energy stores in plants), cellulose (is a major component of plant cell walls), and chitin (forms the exoskeleton of insects).

(a) Components of a fat molecule

(b) Synthesis of a fat molecule

(c) Product of synthesis

A display of fats showing (a) the composition of a molecule of fat; (b) the synthesis of a fat molecule; and (c) the new fat molecule.

A display of monosaccharides. (a) Glucose is the most frequently encountered monosaccharide in anatomy and physiology and metabolism. It exists both in a chain form and a ring form, as shown. (b) Two other monosaccharides, galactose and fructose, have the same number and type of atoms, but the arrangements are different.

Disaccharides and the polysaccharide starch. (a) The disaccharides maltose, lactose, and sucrose are formed from their constituent monosaccharides. (b) Starch is formed from numerous glucose units. Note that the carbohydrates are shown in their ring forms. Water molecules are formed in the synthesis of disaccharides and polysaccharides.

The structure showing:

Alanine   Valine   Alanylvaline

The linking of the amino acid alanine to the amino acid valine to form a protein consisting of two amino acids. Note that the (-COOH) of one amino acid and the (-NH$_2$) of the second amino acid are involved. Water is a product of the dehydration synthesis. The covalent bond formed is a peptide bond.

Proteins are a very diverse group of macromolecules that are instrumental in almost all processes in an organism. Humans, for example, have tens of thousands of proteins, each with its own specific structure and function. Protein functions include support (keratin in hair), transport (hemoglobin in blood), movement (actin and myosin in muscle), and hormonal coordination (insulin in the pancreas). The architecture of protein molecules is highly variable and very complex. First, proteins are constructed from amino acids, simple carbon compounds that link together to form polypeptide chains. The sequence of amino acids in the polypeptide chain is programmed in the genes and is called the primary structure. The secondary structure refers to the folding and twisting of a polypeptide chain into a structure such as a helix. The tertiary structure is the large-scale folding pattern of the protein that results in its three-dimensional shape. Finally, in the quaternary structure the subunits of a protein bind together in a specific way.

Nucleic acids are macromolecules that carry genetic information. There are two types of nucleic acids: deoxyribonucleic acid (DNA) and ribonucleic acid (RNA). Nucleic acids are made up of chains of nucleotides, each of which is composed of a five-carbon sugar covalently bonded to a phosphate group and a nitrogen-containing base.

II. ORIGINS OF LIFE

A. First Living Cells

How did life begin on Earth? There are many scientific theories and much disagreement. Most biologists agree, however, that because there was no free oxygen in the ancient atmosphere, the first living cells were anaerobic; that is, they lived in the absence of oxygen. These cells were autotrophs, able to capture energy from their environment, and were one-celled and prokaryotic, similar to the bacteria of today.

B. Theories

Spontaneous generation, the theory that living organisms arise from nonliving material, was adhered to for thousands of years. For instance, it was widely believed that frogs came from soil and that maggots arose from rotting flesh. In 1668, however, Francseco Redi challenged the theory of spontaneous generation by showing that larvae appear only on carcasses that have been exposed to air, thereby demonstrating that maggots cannot originate solely from meat.

A more modern hypothesis is that, under primordial conditions, inorganic material accumulated and synthesized to form organic molecules, such as amino acids. These organic molecules joined to form larger molecules, for example, proteins or nucleic acids, which isolated themselves from their environment, developed heredity, and slowly evolved into many other types of molecules. Stanley Miller demonstrated this synthesis in 1953, when he showed experimentally that inorganic materials organized themselves into amino acids when maintained under ancient atmospheric conditions.

III. CELL METABOLISM

A. Chemical Pathways

As cars need fuel to run, so cells need energy to survive. Cells create, store, and release energy in various forms through carefully arranged reactions called chemical pathways. These pathways continuously transfer energy from one form to another to be used by the cell in life-giving processes. There are thousands of reactions and many pathways within the cell; metabolism can be thought of as a map that tracks the movement of energy through these transformations.

There are two main types of reactions: anabolic and catabolic. Anabolic reactions require energy in assembling larger molecules from smaller ones. Catabolic reactions, on the other hand, release energy by breaking down large molecules into smaller ones. Cells, for instance, use catabolic reactions to break down the organic molecules in food to simpler products. In the process, the cell harvests some of the potential energy stored in the food for use in cellular work (the rest is released as heat). The following subsections provide a summary of the catabolic pathways that provide energy for cellular life.

B. Cellular Respiration

We usually associate respiration with breathing. On the cellular level, respiration takes place in and around the mitochondrion and refers to the series of pathways that free energy from organic molecules. The stages of respiration are glycolysis, the Krebs cycle, and the electron transfer chain.

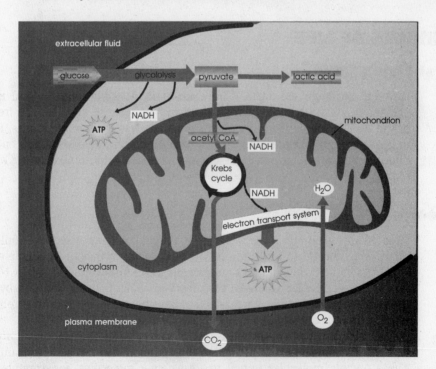

Overview of Cellular Respiration

The types of energy in organic compounds vary, but the most representative source of energy is the simple sugar glucose. Respiration breaks down the C–H bonds of glucose, releasing energy to change adenosine diphosphate (ADP, a low energy molecule) into adenosine triphosphate (ATP, a high energy molecule). ATP is a nucleotide that is an excellent source of immediate energy for the cell. Aerobic respiration, or respiration that uses oxygen as a fuel, can be summarized by the equation:

$$\text{Glucose} + \text{Oxygen} \rightarrow \text{Carbon Dioxide} + \text{Water} + \text{Energy}$$

Aerobic respiration is many times more efficient in producing energy than anaerobic respiration (respiration in the absence of oxygen), which is why plants and animals primarily use aerobic respiration to produce energy. Anaerobic respiration is the sole source of energy only for certain types of bacteria and fungi.

Glycolysis, the Krebs Cycle, and the Electron Transfer Chain

Glycolysis occurs in the cytoplasm of all living cells and is the first chemical pathway in cellular respiration. This reaction converts glucose (a 6-carbon sugar) into pyruvate (pyruvic acid, a 3-carbon compound) and produces ATP and high-energy electrons to be passed on to a carrier (NAD+) and the electron transfer chain.

Glycolysis

The Citric Acid Cycle (Krebs Cycle, Tricarboxcylic Acid Cycle)

If oxygen is present in the cell, the Krebs (or citric acid) cycle is the second step in glucose energy release. Pyruvate (produced in glycolysis) enters the mitochondrion, where it is further broken down to produce high-energy electrons (NADH and $FADH_2$), CO_2, and GTP (an ATP-like compound).

The last step in respiration is the electron transfer chain, which also occurs in the mitochondrion and results in the greatest production of ATP molecules. In this step, the high-energy electron products of the Krebs cycle (NADH and $FADH_2$) are passed down a series of electron acceptors. The energy levels of the electrons are reduced at every step and end with the final acceptor of electrons—oxygen. The series of reactions in the electron transfer chain are called redox (short for "reduction-oxidation") reactions. Reduction refers to the acceptance of electrons by one compound in the reaction. The donating of electrons by the other compound is called oxidation. The electron energy released from these cascading reactions drives a highly efficient production of ATPs from ADPs, called oxidative phosphorylation.

As previously mentioned, oxygen is important in respiration as an oxidizing agent and as the final electron acceptor. In the absence of oxygen, however, cells can break down sugars anaerobically, a process called fermentation. Fermentation breaks down sugars through glycolysis, the only step in glucose catabolism that does not require oxygen. The later stages of energy release are absent, so that very few ATPs are produced in comparison to aerobic respiration. Fermentation occurs in simple organisms, such as yeast and bacteria, in oxygen-deficient environments, and in vertebrate muscle cells after strenuous activity has exhausted oxygen resources.

Q   uniquinone (coenzyme Q)
FeS   iron-sulfur center
CYT C   cytochrome C
Fd   ferredoxin

Electron Transport and Oxidative Phosphorylation in Mitochondria

C. Photosynthesis

An autotroph is an organism that sustains itself by making its own organic materials (e.g., sugars, amino acids, and fats) from inorganic resources. This mode of acquiring energy is different from that used by a heterotroph, which relies on the consumption of other organisms for food. Plants are autotrophs, synthesizing organic compounds from light and CO_2 in a process called photosynthesis. Photosynthesis can be considered the opposite of respiration. The reaction of photosynthesis is:

$$6H_2O + 6CO_2 \rightarrow C_6H_{12}O_6 + 6O_2$$

$$6CO_2 + 12H_2O \longrightarrow C_6H_{12}O_6 + 6H_2O + 6O_2$$

atmospheric   water vapor   sugar   water   oxygen gas
carbon dioxide   from water

Overview of Photosynthesis

During photosynthesis, CO_2 reduces to form a sugar; in respiration, a sugar oxidizes to form CO_2.

    Photosynthesis occurs in the chloroplasts of plant cells, where the sun's energy is trapped by a photosynthetic pigment called chlorophyll. Chlorophyll, which gives plants their green color, absorbs light and releases its energy as high-energy

Electron Transport and Photophosphorylation in Chloroplasts

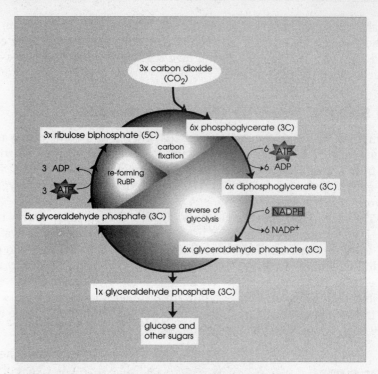

The Calvin-Benson Cycle (Light Independent)

electrons, which need to be replaced in the pigment. Water acts as a source of low-energy electrons (extracted from hydrogen) to replenish the supply in chlorophyll. When water is split, the by-product is oxygen. Finally, the high-energy electrons released by chlorophyll convert ADP to ATP (a process called photophosphorylation) and NADP+ to NADPH, both of which are excellent energy sources for the cell.

The steps of photosynthesis that convert solar energy into chemical energy for use by the plant cell are referred to as the light reactions of photosynthesis (because they must take place in light). The second stage in photosynthesis is the dark reactions, so named because they do not need light to occur. Dark reactions use the products of light reactions to power a process known as carbon fixation. Carbon fixation is the series of reactions that takes CO_2 from the atmosphere and converts it into organic compounds (carbohydrates, lipids, and oils) for use by the cell. There are two ways that a plant can fix carbon. Most plants use the Calvin-Benson (or C_3) cycle, a pathway that uses the energy from ATP and NAPH to produce fructose (a 6-carbon sugar), which is a versatile source of energy for the plant. Several types of plants, especially desert plants, also use water-conserving C_4 photosynthesis, which first produces malate (a 4-carbon compound) to enter the Calvin-Benson cycle.

IV. THERMODYNAMICS

A. Kinetic and Potential Energy

Energy, defined as the capacity to do work, comes in many forms. Kinetic energy is the energy of a moving object. For instance, water flowing down a stream contains energy that can turn a turbine that powers a windmill. Energy also can be stored as potential energy. A pencil lying on a desk has potential energy. It is not moving, so it does not have kinetic energy. If the pencil falls off the desk, however, its energy will be released as it falls to the ground. In biology, potential energy comes in a special form called chemical energy, which is the energy contained in the bonds that hold molecules together. As seen in metabolic pathways, energy can be converted from one form to another and then back again. Energy changes are studied in a field called thermodynamics.

B. First and Second Laws of Thermodynamics

The first law of thermodynamics states that energy in the universe is neither created nor destroyed. Energy stays constant; it just changes forms. When a bullet is fired from a gun, the chemical energy of the gunpowder is converted into the kinetic energy of the moving bullet. The gunpowder's potential energy converts to the work of moving the bullet.

The second law of thermodynamics is involved with such energy transformations. It states that, once energy is used to do work, less energy is available to do more work. In other words, the small amount of gunpowder in a gun cannot fire an infinite number of bullets. Once a bullet fires, the chemical energy in the gunpowder disperses, becomes less available and more disorderly. The term *entropy* describes the movement of energy toward disorder. In fact, an alternative way to state the second law of thermodynamics is to say that in the universe the entropy of any energy transformation always increases.

V. ENZYMOLOGY

A. Chemical Reaction

When chemical energy is converted, the process is called a chemical reaction. During a reaction, chemical bonds are either broken or made. Reactions that release energy are exergonic; those that require energy are endergonic. In living cells, the exergonic reactions usually provide the energy to perform the endergonic reactions. However, even exergonic reactions require a small amount of energy, called activation energy, to get them started. Often activation energy comes as heat, which, if not available, prevents the reaction from taking place.

B. The Lock and Key Model

In chemistry, catalysts are the chemical compounds that lower the activation energy to make it easier for a reaction to occur. Catalysts do not affect the energy transfer of the reaction. Enzymes are proteins that act as biological catalysts. They are very important for the functioning of cells because they allow necessary reactions to take place at ordinary temperatures. Enzymes can also speed up or slow down reactions.

The lock and key model describes how enzymes work. The "key" is the substrate, or the reactant, which binds tightly to or "fits into" the "lock," the enzyme. The place where the binding takes place is the active site. Like a lock, an enzyme has a very specific shape, allowing only one type of molecule to fit into its active site. There are thousands of enzymes in the living cell, each specific to a certain compound. As binding takes place, the active site of the enzyme can change shape to better fit the substrate, resulting in a tighter fit, called an induced fit. At this binding point, the substrate converts to the product of the reaction at a highly accelerated rate.

Many enzymes require an additional molecule to function. If this helper is inorganic, it is called a cofactor. A cofactor usually is an atom of metal such as zinc, copper, or iron. If the helping molecule is an organic molecule, it is a coenzyme. Vitamins are examples of coenzymes that aid in various enzymatic reactions in the

Active site — **Enzyme**

Substrates bind to enzyme

Substrates interact to form product with the assistance of enzyme

Product detaches from enzyme

Product

S₁ S₂

The activity of enzymes. An enzyme has a specific active site where a pair of substrate molecules bind. The product detaches, and the enzyme is freed to participate in another reaction.

body. On the other hand, certain compounds inhibit enzyme function. Molecules that mimic the enzyme shape and block the active site are called competitive inhibitors. Noncompetitive inhibitors are molecules that change the shape of the active site without actually entering it. Sites other than the active site that are involved in enzyme activity are called allosteric sites.

Enzymes can be thought of as reaction machines. It is important to control these machines in order for metabolic pathways to operate correctly. Enzyme regulation is based on the principle that an enzyme pathway can fluctuate between active and inactive. The most common mode of enzyme regulation is feedback inhibition, where the product of the reaction also acts as an inhibitor. As a result, when low amounts of a compound, such as an amino acid, are present, the enzyme pathway switches "on." When there are sufficient amounts, the pathway switches "off." Feedback inhibition is an example of allosteric regulation, in which varying concentrations of allosteric activators—molecules that stimulate enzyme function—and allosteric inhibitors—those that inhibit enzyme function—can determine the rate and duration of enzyme activity.

VI. ORGANELLE STRUCTURE AND FUNCTION

A. Prokaryotic Cells—Bacteria

Every organism is composed entirely of either prokaryotic or eukaryotic cells. Prokaryotic cells have no true nucleus and no membrane-bound organelles. They are found only in the kingdom Monera, which consists of bacteria and cyanobacteria. All other

DNA

ribosomes

pilli

cell wall

capsule

plasma membrane

flagellum

**Generalized Prokaryotic Cell
(One type of bacterium)**

organisms are made up of eukaryotic cells, which have true nuclei and organelles that have membranes. Prokaryotic cells are far simpler and smaller than eukaryotic cells and therefore are thought of as more primitive.

B. Eukaryotic Cells

This section describes the structures and functioning of eukaryotic cells. Many structures in the cell are known as organelles, which are like little organs within the cell. Many organelles are surrounded by membranes and perform specialized tasks for cell processing.

These are the structures of eukaryotic cells:

Cytoplasm

The cell's interior, except for the nucleus, is composed of a mixture called the cytoplasm. The cytoplasm can change from a liquid (sol) state, in which the cell's macromolecules disperse, to a semisolid gel state, where the particles interact to form a network.

Nucleus

The nucleus is the organelle that contains almost all of the cell's DNA and is responsible for several cellular activities, such as cellular reproduction, DNA replication, RNA synthesis, and responding to changes in the cell's environment. The condensed material inside the nucleus, called chromatin, consists mostly of protein and DNA.

Ribosomes

Ribosomes are small particles that produce the cell's proteins and enzymes. A ribosome consists of a small and a large subunit and is either bound to the membrane of the endoplasmic reticulum or free in the cytoplasm. Ribosomes are found also in prokaryotic cells.

Endoplasmic Reticulum

The endoplasmic reticulum (ER) is a highly convoluted membrane that secretes enzymes and produces other membranes. The ER occurs only in eukaryotic cells. There are two portions to the ER: rough and smooth. Ribosomes cover

A diagram of a "typical" human cell showing certain organelles. Some of the smaller organelles have been drawn larger than their normal relative size to show their detail.

the rough ER, the site of enzyme and protein synthesis. The smooth ER has no ribosomes and has varied biochemical functions, such as specialized enzyme secretion or ion pumping.

Golgi Apparatus

The Golgi apparatus (or complex), made up of many flattened membrane-bound vesicles, is closely linked with the ER. The Golgi apparatus stores and adjusts the proteins synthesized in the ER and secretes the protein.

Secretory Vesicles and Exocytosis

Some proteins synthesized in the Golgi apparatus are released by the cell into the surrounding environment. Such proteins travel from the Golgi to the secretory vesicles, which store the proteins until release. The process of releasing an enzyme is called exocytosis; the secretory vesicle membrane fuses with the cell membrane and expels its contents.

Lysosomes and Endocytosis

Some lysosomes are produced by the Golgi complex. They are small membrane-bound bags that are filled with enzymes. These enzymes break down and digest macromolecules into smaller compounds that the cell can more easily use. The process of bringing substances into the cell is called endocytosis. In some cells, the substance that is endocytosed may be digested by lysosomes.

Vacuoles

Vacuoles are large membranous sacs that store food, waste, and other chemical products. The number of vacuoles in a cell and the compounds stored vary from cell to cell. Vacuoles can contract and expel water out of the cell, or expand and play a role in cellular elongation.

Mitochondria

Mitochondria are the sites of many of the steps of cellular respiration. For example, ATP synthesis occurs in the mitochondria. Since ATP is an essential, high-energy molecule, the mitochondria are regarded as the energy powerhouses of the cell. The number of mitochondria in a cell varies from one to thousands, depending on the cell's energy needs. These organelles are composed of a deeply folding inner membrane surrounded by an outer membrane.

outer membrane
inner membrane
outer compartment
crista   matrix

Mitochondrion

Chloroplasts

In plants and photosynthetic cells, solar energy is converted into chemical energy by organelles called chloroplasts. Chloroplasts contain chlorophyll and other molecules that absorb the radiant energy of sunlight. This energy drives the light-dependent reactions of photosynthesis, which produce high-energy compounds for use by the cell.

granum
thylakoid disk
outer membrane
stroma
inner membrane

Chloroplast

Cytoskeleton and Microfibers

The cytoskeleton is the support structure of the cell. It is a network of criss-crossing fibers that help to maintain and change the cell's shape. The cytoskeleton is associated with three types of fibers: microtubules, intermediate filaments, and microfilaments. Microtubules are thick, hollow rods found mostly in the cytoplasm. Cilia and flagella are specialized organelles, composed of microtubules used for locomotion in some cells. Cilia and flagella are rooted in the cytoplasm to basal bodies; these are identical to structures called centrioles, which line up and separate the chromosomes during cell division. Intermediate filaments are midsize protein fibers. The smallest fibers are microfilaments; an example is actin, a contractile filament in muscle (see Muscular System in Section VIII for similarities).

C. Cell Membranes

Membranes are extremely important to the functioning of the cell. They separate the cell from its environment, divide the cell into different compartments, and control the passage of substances. The basic structure of a membrane is a lipid bilayer. The lipids that compose the bilayer, called phospholipids, have a hydrophilic polar group (water-loving head) on the outside of the membrane, and an oily hydrocarbon chain (water-fearing tail) in the membrane's center. Dispersed throughout the lipid bilayer are membrane proteins, which may serve as selective transporters of molecules.

Membranes are not rigid bodies with their many components locked into place. Rather, they are fluid, flexible, and changing, with proteins, lipids, and other elements able to move about freely in the plane of the membrane. This dynamic model of membrane structure is called the fluid mosaic model. Membrane fluidity is important for the membrane to work properly, and can change with such factors as temperature, electrical charges, and the presence of various electrolytes (e.g., sodium and calcium) in the immediate environment.

Pores
Globular protein
Lipid layer #1
Lipid layer #2
Globular protein
Pore

The fluid mosaic model of the plasma membrane at the cell border. The membrane consists of two lipid layers in which globular proteins float about.

(a) Isotonic   (b) Hypotonic   (c) Hypertonic

The process of osmosis in three different environments. (a) In an isotonic solution, the concentrations of solute are equal on both sides of the plasma membrane and no water movement occurs. (b) In a hypotonic environment, the higher solute concentration exists inside the cell, and water moves into the cell, causing it to swell and explode. (c) In a hypertonic environment, the higher solute concentration exists outside the cell, and water moves out of the cell, causing it to shrivel.

Membranes are selectively permeable; that is, some molecules can pass through them easily and some cannot. The passage of molecules through a membrane on their own, without any energy exerted by the cell, is called passive transport. One type of passive transport is diffusion, which is the tendency of particles to spread from areas of higher concentration to those of lower concentration. A second type of passive transport is osmosis, which is the movement of water across a semipermeable membrane. As with diffusion, a concentration gradient has to exist for osmosis to take place. Water will flow from areas of high water concentration (hypotonic solutions) to areas of low water concentration (hypertonic solutions) until the solution reaches equilibrium. For instance, if a bag of salt water is placed in a beaker of fresh water, the fresh water (higher water molecule concentration) will flow into the bag of salt water (lower concentration of water molecules). However, equal salinity may only be reached between the bag of salt water and its environment if salt can cross through the bag.

The force generated by the osmotic movement of particles is called osmotic pressure. Cells must counteract this osmotic pressure; otherwise, they will keep taking in water and burst in a hypotonic environment or lose water and shrivel in a hypertonic environment. The cell's process of balancing its water concentrations, called osmoregulation, is extremely important to cell functioning. Some cells "bail out" excess water through specialized contractile vacuoles. In larger organisms, the microenvironment around the cell is maintained as an isotonic solution, one having water concentration equal to that within the cell. For many plants, bacteria, and algae, the answer is to have a cell wall, which is a rigid layer surrounding the membrane that prevents the cell from expanding. Only plants have cell walls.

Some molecules diffuse through membranes with the help of transport proteins. In a process called facilitated diffusion, these molecules are "carried" through the membrane by the action of carrier proteins. It is important to note that facilitated diffusion speeds up particle movement, but does not change the direction of transport. The direction can be changed, however, in a process known as active transport, which uses the energy of the cell to move particles against a concentration gradient, or from low concentrations to higher concentrations. An example of active transport is the sodium-potassium pump, which uses energy from ATP molecules to pump sodium ions out of the cell and potassium ions in.

D. Cellular Reproduction

Cells have several stages in their life history. These stages repeat, leading to the term cell cycle. Ninety percent of the total time in the cell cycle is spent in interphase, a time when the cell grows, maintains itself, and metabolizes energy sources. There are three parts to interphase: the S phase, when DNA synthesis occurs, and two gaps (G_1 and G_2) before and after the S phase, during which there is no DNA synthesis. The remaining 10 percent of the life cycle is the period of cell division.

All cells reproduce to make new cells. Prokaryotic cells (e.g., bacteria) divide through a process called binary fission, in which DNA is replicated and there is a systematic compartmentalizing of DNA into two cells. The genetic material disperses throughout the cytoplasm, and a membrane forms in the middle of the cell and continues to extend until there are two daughter cells. Eukaryotic cells divide through either mitosis or meiosis, depending on the type of cell. Mitosis and meiosis are processes that include the mechanics of nuclear disassembly and reassembly, and are more complicated than simple fission because of the presence of nuclei and chromosomes.

Mitosis

In mitosis, there are several stages that prepare, line up, replicate, and separate the genetic material of the cell for reproduction:

Prophase

During this stage, the nuclear envelope begins to disintegrate and the chromosomes condense. Each chromosome consists of two duplicated DNA strands called chromatids. These strands are held together at the center by the centromere, forming an X-shaped structure. Microtubules appear, forming the mitotic spindle near the centrioles.

Metaphase

During this stage, the centrioles gravitate to opposite ends of the cell. The centromeres of each chromosome line up in the middle of the cell.

Anaphase

When the chromosomes begin to separate, anaphase begins. The centromeres split, and spindle fibers pull the chromatids apart to opposite ends of the cell.

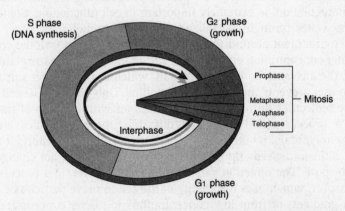

The cell cycle. The two major periods of interphase and mitosis are shown. Three phases are contained in interphase, and four compose mitosis.

Telophase

When the chromatids are in place, telophase begins. The daughter nuclei start to form, the chromosomes disperse within each new nucleus, and the mitotic spindles disappear.

Cytokinesis

In this stage a cleavage furrow develops and progresses to split the cell into two distinct daughter cells. The cell membrane develops around the two new cells, each containing identical genetic information.

Control of Cell Division

Contact inhibition is one method of regulation, where physical contact with neighboring cells signals a halt to reproduction. Mitogens also regulate cell replication; these chemicals, produced by the body, can stimulate or inhibit cell division. Cancer is a disease in which uncontrolled or abnormal cell replication occurs.

Meiosis and Gametes

Mitosis and fission are examples of asexual reproduction, where there is no genetic mixing in the making of a new organism. Meiosis takes place only in reproductive cells. The testes and ovaries are reproductive organs specialized for producing sex cells. Meiosis is a two-phase process that produces daughter cells, called gametes, with half of the original chromosome material. These gametes meet and combine the genetic material in sexual reproduction. Meiosis and sexual reproduction are described in detail under Reproductive System in Section VIII.

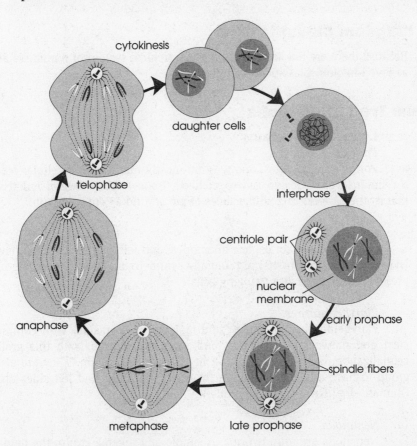

Mitosis in Animal Cells

VII. BIOLOGICAL ORGANIZATION AND RELATIONSHIP OF MAJOR TAXA

A. Binomial Nomenclature

Life comes in many diverse forms. To name all of these forms, Carolus Linnaeus (1707–1778) devised binomial nomenclature, a system designed to give each organism a unique scientific name. The names are in Latin, and each has two parts. The first part is the genus name, which denotes a group of similar life forms. For instance, all cats are in the genus *Felis*, and all dogs are in a different genus, *Canis*. The second part of the name is the species name, which is specific to a population of organisms that have similar characteristics, interbreed, and are reproductively isolated. In other words, a species can reproduce within its own species, but not with other species. The full names of the common house cat (*Felis domestica*) and Florida panther (*Felis concolor coryi*) indicate that both animals are cats but the two belong to different species.

B. Taxa

Organisms are also classified into other categories, known as taxa, which group similar species on different levels. The range of classification from largest to smallest is as follows: kingdom, phylum, class, order, family, genus, species. For instance, the full classification for humans is Animalia, Chordata, Mammalia, Primates, Homonidae, *Homo sapiens*.

C. Five Kingdom Classification

Because there are five kingdoms, the hierarchical system of naming is also known as Five Kingdom Classification.

D. Phylum Tree of Animalia

Lower Invertebrates

Porifera

Porifera are sponges. Sponges are mostly marine, multicellular feeders, with a cellular level of design (no specialized tissues). They exhibit radial symmetry; that is, they are organized like slices of pie around a central mouth.

Cnidarians

Cnidarians are corals, sea anemones, and jellyfish. Cnidarians have a tissue level of design (no organs), are radially symmetrical, and are characterized by the presence of nematocysts (stinging cells).

Platyhelminthes

Platyhelminthes are flukes and tapeworms (parasitic, with complex life cycles) and flatworms (free-living and wormlike). Animals in this group exhibit cephalization, or the presence of a head and a tail region. They are also the first group to have bilateral symmetry, in which the right and left sides are identical (humans are bilaterally symmetrical).

Nematoda

Nematoda are roundworms. A simple and diverse group, the nematodes are among the most abundant animals on the earth today.

Higher Invertebrates

The higher invertebrates have a coelom at some stage of development. A coelom is a lined body cavity that aids in movement, nutrient transport, and gamete maturation. Coelomate animals are divided into two evolutionary lineages, the protostomes and the deutorostomes. During embryonic development, the mouth develops first in protostomes and second in deutorostomes. Also, cells divide at an angle, a process called spiral cleavage, in protostomes, with each cell determined to become a specific part of the organism. In duetorostomes, cell division is vertical, called radial cleavage, and cell fate is not determined.

SOME GENERAL CHARACTERISTICS OF THE FIVE KINGDOMS

	Prokaryotes	Protoctists (Protists)	Fungi	Plants	Animals
cell size	small ~1 - 10 μm	large ~10 - 100 μm	large ~10 - 100 μm	large ~10 - 100 μm	large ~10 - 100 μm
cell type	prokaryotic	eukaryotic	eukaryotic	eukaryotic	eukaryotic
nucleus	absent	present	present	present	present
chromosomal structure	nucleoid—single naked circle of DNA	chromosomes made of DNA, RNA, and protein	chromosomes made of DNA, RNA, and protein	chromosomes made of DNA, RNA, and protein	chromosomes made of DNA, RNA, and protein
mitochondria	absent	sometimes present	sometimes present	present	present
respiration	range from obligate anaerobes to obligate aerobes, included facultative forms of both	most obligate aerobes	most obligate aerobes	most obligate aerobes	most obligate aerobes
photosynthesis	if present, enzymes bound to cell membrane, large variation in metabolic raw materials and end-products	if present, enzymes packaged into plastids, all generate oxygen	absent	generally present, enzymes packaged into chloroplasts, all generate oxygen	absent
metabolism	many variations	oxidative metabolism: glycolysis, Krebs cycle, electron transport	oxidative metabolism: glycolysis, Krebs cycle, electron transport	oxidative metabolism: glycolysis, Krebs cycle, electron transport	oxidative metabolism: glycolysis, Krebs cycle, electron transport
cell wall	polysaccharide-amino acid	some forms, various types	chitin and/or polysaccharides	cellulose and/or polysaccharides	absent
genetic recombination	rare: conjugation transduction transformation	common: fertilization and meiosis	common: fertilization and meiosis	common: fertilization and meiosis	common: fertilization and meiosis
nutrition	autotrophic (photo- or chemosynthetic) and/or heterotrophic	autotrophic (photosynthetic) and/or heterotrophic	heterotrophic: absorption	autotrophic photosynthetic	heterotrophic: digestion
motility (single cell)	bacterial flagella composed of flagellin	9+2 undulipodia, ameboid	nonmotile	9+2 undulipodia only in some gametes	9+2 undulipodia
cellularity	unicellular	various	various	multicellular	multicellular
cell division	mostly binary fission no centrioles, mitotic spindle or microtubules	varies	mitosis mitotic spindle centrioles absent	mitosis mitotic spindle centrioles absent	mitosis mitotic spindle centrioles absent
development	N/A	varies	spores	multicellular embryo enclosed in maternal tissues	blastula

Mollusca

Mollusca are snails, clams, and squid. Mollusks are the earliest protostome phylum. Many are soft-bodied organisms with a hard outer covering.

Annelidae

Annelidae are segmented worms (e.g., the common earthworm). Annelid bodies are made up of many identical segments.

Arthropoda

Arthropoda are spiders, insects, and lobsters. The many species in this phylum are characterized by jointed appendages and an exoskeleton (external skeleton).

Lophophorates

Lophophorates are bryozoans, ectoprocts, and brachiopods. Lophophorates share characteristics of both the protostomes and deutorostomes and are therefore placed between the two groups. They have free-swimming larvae that settle and grow into sedentary adults. The group is characterized by a U-shaped gut and a specialized feeding apparatus called a lophophore.

Echinodermata

Echinodermata are starfish, urchins, and sea cucumbers. One of two deutorostome phyla, echinoderms have pentaradial symmetry (five arms). Their larval stages are similar to those of chordates, suggesting that the phylum Chordata arose from the echinoderms.

Chordata

Chordata are sea squirts, mammals, fish, reptiles, and birds. These are animals that have backbones. More specifically, every chordate has, in some stage of development, a notochord, a nerve cord, and pharyngeal slits.

E. Taxonomy

The systems of classification help us to understand the world around us but are by no means definite. Many taxonomic debates are raging about such issues as which species belongs where, and whether a so-called species is indeed one species or includes several species. In general, there are two schools of taxonomy, the phenetic and the cladistic views. The phenetic view groups organisms by similarity of characteristics. For instance, all animals with hair belong to the class Mammalia. The cladistic view, on the other hand, groups organisms according to their evolutionary lineages. According to cladistics, Mammalia is its own class because, at some point in the evolutionary history of chordates, animals with hair branched away from such other chordates as fish and reptiles.

VIII. STRUCTURE AND FUNCTION OF VERTEBRATE SYSTEMS

A. Integumentary System

The integumentary system, or skin, is divided into two sections, the epidermis and the dermis. The epidermis is the thin outer layer. It has no blood vessels. Its outermost layer is composed of dead cells, which are continuously being lost and replaced. The inner layer of the epidermis contains epithelial cells, which produce keratin, a structural protein that toughens the skin (keratin is also present in hair

A general overview of the skin and the subcutaneous layer beneath it.

and nails). The dermis is the deep layer and is mostly composed of connective tissue. It produces melanin, the pigment that absorbs ultraviolet rays from the sun. The level beneath the dermis, called the subcutaneous layer, is filled with fatty deposits that help to store heat. Scattered throughout the skin are sweat glands and hair follicles.

Functions of the Skin

The skin has two major functions, thermoregulation and protection. Thermoregulation is the process of keeping the body at a constant temperature. Most of the body's heat diffuses through the skin. The amount of heat lost can be changed by varying the blood supply to the capillaries, small blood vessels in the skin. If the body temperature is high, perhaps because of exercise or hot weather, the blood supply increases and the capillaries dilate, allowing heat to be lost. When the body temperature is low, the blood supply to the skin decreases and the capillaries close, thereby conserving heat. Also, high body temperature stimulates the sweat glands to produce sweat, which evaporates and thus helps the body to cool. Sweat also contains metabolic wastes and therefore has an excretory function.

There are several ways in which the skin protects the body. First, the skin is a physical barrier against infection. Usually, disease-causing agents cannot enter the body where the skin is intact (entry occurs mostly through orifices or broken places in the skin). For this reason, burn victims have a very high risk of infection. The skin is also part of the inflammatory and immune systems, producing scabs, blisters, and rashes that inhibit the growth of an infection. Finally, the skin's absorption of ultraviolet rays protects other layers of tissue from damage.

B. Skeletal System

The skeletal system protects organs, offers structural support, and provides sites for muscle attachment. The skeletal system is made up of bones, which work together with skeletal muscles to generate movement. Bone is mineralized connective tissue, a mix of cells, fibers, and minerals (calcium and phosphate). These materials are assembled in a way that makes bone rigid and strong, yet remarkably flexible.

Types of Bone

There are basically four types of bones in the body: long, flat, short, and irregular. Long bones are in the arms, legs, toes, and fingers. They curve slightly to absorb shock and have large ends. The skull, ribs, hips, sternum, and scapula consist of broad plates of bone called flat bones. Short bones are present in the kneecap, wrist, and ankle. Finally, irregular bones make up the vertebrae and parts of the face.

Bone Tissue

Most bones contain several forms of bone tissue. The outer layer is composed of compact bone, a dense matrix made up of structural units called Haversian systems. Haversian systems are cylindrical sections. At the center of each is a Haversian canal, a tube that houses bundles of blood vessels and nerves. Surrounding the canals are concentric rings of bony tissue, which contain osteoblasts that lay down the bony matrix. The inner portion of bone is spongy bone, which is less dense than compact bone. Spongy bone contains no Haversian systems. Rather, it consists of a network of supporting elements called trabeculae. At the center of long bones is the bone marrow, composed of fatty soft tissue and cells that produce red and white blood cells.

Connective Tissues

Cartilage is a dense connective tissue essential to the skeletal system. It is more flexible than bone and functions well in absorbing shock, lubricating joints, and providing support. At birth, most of the skeleton is cartilage, later replaced by bone. In adults, cartilage remains in joints, the nose, and ears. Other connective tissues are the tendons, which attach muscle to bone, and the ligaments, which attach bones together at the joints.

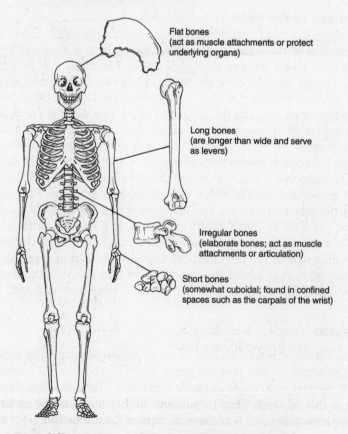

Flat bones
(act as muscle attachments or protect underlying organs)

Long bones
(are longer than wide and serve as levers)

Irregular bones
(elaborate bones; act as muscle attachments or articulation)

Short bones
(somewhat cuboidal; found in confined spaces such as the carpals of the wrist)

Four different types of bones and their locations.

Skeletal Structure

The axial skeleton consists of the inner supportive elements of the body: the skull, vertebral column, ribs, and sternum. The cranium, the part of the skull that protects the brain, is composed of several bones that fuse together at the sutures. The appendicular skeleton consists of the arm bones, the leg bones, and their attachments to the axial skeleton. The largest bone in the body is the femur, the bone of the thigh.

The structure of a typical long bone of the human body and its important parts.

The bones of the axial skeleton in humans. Eighty bones make up this portion of the complete skeleton. Numbers in square brackets indicate number of bones for each item.

Bones come together at joints. Some joints are immovable, like sutures. Others, namely cartilagenous and synovial joints (e.g., the knee), are movable. Cartilagenous joints are found throughout the axial skeleton, for example, between the vertebrae. These joints absorb shock and are able to move slightly. Synovial joints are present in the appendicular skeleton and vary in form, depending on the location. Synovial joints are strong and have free movement. They are lubricated by synovial fluid, which reduces friction between tendons, ligaments, muscles, and bones.

The bones of the appendicular skeleton in humans. One hundred twenty-six bones make up this portion of the complete skeleton. Numbers in square brackets indicate number of bones for each item.

(a) Synarthrosis

(b) Amphiarthrosis

(c) Diarthrosis

Three basic types of joints found in the human body. (a) An immovable joint such as found between bones of the skull. (b) A slightly movable joint such as found between vertebrae in the vertebral column. (c) A freely movable joint known as a synovial joint, such as found at the hip joint. Note the structural parts of the synovial joint.

C. Muscular System

The muscular system is responsible for converting electrical impulses and chemical elements into mechanical movement. Muscles control body movement and the transport of fluids within the body.

Types of Muscle

There are three types of muscle tissue: smooth, cardiac, and skeletal. Smooth muscle, also called visceral muscle, lines the walls of arteries and organs. It is called "smooth" because, on microscopic examination, it lacks the striations, the dark and light bands, of skeletal muscle. Because smooth muscle is generally not under conscious control (e.g., you cannot constrict your arteries at will), this type of muscle is called involuntary. Cardiac muscle is found only in the contractile walls of the heart. This tissue is striated (like skeletal muscle), but is controlled by the autonomic nerve system (like smooth muscle). Also, between cardiac muscle cells there are electrical connections called intercalated discs, which relay impulses during a heartbeat.

Skeletal muscle is responsible for voluntary movement. If you lift this book, skeletal muscles are at work. Red muscle, also called slow-twitch, is skeletal muscle that contains many mitochondria to supply energy for movement. The mitochondria give the red color and enable the muscle to work for extended periods without fatigue. When you take a long walk, for instance, you use slow-twitch fibers in the legs and arms. A sprint to the bus, however, calls for white, or fast-twitch, muscles. These muscles contract with more force than red muscle but fatigue more rapidly.

Structure of Skeletal Muscle

Skeletal muscle is attached to other muscle or bone by tendons. The muscle itself consists of many long parallel units called fibers, or muscle cells. Many closely packed myofibrils make up each fiber. Myofibrils have thin and thick filaments that slide across each other during muscle contraction. Thin filaments are composed mostly of three types of actin. Thick filaments are made of the protein myosin. Surrounding the filaments are two types of networks: sarcoplasmic reticulum, which stores calcium ions, and T-tubules, which help to conduct nerve impulses. Units of overlapping thin and thick filaments are called sarcomeres. Z-lines bind these units together.

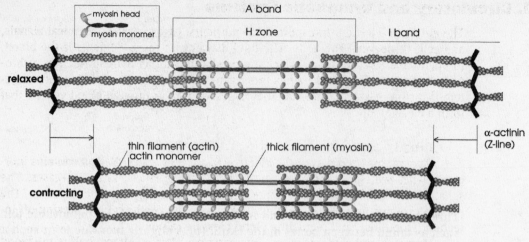

Sarcomere

Sliding Filament Model

Contraction of muscles begins with a nerve impulse, which triggers the release of stored calcium ions. What follows is best described by what is called the sliding filament model. The calcium ions expose binding sites in the actin filament. At these sites, a "head" of the myosin filament attaches and pulls the thinner actin filament inward. ATP in the muscle triggers the release of the myosin head, which now is free to attach again. The repeated attachment and release of many heads and binding sites brings the two filaments together. Contraction of the muscle continues as long as there is stimulation or until the muscle fatigues.

Fatigue is defined as the muscle's inability to sustain contraction. Two factors lead to fatigue: the depletion of ATP stores and the buildup of lactic acid. Lactic acid is produced when muscle cells are starved of oxygen and begin to function anaerobically.

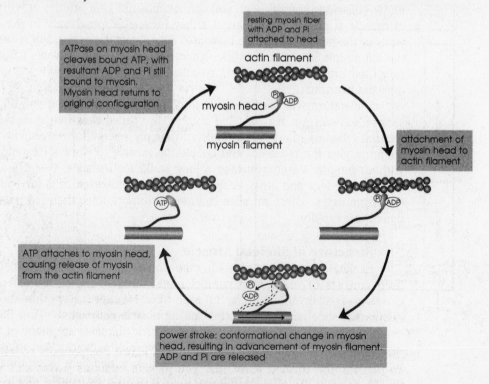

Molecular Basis of Muscle Contraction

D. Circulatory and Lymphatic Systems

The circulatory system transports vital nutrients, gases, wastes, chemical signals, and cells throughout the body. The fluid that houses these elements is the blood. In open circulatory systems, which are present in simpler animals such as arthropods and mollusks, blood bathes the organs directly. The human circulatory system is a closed system, meaning that the blood travels through blood vessels that form a closed loop.

Blood

Plasma, the fluid part of the blood, is 92 percent water. Plasma contains inorganic salts, proteins, hormones, nutrients, waste products, fats, and gases. The salts, called electrolytes, are important in maintaining osmotic balance. The plasma proteins function in clotting (fibrinogen and prothrombin), staving off infection (globulins), and regulating blood pressure (albumins).

Human blood contains many different types of cells. Almost half of the blood is made up of two types of blood cells: red blood cells, which carry oxygen, and white blood cells, which fight infection. Platelets are cell fragments that function in blood clotting. Red blood cells (erythrocytes) produce hemoglobin, the oxygen-carrying protein. Some white blood cells (leukocytes) are phagocytic in that they engulf invading microbes. Other white blood cells, called lymphocytes, produce antibodies that either latch on to invading cells and help disable them (B-cells) or directly attack and destroy foreign cells (T-cells). Both white and red blood cells are formed in bone marrow. Platelets are not actually cells, but rather are fragments of cells. These fragments attach to fibrin at the site of a cut; the result is a blood clot, which seals up the injury.

The composition of human blood. The two major components of whole blood are plasma and formed elements. The plasma contains water and numerous dissolved materials, including proteins, metabolites (nutrients and waste products), and ions. The great majority of formed elements are red blood cells.

Side view

2.6 μm

7.8 μm

Top view

Red blood cells (erythrocytes) and their structure.

Arteries and Veins

Blood travels through vessels called arteries and veins. Arteries carry blood away from the heart and have muscular walls that pulsate with every heartbeat. Systolic pressure is the maximum pressure attained during an arterial pulse, and diastolic pressure is the lowest. Arteries branch off into smaller vessels, the arterioles and capillaries. Capillaries, the smallest vessels, are about as thick as a single cell. Nutrients, gases, and other molecules in the blood diffuse through the thin capillary walls and surround the cell in a medium called interstitial fluid. Veins collect blood from the tissues and carry it back to the heart. Most veins have valves that prevent the blood from flowing backward.

Capillary beds where gas exchange occurs in lungs

Pulmonary circuit

Pulmonary veins

Pulmonary arteries

Aorta and branches

RA LA
RV LV

Vena cava

Systemic circuit

Capillary beds where gas exchange occurs in all body tissues

The two main cardiovascular circuits in the human body. In the pulmonary circuit, blood travels from the right ventricle to the lungs and returns to the left atrium. In the systemic circuit, blood travels from the left ventricle to the body and returns to the right atrium.

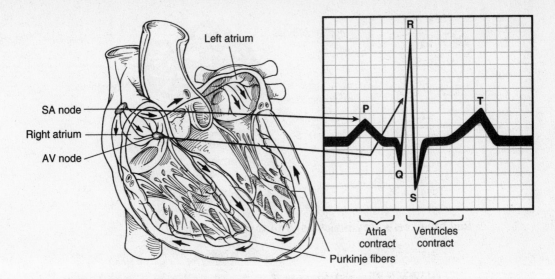

The cardiac cycle as seen in the waves of an electrocardiogram. Impulses from the SA node cause the atria to contract and are reflected in the P wave. After a momentary pause, the impulses from the AV node cause the ventricles to contract. These contractions are shown in the QRS wave. The T wave represents the time that the muscles are recovering from the contraction.

The Heart

The heart is the center of the circulatory system. Through several steps, called a heart cycle, the heart pumps blood to the lungs, where it is oxygenated, then pumps the oxygenated blood back into the circulatory system.

These are the events of a heartbeat:

1. Deoxygenated venous blood enters the first chamber of the heart, the right atrium, through the superior vena cava.
2. Blood flows to the right ventricle and out to the lungs through the pulmonary arteries.
3. The oxygenated blood returns from the lungs via the pulmonary veins and enters the left atrium.
4. The heart pumps the blood to the left ventricle and out into the circulatory system through the aorta. The force exerted by the heart on the walls of the vessels is the blood pressure. The coronary arteries supply the heart itself with nutrients.

The Lymphatic System

The lymphatic system is the link between the circulatory system and the immune system. As mentioned, molecules in the blood flow through the capillaries into the interstitial fluid. However, more fluid leaves the blood vessels and enters the body tissues than the reverse. What happens to the extra interstitial fluid? Unless collected, fluid would continue to build up in the tissues. Therefore, one of the functions of the lymphatic system is to absorb the excess fluid. Tiny tubes called lymph vessels collect the interstitial fluid, which passes though the lymph nodes and eventually cycles back into the circulatory system. The lymphatic system also plays a critical role in the body's defenses by producing lymphocytes and transporting white blood cells.

The lymphatic system as it relates to the circulatory system. Fluid seeps out of the circulatory system in the tissues and, while much of the fluid returns to the system, some fluid enters the lymph capillaries and returns to the circulation by this method. The lymphatic system is therefore a one-way system.

E. Immune System

Pathogens

The most common pathogens (microorganisms that invade the body and cause disease) are bacteria, viruses, and protozoans. Most types of these microorganisms are not harmful. In fact, our digestive tract is populated by billions of non-harmful bacteria. However, some species can cause serious diseases in humans by secreting toxins, attacking cells, or multiplying rapidly. Tuberculosis, syphilis, and leprosy are examples of bacterial diseases. Protozoans, single-celled eukaryotic organisms, can also be pathogenic, causing such diseases as malaria and African sleeping sickness.

Viruses are entirely different from bacteria and protozoans. Viruses cannot function on their own because they lack the mechanisms for respiration and protein synthesis that living cells possess. In fact, scientists debate as to whether

A T$_4$ Bacteriophage

viruses are even alive. Simply put, viruses are protein-coated genes. They can re-produce only by penetrating a cell and changing it into a virus factory. In the process, the virus destroys the host cell, which is why an uncontrolled viral inva-sion can be so harmful to an animal. Smallpox, herpes, measles, and AIDS are ex-amples of viral diseases.

A virus enters the cell and changes its biochemistry to produce thousands of viral progeny. Generally, when viruses infect a cell, they use its resources to copy its DNA and produce viral RNA. Retroviruses, such as the AIDS virus, operate slightly differently. They have RNA gene material and can create an intermediate copy of DNA within the host. This DNA copy is then copied to form viral RNA.

Humoral versus Cell-mediated Response

The role of the immune system is to protect the body from foreign sub-stances. Foreign molecules in the body are called antigens. The body has two types of defense mechanisms to combat antigens: humoral immunity and cell-mediated immunity. Humoral immunity involves the production of antibodies, which are a diverse group of proteins that recognize and bind to specific antigens. A cell-mediated response involves specialized cells to combat foreign cells.

Cells of the Immune System

Before discussing the immune response, it is necessary to describe the cells and proteins involved. Macrophages are cells that recognize the presence of an antigen, engulf it, and initiate the cell-mediated immune response. Antibodies, also called immunoglobulins, are Y-shaped proteins with two regions: variable re-gions, which act as very specific antigen-binding sites, and constant regions, which determine the method of antigen elimination. In a humoral immune re-sponse, antibodies either bind antigens together to be ingested by other cells, or designate an antigen as highly attractive to other phagocytic cells. Also, an anti-body has four polypeptide chains, called light chains and heavy chains, which, through variation, lead to the tremendous diversity in antibody types.

The major cell type of the immune system is the lymphocyte. Lymphocytes originate in bone marrow and are found throughout the body. Large numbers are present in the lymph vessels and lymph nodes, spleen, thymus, and blood vessels. There are two types of lymphocytes, B-lymphocytes, or B-cells, and T-lymphocytes, or T-cells. B-cells produce antibodies, and therefore play a key role in humoral im-munity. T-cells are involved in the cell-mediated response and come in three forms: helper T-cells, which stimulate the activity of other cells; killer T-cells (also cyto-toxic cells), which destroy target cells directly; and suppressor T-cells, which de-crease the activity of other B- and T-cells after infections are brought under control.

After encountering an antigen, the immune system "remembers" it through storing some of the lymphocytes that were mobilized for the attack. These cells are

Antibodies. (a) The structure of antibody molecule showing the four chains that make up the molecule. (b) The structures of five different types of antibodies. (c) The reaction between antibody molecules and antigens on the surface of a microorganism. Antibody molecules bind the microorganisms together and assist phagocytosis.

memory B- and T-cells, stored in the spleen and ready to react quickly should the antigen present itself again. When there is a large immune response, many memory cells remain. The result is permanent immunity, which occurs, for example, in the case of measles. After a mild response, there is a temporary immunity, such as is experienced after a bout with the flu.

Events of an Immune Response
The following are the events of an immune response:

Self versus Nonself
The immune system must be able to distinguish between intruders and non-intruders. The proteins that identify the body's own cells are called major histocompatibility markers (MHC). These proteins are unique to each individual and occur in every cell. They signal the immune system that a cell belongs to the body. Autoimmune diseases occur when the body is unable to differentiate between self and nonself, and the immune system attacks its own cells.

Recognizing the Antigen
Macrophages and B-cells travel throughout the body searching for foreign MHC markers. If one is found by either type of cell, the cell will sound an "alarm" that an antigen has entered the body. The macrophage engulfs the antigen and displays pieces of the antigen's proteins on its surface. When a B-cell encounters an antigen, it binds to the antigen and becomes activated. Like the macrophage, the activated B-cell digests the antigen and displays its proteins.

Mobilization
The immune response comes in two forms. In a cell-mediated response, a helper T-cell encounters a macrophage and binds to it. The macrophage-produced molecule interleukin then activates a helper T-cell, which signals other T-cells to begin multiplying. In a humoral response, the activated B-cell begins to clone itself and multiply.

Attack

Some B-cells will differentiate into plasma cells, which produce large numbers of antibodies. These roaming antibodies attract phagocytic cells to destroy the antigens, or the antibodies cause the antigens to clump together for easier removal. Also, killer T-cells arrive and destroy either the antigen, or the infected cells.

Halt

Suppressor T-cells send the message to plasma cells and T-cells to halt their replication and activity.

Memory

Some T-cells and B-cells become memory cells, stored in the spleen and ready for future encounters with the antigen.

Cell-Mediated Immune Response

Humoral Immune Response

F. Digestive System

The roles of the digestive system are to convert material from food into nutrients that the body can use and to eliminate products that cannot be absorbed.

Mouth

Digestion begins in the mouth, where several types of teeth break up the food. The incisors have sharp edges that cut food. The cuspids, which have one point (cusp), and the bicuspids, which have two points, grasp and tear food. Molars, with flat surfaces, grind the food.

Teeth are composed mostly of dentin, a calcium substance similar to bone. On the crown, the part of the tooth that is exposed, there is an outer thin coat of enamel, the hardest substance in the body. The middle of the tooth is composed of nerves and blood vessels.

Salivary glands secrete saliva into the mouth. Saliva increases moisture and begins to break down carbohydrates. Salivary amylase, a digestive enzyme in saliva, splits starch bonds and releases certain sugars of the carbohydrate. The tongue is a large muscle that tastes and manipulates food.

Pharynx and Esophagus

From the mouth, food is swallowed and travels to the pharynx, commonly called the throat. The pharynx is a passageway that channels food to the esophagus and air to the trachea. Once in the esophagus, food is forced down to the stomach by muscular contractions of the esophageal wall, called peristalsis.

Stomach—Chyme

The stomach is a large muscular organ, where considerable amounts of food can be stored before being shunted to other parts of the digestive system. In the stomach, digestive enzymes and high concentrations of hydrochloric acid (HCl, pH of about 2) begin to digest proteins in the food, as well as break down the food into smaller and smaller particles. After a while, the food becomes a nutrient-rich acid broth known as chyme. This chyme is slowly released into the duodenum (the upper portion of the small intestine), where most of the breakdown of macromolecules occurs.

Pancreas, Liver, and Gallbladder

Two glands, the pancreas and the liver, secrete into the duodenum substances that are crucial for digestion. The exocrine pancreas secretes molecules via ducts into the duodenum, as opposed to the endocrine pancreas, which secretes products (i.e., insulin) directly into the bloodstream. The exocrine pancreas delivers

THE CHARACTERISTICS OF SEVERAL COMPONENTS OF GASTRIC JUICE

COMPONENT	SOURCE	FUNCTION
Pepsinogen	Chief cells of the gastric gland	Converts to pepsin
Pepsin	Formed from pepsinogen in the presence of hydrochloric acid	Protein-digesting enzyme capable of breaking down nearly all types of protein
Hydrochloric acid	Parietal cells of the gastric glands	Provides acidic environment; needed for converting pepsinogen into pepsin
Mucus	Goblet cells and mucus glands	Provides viscous, alkaline protective layer on the stomach wall
Intrinsic factor	Parietal cells of the gastric glands	Encourages the absorption of vitamin B_{12}

to the duodenum powerful hydrolytic enzymes that break down proteins, fats, and carbohydrates. It also delivers a strongly alkaline bicarbonate solution, which neutralizes the highly acidic chyme. The liver produces bile, a mixture that contains no digestive enzymes but does contain salts and lipids that aid in fat processing. Bile also has pigments, by-products of the liver's breakdown of red blood cells, that are removed from the body with the feces. The gallbladder, a small sac attached to the liver, stores the bile until it is needed.

Small Intestine

Food is broken down in the duodenum, but the nutrients of the food are absorbed in the other parts of the small intestine, the jejunum and the ileum. The lining of the lower small intestine has many folds and is covered with projections called microvilli, which maximize the surface area for the diffusion and active transport of molecules. The network of blood vessels surrounding the lower small intestine collects the nutrients and transports them to the liver, which regulates their release to the heart and the rest of the body.

Large Intestine—Feces

In the large intestine, or colon, water is reabsorbed from the chyme. Salts are actively transported from the large intestine, and water follows by osmosis, leaving dense feces. The feces, consisting mainly of undigested roughage, travel to the rectum, where they are stored before being eliminated via the anus.

G. Respiratory System

The role of the respiratory system is to transport gases between the cells of the body and the environment. In humans, cellular respiration produces carbon dioxide, which is exchanged for oxygen, a necessary ingredient of respiration. Air (20% oxygen, 80% nitrogen) enters the body through the trachea and travels to the lungs. The lungs are made up of small passageways that end in air sacs called alveoli, where gas exchange occurs with the circulatory system. Alveoli have extremely thin walls and are surrounded by a network of pulmonary capillaries. Oxygen molecules diffuse across the thin walls and into the blood, while carbon dioxide in the blood diffuses into the air of the lungs. After gas exchange, the protein hemoglobin carries the oxygen in the blood, where it travels to the heart and the cells of the body. The deoxygenated air containing CO_2 waste is exhaled.

H. Urinary System

The urinary system has two functions: (1) to remove metabolic wastes from the body and (2) to osmoregulate, or balance the amounts of salts and water in the circulatory system. The kidneys, a pair of bean-shaped organs, are the sites of urinary function. Blood enters the kidneys through the renal artery. The kidneys filter out waste products and water, forming a concentrated excretory fluid called urine. The filtered blood returns to the circulatory system through the renal vein. The bladder stores the urine, which eventually passes through the urethra and is eliminated from the body.

An important function of the urinary system is the removal of ammonia (NH_3), a nitrogenous by-product of cell metabolism that is highly toxic to the cells of the body. Because of its poisonous qualities, ammonia must be removed from the blood quickly or changed into a less toxic substance. In humans, the liver converts ammonia to a soluble form called urea. Urea can travel in the blood safely for longer periods than ammonia. The kidneys remove urea from the blood, where it becomes a major component of urine.

A summary of transport and gas exchange mechanisms in the human body. (a) At the alveoli, CO_2 is released and oxygen is picked up. The gases pass across the membranes of the alveolus and the capillary. (b) At the body cells, the opposites occur for the two gases. Note that oxygen is carried bound to the hemoglobin (Hb) of RBCs, while CO_2 is carried dissolved in plasma, bound to hemoglobin molecules, and as bicarbonate ions in sodium bicarbonate.

The hemoglobin molecule of red blood cells. Two alpha chains and two beta chains of polypeptides make up the bulk of the molecule. A heme group is attached to each of the four polypeptide molecules. Note the iron ion (Fe) at the center of the heme group. This is where the oxygen molecule binds for transport.

Structure of the kidney and its fine structures. (a) A sagittal section of the kidney showing the entry and exit of the renal artery and renal vein, respectively. Note the minor calyx leading to the major calyx, then to the renal calyx and the renal pelvis and ureter for the elimination of urine. (b) The renal cortex and renal medulla are enlarged and the nephron can be seen. The swollen portion is Bowman's capsule. Tubes lead down into the renal medulla, then turn up back toward the cortex. Here they join with ducts leading down to the minor calyx. (c) A nephron expanded to show its details. Note the location of the capsule and how it leads to the proximal tubule, Henle's loop, the distal tubule, and the collecting duct. The peritubular capillary is not shown.

The kidney is made up of about one million functional units called nephrons. The nephrons perform three processes in controlling the salt and water concentrations of the blood.

Filtration, Secretion, and Reabsorption
Filtration
Filtration occurs in the cortex, when much of the blood plasma and many small molecules, such as amino acids, salts, and waste, are strained out of the blood.

Secretion
To maintain pH and salt concentrations in the blood, the nephrons take out certain amounts of acids, bases, and ions (especially hydrogen ions in order to control pH) and secrete them into the filtrate.

A detailed view of activity at the nephron. Note the arrow indicating the flow of blood from the artery to the afferent arteriole, through the glomerulus, and out the efferent arteriole. The blood then flows through the peritubular capillary network before leaving at the vein. Meanwhile, plasma enters the wall of Bowman's capsule, then flows through the proximal convoluted tubule, loop of Henle, and distal convoluted tubule before entering the collecting duct. Modifications of the plasma in the tubules results in urine. Note the intertwined peritubular capillary and nephron tubules that make the transfers possible. Also note that the collecting duct receives urine from other nephrons in the area. Portions of the nephron are in the cortex of the kidney, as indicated, while other portions are in the medulla.

Reabsorption

Many substances such as sugars, nutrients, and amino acids must return to the blood at their proper levels. Reabsorption is regulated, in part, by antidiuretic hormone (ADH) secreted by the pituitary gland.

After these steps, the waste products remaining in the nephron are excreted.

Flow of Filtrate

The flow of filtrate is as follows:

1. Blood enters the kidney and travels to the glomerulus, a network of capillaries. The bulb-shaped Bowman's capsule surrounds the glomerulus. Much of the blood plasma and small molecules in the blood, such as amino acids, salts, and waste, filter through the thin walls of the capillaries to form a fluid called the filtrate. Large molecules, such as proteins and blood cells, remain in the blood.
2. The filtrate travels from the Bowman's capsule through the proximal convoluted tubule to the loop of Henle. During the descending journey, water diffuses out of the tubule through the permeable membrane, concentrating the filtrate.
3. The tubule ascending from the loop of Henle is impermeable to water but is permeable to salts. As the filtrate passes through this section, salt ions are pumped out of the filtrate, diluting the fluid.
4. The urine travels to the collecting duct, which is permeable to water but not salts. More water is reabsorbed, leaving a concentrated filtrate.

I. Brain and Nervous System

The nervous system enables the body to receive and respond to stimuli from the environment. The primary cell of the nervous system is the neuron. Neurons process a stimulus and transmit it as an electric charge to other cells.

Anatomy and Function of the Neuron

A neuron consists of (1) a cell body (soma), which contains the nucleus and organelles; (2) dendrites, which are extensions of the cytoplasm that carry signals to the soma; and (3) the axon, which is a long nerve fiber that carries the electro-chemical signal to other cells. The gap between two adjacent neurons or between a neuron and a target cell (i.e., muscle) is called a synapse. Most axons are covered with myelin sheaths, fatty insulating coats that speed up the conduction velocity of the axon. Myelin sheaths are made of Schwann cells, with gaps between them called nodes of Ranvier. Schwann cells are examples of glial cells, that is, cells that are closely associated with neurons but do not transmit signals. Glial cells have very important supportive roles in the nervous system.

An illustration of the three types of neurons found in the nervous system. Multipolar neurons (a) have numerous extensions, while bipolar neurons (b) have two extensions, and unipolar neurons (c) have one. The details of a neuron are shown in the multipolar neuron.

How the myelin sheath forms as the Schwann cell wraps itself around the axon in successive diagrams (a), (b), and (c). Myelin is the white, lipid-rich substance in the plasma membrane of the Schwann cell.

Types of Neurons

There are three types of neurons: sensory neurons (afferent), which interpret stimuli from the environment; interneurons, which relay the information received; and motor neurons (efferent), which control muscular movement. The axons and dendrites of these neurons are grouped together in bundles called nerves. For instance, a baseball player sees the ball coming toward him with sensory neurons. Interneurons process the speed and trajectory of the ball, and motor neurons control the muscles in the baseball player's body as he swings the bat. This information travels great distances along the three types of neurons.

Transmission of Information

Several steps are involved in transmitting information through a nerve cell and to other cells.

Resting Potential

A neuron works because its membranes have electrical potential, or the force to move charged particles. When the neuron is not active, it is polarized, meaning that the electric charge inside the cell differs from the charge outside it. Specialized proteins in the membrane make up the sodium-potassium pump and create the difference in charge. Na^+ ions are pumped outside the neural membrane, and K^+ ions are pumped inside. The membrane is also selectively permeable, allowing K^+ ions to leak through much more readily than Na^+ ions. The result is that the inner surface of the nerve cell membrane is negatively charged relative to its outside. When the neuron is not firing, this difference in charge is called a resting potential.

Action Potential

Information in the nervous system is carried through electrical signals. These signals among nerve cells are sent as action potentials, or disturbances in the membrane's electrical potential that travels along the axon. An action potential begins with a stimulus, which changes the permeability of the nerve cell's membrane and upsets the normal balance of ions. Na^+ ions leak in, making the charge inside the cell more positive. Small changes in ion concentrations have no effect.

If, however, the stimulus is strong enough, the membrane potential becomes more positive and reaches the threshold potential (the potential that generates an action potential). The moment the charge reaches threshold potential, the proteins that control the entry and exit of sodium through the membrane (gated sodium channels) swing open. Sodium ions rush into the cell, briefly reversing the potential of the cell from negative (–40 mV) to positive (+70 mV) in a small segment of

The Sodium-Potassium Pump

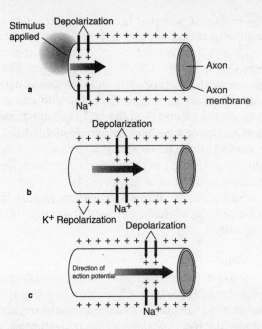

The action potential in a nerve cell. (a) A stimulus is applied to the membrane, and sodium ions (+) rush into the cell; the membrane loses its polarity, thereby generating an action potential. (b) The adjacent membrane area is depolarized by this action, and the action potential is propagated; meanwhile the original area undergoes repolarization with the accumulation of potassium ions (+) so it can "fire" again. (c) The action potential continues down the axon as successive areas undergo depolarization. Eventually, the action potential will pass into another nerve cell or a muscle cell.

the axon. Just as quickly, those channels close, other channels open, and the resting potential is restored. The opening, then closing, of the channels constitutes the action potential. It is important to note that a stronger stimulus does not increase the level or duration of the action potential; it only creates more frequent action potentials. After a segment of an axon is activated to produce an action potential, there is a period of time, called the refractory period, before this segment can be activated again.

An action potential is an example of an all-or-nothing response. If the stimulus is too low to cause critical changes in the permeability of the membrane, nothing

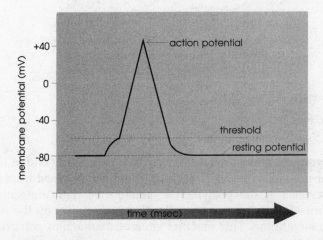

Action Potential

will happen. If, however, the threshold potential is exceeded, an action potential is fired and is propagated along the axon and to other cells.

Propagation of the Impulse

Action potentials move along the membrane as a wave moves across a pool. An action potential fires only in a short portion of the axon. The sodium ions that rush into that portion also cause the electrical potential to change in the adjacent portion. The adjacent portion reaches a threshold potential, which quickly initiates an action potential in that area. Meanwhile, the original area returns to its resting potential. This pattern continues as the action potential moves along the axon. The wider the axon, the greater the speed of the action potential. Also, myelin sheaths speed up the conduction velocity of the impulse. They insulate sections of the membrane, making the impulse jump quickly between the nodes of Ranvier (a process called saltatory conduction).

Transmission between Cells

As stated previously a synapse is the junction between two nerve cells or between a nerve cell and an effector membrane, such as muscle. More specifically, a synapse occurs between the axon of the presynaptic neuron and the membrane of a postsynaptic cell. There are two types of synapses: electric synapses, also called gap junctions, and chemical synapses. Gap junctions are protein channels that allow ions to flow freely from one cell to another, and thus to function as a unit. The transmission is virtually instantaneous, a feature that is important for some functions.

The more complex synapse is the chemical synapse, where a cell relays an impulse to another cell by converting the impulse into a chemical message. The chemical signals are called neurotransmitters. When an impulse travels to the synaptic knob of the presynaptic neuron, mitochondria and synaptic vesicles re-

Activity at the synapse. When an action potential reaches the end of the axon, neurotransmitter molecules (such as acetylcholine) are released from synaptic vesicles by exocytosis at the presynaptic membranes. The molecules move across the synaptic cleft (space) and react with receptor sites on the surface of the postsynaptic membrane. This reaction generates an action potential in the postsynaptic neuron.

lease the neurotransmitters into the synaptic cleft, the gap between the two cells. The neurotransmitter binds to receptor sites on the postsynaptic membrane, thereby triggering a change in its permeability. The change either promotes or inhibits the propagation of the impulse. Very quickly, the neurotransmitter is eliminated from the synaptic cleft, and the system is ready for the next impulse.

Processing Information

Nerve cells can receive impulses from thousands of axons. One impulse does not necessarily trigger the transmission of an action potential. Many impulses come together to make the cell fire, a process called summation. Remember that certain impulses can have an inhibitory effect, so that impulses can also neutralize each other. The integration of the various sources by the nerve cell is the key to processing information.

Central and Peripheral Nervous Systems

The human nervous system is divided into two continuously interacting parts, the central nervous system and the peripheral nervous system.

The central nervous system, which processes information, consists of the brain and spinal cord. The spinal cord has two functions in the central nervous system: to relay information to and from the brain and to process simple stimuli. The spinal cord primarily integrates by way of a reflex, a connection of two or three neurons that unconsciously reacts to a simple stimulus. The knee jerk—the kicking response to a doctor tapping below the knee—is an example of a reflex.

The brain is the center of complex nerve integration. The outer part of the brain is composed of gray matter, a grouping of cell bodies. The interior consists of white matter, a network of axons. The brain is made up of three main parts. The forebrain is the largest part of the brain and has various sections that control memory and thought (cerebral cortex), integrate spinal cord information (thalamus), and regulate various autonomic functions such as those involved with sex, hunger, and temperature (hypothalamus). The midbrain relays impulses from the eyes and ears. It also contains the limbic system, which controls emotions. The hindbrain has three parts, which control movement and coordination (cerebellum) and maintain body homeostatic functions such as breathing, heart rate, and digestion (medulla and pons).

Organization of the Vertebrate Nervous System

Interneuron

Cell body of sensory neuron

Cell body of motor neuron

Effector muscle

Pain receptors in skin

A typical reflex arc as shown by the withdrawal reflex. Impulses arise at the pain receptor and travel to the spinal cord by the sensory neuron. The interneuron interprets the impulse and dispatches a response via the motor neuron to the effector muscles that withdraw the foot from the pain. Note the position of the cell body of the sensory neuron outside the spinal cord in a ganglion and the cell body of the motor neuron within the cord.

The peripheral nervous system collects and distributes information and is made up of the sensory organs, motor (efferent) neurons, and sensory (afferent) neurons.

The motor division is divided into the somatic nervous system, which controls voluntary movements and reflexes, and the autonomic nervous system, which regulates smooth and cardiac muscles and organs of the digestive, cardiovascular, urinary, and endocrine system (involuntary actions).

The autonomic nervous system is further divided into the sympathetic and parasympathetic divisions. When there is danger, the sympathetic division is responsible for the "fight or flight response," including responses such as increased heart rate, hormone release, decreased digestion, and dilation of blood vessels to muscles. When no danger is perceived, the parasympathetic division controls responses that conserve energy, including decreased heart rate and increased digestion.

J. Endocrine System

The endocrine system is a system of internal communication, regulating the activities of various tissues of the body. Unlike the nervous system, which uses electrical impulses to trigger rapid response, the endocrine system relies on chemical signals to coordinate longer lasting activities, such as growth, reproduction, tissue repair, and nutrient balance in the blood.

The endocrine glands in relation to some of the other major body organs.

Hormones

Biochemical signals are mediated by hormones, which endocrine glands secrete directly into the bloodstream. These hormones travel to target cells, where they bind to appropriate receptors and can cause dramatic changes in the cells' functioning. It is interesting that one hormone can have varied effects on different types of cells, as well as on several processes in one cell.

There are three main types of hormones in the body. Steroid hormones, such as estrogen and testosterone, are lipids and can travel easily through cell membranes to bind with interior cell receptors. Polypeptide hormones and amino acid derivatives do not actually enter the cell but bind to receptors on the cell surface.

Secondary Messengers and the Cascading Effect

Secondary messengers are substances that are activated by a hormone. They, in turn, activate enzymes, which activate more enzymes, which activate still more enzymes, and so on. This amplified effect of the hormone is called the cascading effect and is one reason why very small amounts of a hormone in the blood can cause dramatic changes in physiology.

K. Reproductive System

The reproductive systems of humans are designed to manufacture male and female germ cells, then provide a way for them to come together during sexual reproduction. In males, gametes called sperm are produced in the testes. The testes are composed of tightly wound seminiferous tubules, where sperm are formed in a three-stage process called spermatogenesis, that includes one mitotic and two meiotic divisions. The result is a sperm containing 23 chromosomes, half the full complement of 46. Dispersed throughout the sperm-producing tubules are interstitial cells. These cells secrete androgens, male sex hormones that, among other functions,

Spermatogenesis

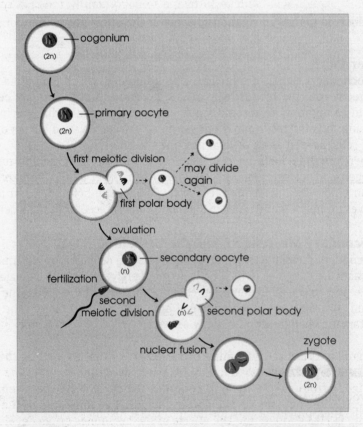

Oogenesis

regulate the rate of sperm production. From the testes, sperm travel through what is collectively known as the male reproductive tract—the epididymis, to the vas deferens, through the urethra, and finally out the tip of the penis.

The female germ cell, the egg or ovum, is produced in the ovaries, which are made up of many follicles, each containing a single egg. The follicle is a sac that nourishes and protects the egg during its development. At birth, a female baby has her lifetime supply of follicles, some of which will later develop into egg producers. The cells of the follicle produce estrogen, the female sex hormone that is responsible for secondary female sex characteristics and plays a significant role in regulating the menstrual cycle.

Gamete Production

At puberty, oogenesis, or gamete production, begins. The egg undergoes a single meiotic division. This produces a secondary oocyte, now with 23 chromosomes. Subsequently, once a month at ovulation, the follicle ruptures, releasing the oocyte. The egg moves through the oviduct, or Fallopian tube, where it will undergo a second meiotic division only if it is fertilized there by a sperm.

Hormones and the Reproductive Pattern

Sex hormones called androgens regulate the pattern in male reproduction. Testosterone is the most important androgen. It accounts for secondary male sex characteristics (e.g., pubic hair, facial hair, and muscle growth) and determines certain sexual behaviors, such as sex drive and aggressiveness. The testes are stimulated to produce testosterone by luteinizing hormone (LH), which is secreted by the anterior pituitary gland. Also secreted by this gland is follicle-stimulating hormone (FSH), which acts with testosterone to continuously produce sperm. FSH and LH are gonadotropins, as they regulate function in the gonads.

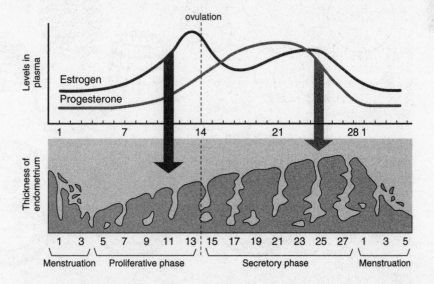

The menstrual cycle. Menstruation proceeds for several days, then the proliferative stage extends from day 6 to day 14, when ovulation occurs. The secretory stage extends from day 15 to 28 to complete the cycle. Note the levels of estrogen and progesterone during the various stages. The thickness of the endometrial lining is also shown, and the effects of the hormones on its development is illustrated by the vertical arrows.

The same gonadotropins play key roles in the female reproductive pattern, which is a 28-day cycle of egg release that differs greatly from the male's continuous gamete production. At the beginning of the hormone-controlled process known as the menstrual cycle, the anterior pituitary gland produces FSH and LH. Together, these hormones trigger the production of estrogen, which stimulates the thickening of the lining of the uterus, a muscular organ commonly called the womb, to make it suitable for egg development. At the same time, FSH triggers follicle growth and egg maturation. About halfway through the cycle, a surge of LH triggers ovulation and the egg is released to be fertilized. If fertilization does not occur within 24 hours, the oocyte is discarded, hormone secretions decline, and the lining of the uterus disintegrates. Blood vessels rupture as the lining of the uterus retreats, and menstrual bleeding begins. Menstruation marks the beginning of a new cycle.

Conception is the point at which the egg becomes fertilized by a sperm cell. The fertilized egg, or zygote, travels via the oviduct to the uterus, where it implants on the endometrium and develops into a fetus.

IX. DESCRIPTIVE EMBRYOLOGY AND DEVELOPMENTAL MECHANICS

A. Cleavage

After fertilization, the zygote develops by rapid cell divisions. The first divisions are called cleavages. In mammals and other animals along the deutorostome evolutionary line, cleavage is indeterminate, meaning that each cell can develop into a

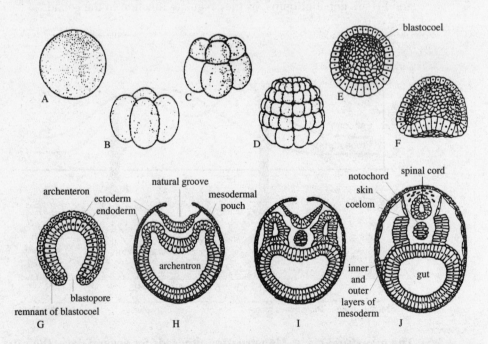

Early embryology of amphioxus. (A) Zygote. (B–D) Early cleavage stages forming a morula (C) and then a blastula (D). (E) Longitudinal section through a blastula, showing the blasticoel. (F–G) Longitudinal sections through an early and a late gastrula. Notice that the invagination is at the vegetal pole of the embryo, where the cells are largest. (H–I) Cross sections through an early and a late neurula. Invagination of the dorsal ectoderm is giving rise to the spinal cord, and pouches off the endoderm are giving rise to the mesoderm. (J) A later embryo in which both the spinal cord and the mesoderm are taking their definitive form. Notice that there is a cavity (the coelom) in the mesoderm.

separate organism. For instance, indeterminate cleavage results in identical twins. Determinate cleavage occurs in the protostome evolutionary line (insects, crabs, and snails), in which cells specialize early in development.

B. From Morula to Gastrula

As the cells divide, a morula, or tight bunch of cells, forms. The morula gradually becomes hollow, as if inflated with fluid, in a process called blastulation. When this process is finished, the hollow sphere of cells is termed a blastula. Inside the blastula is a fluid filled cavity called a blastocoel. The blastocoel develops two specialized parts: the inner cell mass, which will later become the embryo, and the trophoblast, which will become the placenta.

In a process called gastrulation, the cells of the blastula separate into three distinct layers. The outermost layer, the ectoderm, later becomes the skin and the nervous system. The middle layer, the mesoderm, develops into the internal organs and the musculoskeletal, circulatory, and excretory systems. The innermost layer, the endoderm, forms the lining of the digestive tract and the organs of the digestive system. When the three layers have become apparent, the assemblage is called a gastrula. Gastrulation differs among different embryo types. In amphibians, the ball of cells invaginates like a racquetball being pushed in by a thumb. This creates an inner space, the archenteron, which becomes the digestive tract, and an opening called a blastopore, which becomes the anus. In mammals, the mesoderm forms from the rapid inward migration of cells from the ectoderm and endoderm.

At the end of gastrulation, the nervous system begins to develop in a process called neurulation. A hollow cord of cells in the mesoderm develops into the notochord, which later becomes part of the spinal column (every vertebrate has a notochord in some stage of development). Ectodermal cells above the notochord fuse to form the neural tube, which gives rise to the brain and spinal cord. Some ectodermal cells break off the neural tube and become neural crest cells. These cells

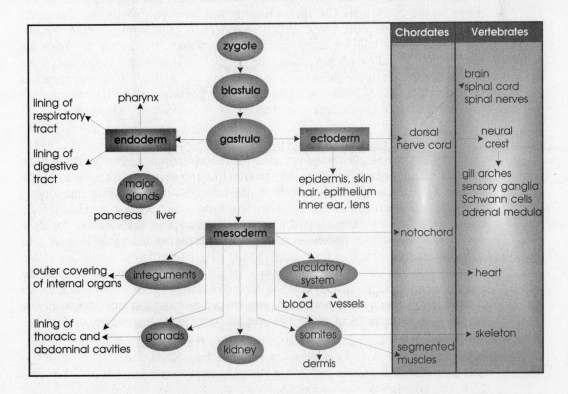

Derivation of Major Tissues and Organs

move throughout the body and develop into many parts of the peripheral nervous system, such as sensory neurons and glial cells.

C. Development of the Fetus

After 8 weeks of growth, the embryo is known as a fetus. In the first few weeks of development, the placenta and the umbilical cord form and become the specialized circulatory system between mother and fetus. This system provides the fetus with nourishment and removes metabolic wastes. The umbilical cord develops from two embryonic sacs, the yolk sac (the site of early blood vessel development) and the allantois (an outpocketing of the gut that contains many blood vessels). The placenta is formed when part of the chorion (a membrane that surrounds the amnion, which is the strong sac that houses the fetus and contains shock-absorbing fluid called amniotic fluid) fuses to the uterine walls. In addition to supplying nutrients and removing wastes, the placenta prevents toxins and drugs from entering the fetus and functions as an endocrine gland, producing the essential hormones progesterone, estrogen, and human chorionic gonadotropin (HCG).

X. MENDELIAN INHERITANCE

A. Genes

The traits passed from parent to offspring are carried by units of information called genes. Genes, studied in the field of genetics, are coded in fragments of DNA found in the chromosomes. Gregor Mendel (1822–1884) described several basic principles of inheritance, two of which are the principle of segregation and the principle of dominance. The principle of segregation states that there are alternative forms, called alleles, of a single gene. For an inherited trait, an animal possesses an allele from each parent. During meiosis, these alleles segregate from each other, resulting in gametes that carry one allele for each trait. For instance, if a white female cat mates with a black male cat, their offspring will have two alleles for coat color, one white and the other black. When reproductive cells mature within the offspring, the alleles will separate, resulting in eggs that carry either the allele for white hair or the allele for black hair. The principle of dominance states that, if the two alleles for a trait are different, one allele will be dominant (fully expressed in the individual) and the other will be recessive (will not show itself). Dominant alleles are written in capital letters, and recessive alleles in lowercase letters.

Genotype versus Phenotype

Modern geneticists also contributed the concepts of the genotype, the genetic makeup of the organism, versus the phenotype, the actual characteristic of the organism. In other words, if a woman has brown eyes, that is her phenotype. However, her genotype is not as clear. She may either possess two alleles for brown eyes or dominant allele for brown eyes and a recessive allele for blue eyes. An organism that possesses two matching copies of the same allele is said to be homozygous for that trait; animals that have two different alleles are called heterozygous. To determine the genotype of an individual, Mendel devised the test cross, an experiment that mates a recessive homozygous individual with an individual of unknown genotype. A Punnett square like the one shown below predicts the frequencies of genotypes and phenotypes in the progeny of a cross.

	Genotype	Phenotype
	BB or *Bb*	**Brown eyes**
	bb	**blue eyes**

BB:

	B	B
b	Bb	Bb
b	Bb	Bb

Bb:

	B	b
b	Bb	bb
b	Bb	bb

	Genotype	Phenotype		Genotype	Phenotype
Offspring:	100% *Bb*	Brown eyes		50% *Bb*	Brown eyes
				50% *bb*	blue eyes

If all the offspring express the dominant phenotype, their eye color will be brown; the unknown phenotype is homozygous dominant. If the recessive phenotype appears in the offspring, the individual is heterozygous. If two heterozygous individuals are crossed, the Punnett square predicts that 50% of the offspring will be heterozygous (*Bb*), 25% will be homozygous dominant (*BB*), and 25% will be homozygous recessive (*bb*). In this case, the phenotype ratio would be three brown-eyed offspring to every one offspring with blue eyes.

The Punnett square for a cross of two heterozygous individuals is shown below:

Bb × Bb:

	B	b
B	BB	Bb
b	Bb	bb

Offspring:

Genotype	Phenotype
25% *BB*	Brown eyes
50% *Bb*	Brown eyes
25% *bb*	blue eyes

Independent Assortment

Mendel's third basic principle is the law of independent assortment, which states that unlinked traits separate independently of each other during meiosis. For instance, in pea plants, an allele for a wrinkled seed will have no effect on the color of the seed, that is, whether the seed will be green or yellow. With yellow and round seeds dominant, the Punnett square below predicts that a cross between a round, yellow seeded plant (*RRYY*) and a wrinkled, green seeded plant (*rryy*) will yield a 9:3:3:1 ratio in the second generation. This ratio is characteristic of crosses between individuals that are either homozygous recessive or homozygous dominant for two independently assorting traits.

RRYY × rryy
First Generation (F$_1$):
                   100% *RrYy*

RrYy × RrYy
Second Generation (F$_2$):

	RY	Ry	rY	ry
RY	RRYY	RRYy	RrYY	RrYy
Ry	RRyY	RRyy	RyYy	Rryy
rY	rRYY	rRYy	rrYY	rrYy
ry	rRyY	rRyy	rryY	rryy

Seed phenotype results:
9 Round, Yellow
3 wrinkled, Yellow
3 Round, green
1 wrinkled, green

Punnett Square-Pea Dihybrid Cross

B. Incomplete Dominance

Some traits are inherited in a more complicated manner than can be explained by Mendelian genetics. For instance, two alleles do not always determine a trait. Some traits, such as coat color in rabbits, have multiple alleles with varying degrees of dominance. Also, not all alleles can be categorized as simply dominant or recessive. Incomplete dominance is a situation in which one allele does not completely block the expression of another, and the alleles blend to form the phenotype. Petal color in snapdragon flowers is an example of incomplete dominance. If red (*RR*) and white (*rr*) flowering plants are crossed, the progeny will have pink flowers.

C. Codominance

If a heterozygous phenotype expresses both alleles equally, the inheritance is codominant. A standard example of codominance is the inheritance of blood type. Blood types are determined by the alleles I^A, I^B, and i, corresponding to different types of antigens in the blood. An individual who is homozygous I^A or I^B has an *A* or *B* phenotype and type *A* or *B* blood. If an individual is heterozygous ($I^A I^B$), however, the alleles are codominant and the phenotype is *AB*; this individual has type *AB* blood.

XI. CHROMOSOMAL GENETICS

A. Chromosomes

Mendelian genetics is based on the behavior of chromosomes, the protein and DNA structures that contain the genetic information of an organism. Diploid species have two sets of chromosomes, one from each parent. Chromosome pairs, also called homologues, have an allele for a trait on each chromosome. Gametes have half the chromosome number and are referred to as haploid. In humans, the full complement of genetic material includes 22 chromosome pairs, called autosomes, which do not differ between the sexes, and an additional pair of sex chromosomes.

B. Sex Chromosomes

Sex chromosomes determine the sex of the individual; males are heterologous, XY, and females are homologous, XX. Sex chromosomes segregate like autosomes during meiosis, with each gamete receiving either an X or a Y chromosome from the father. The offspring will receive one of the two X chromosomes from the mother. If the sperm that fertilizes the egg has a Y chromosome, then the offspring will be male. If it has an X, the offspring will be female.

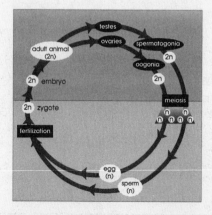

Generalized Animal Life Cycle

XII. MEIOSIS

A. Asexual Reproduction

Many invertebrates produce new individuals through asexual reproduction. This process results in offspring that are genetically identical to the parent. There are three types of asexual reproduction. In *binary fission*, a parent cell literally divides in half through mitosis. The parent cell becomes two daughter cells (bacteria and amoeba). In *budding*, small bud cells are pinched off the parent by cell division (yeast cells). In *fragmentation*, the parent's body breaks up into several pieces, some or all of which develop into complete adults (sea stars reproduce by fragmentaion; they use regeneration to regrow lost body parts).

B. Meiosis versus Mitosis

Sexual reproduction combines genetic material from two sources to create offspring. During sexual reproduction, specialized cells, called germ cells, undergo meiotic cell divisions and come together to form individuals with new genetic

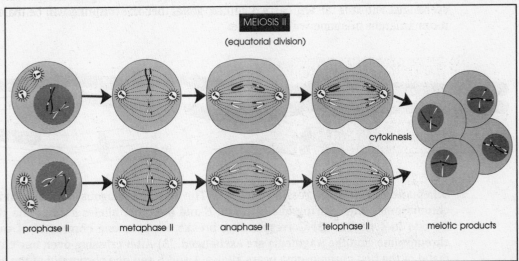

Meiosis in Animal Cells

combinations. Unlike mitosis, which produces diploid cells (paired chromosomes, 2N), meiosis produces haploid gamete cells (single chromosomes, 1N). When the single chromosomes of the gametes meet during sexual reproduction, they produce a diploid organism.

C. First and Second Meiotic Divisions

Meiosis occurs over two cell divisions, resulting in four haploid daughter cells. *Division I*: The chromosomes (single-stranded) double as in mitosis to form chromatids (double-stranded). In meiosis, unlike mitosis, however, the homologous pairs come together to form tetrads. During the formation of tetrads, chromatids exchange material, a process called crossing over or genetic recombination. The chromosomes pull apart, producing two haploid daughter cells. *Division II*: The genetic material does not double. The chromosomes come together, then pull apart into the daughter cells. Each gamete cell receives the full haploid complement of chromosomes unless there is nondisjunction, in which case chromosomes (meiosis I) or chromatids (meiosis II) do not pull apart properly. The result is polyploidy, two copies of the gene in one gamete, and aneuploidy, no copies of the gene, in the other.

XIII. MOLECULAR AND HUMAN GENETICS

A. Independent Assortment

If genes are on different chromosomes, they will segregate independently to the daughter cells during the first meiotic division. This is the basis for classic Mendelian genetics. For instance, if the genetic information for flower color and seed type is on different chromosomes in a certain plant, the inheritance of the traits will not be related in any way in the next generation.

B. Linkage

If purple flowers usually produce long seeds and red flowers usually produce round seeds, it is reasonable to assume that flower color and seed shape are inherited together. This means that genes for these traits are linked on the same chromosome and will not separate during meiosis. Genes that are close to each other on a chromosome are more likely to be inherited together. On the other hand, genes that are farther apart have a higher probability of crossing-over and exchange. The rate at which two linked genes become unlinked is called the recombination frequency.

Schematic diagram of crossing-over. (1) The two homologous doublestranded chromosomes, one bearing alleles *A* and *B* and the other alleles *a* and *b*, lie side by side in synapsis. (2) Corresponding breaks occur in one chromatid of each chromosome, and the fragments are exchanged. (3) After crossing-over, one chromatid of the first chromosome bears alleles *A* and *b* and one chromatid of the second chromosome bears alleles *a* and *B*.

By establishing recombination frequencies, it is possible to make genetic maps that show the locations of the various alleles on the chromosome.

Sex-Linkage

Sex-linked genes are located on sex chromosomes. The X chromosome is much larger than the Y chromosome and carries the sex-linked genes. Because females have two X chromosomes, the dominant sex-linked allele is expressed and the recessive allele is not. In males, however, any allele on the one X chromosome is expressed. Inheritance of sex-linked genes is quite complicated. For example, a woman can be heterozygous for a recessive sex-linked disease, such as hemophilia or color

Patterns of Inheritance

Roman numerals identify generations; the numbers identify individuals within each generation. *(a)* Inheritance of an autosomal dominant trait. Individual I-2 is a male heterozygous for the trait; if he were homozygous, all of the progeny in generation II would show the trait. None of the affected individuals in generations II or III can be homozygotes, because each has received a normal recessive allele from one parent. *(b)* Inheritance of an autosomal recessive trait. If the trait were dominant rather than recessive, then either III-3 or III-4 would have to show the trait in order for IV-2 and IV-6 to have inherited it. III-3 and III-4 are first cousins—their mating is represented by the double horizontal line. There is no indication of sex linkage. *(c)* Inheritance of a sex-linked recessive trait. The affected individuals II-1, III-4, and IV-4 are all males. The carriers are all females. This is the pattern of inheritance for hemophilia.

blindness, and act as a carrier. She is not affected, but half of her sons will suffer from the disease. Also, the male X chromosome is passed only to the female off-spring. Therefore, an affected male cannot pass on a sex-linked disease to his sons but can pass the gene on to his daughters. If a daughter is homozygous for a recessive disease, she will be affected; if she is heterozygous, she will act as a carrier.

Over several generations, it is possible to track the inheritance of genes by means of a pedigree. A pedigree depicts the pattern of inheritance of a particular trait in a family and thus helps geneticists to understand the mechanism of gene transfer.

C. Gene Structure

Genetic information is carried in strands of DNA (deoxyribonucleic acid). DNA is a nucleic acid, made up of four nucleotide bases: adenine (A), cytosine (C), guanine (G), and thymine (T). The structure of DNA is a double helix, a coiled ladder with rungs of paired nucleotide bases. The base-pairing rule is that the purines (A, G), pair up with the pyrimidines (T, C): A-T and G-C.

DNA Duplex

Nucleic Acid Base Structure

Pentose Sugars

DNA Replication

The fundamental significance of DNA is that it is a copyable blueprint for life that can be passed on to future generations. The steps in DNA replication are as follows.

1. Enzymes, called helicases, unwind the two strands of the DNA molecule.
2. Because of the base-pairing rule, the single strands act as templates for the formation of new complementary strands.
3. DNA polymerase moves along the original strands and attaches to the appropriate nucleotide bases.
4. If the incorrect base-pair is inserted, part of the DNA polymerase enzyme will correct the mistake. Through this elegant process, many identical DNA copies can be made from a single molecule.

D. DNA Transcription and Translation

DNA carries information by encoding directions for the synthesis of proteins. Proteins, in turn, synthesize the molecules that make up the organism. As in replication, DNA acts as a template from which new molecules can be formed. However, DNA does not directly determine the sequence of amino acids in the protein. The molecule that performs this function is messenger RNA (mRNA). The differences between RNA and DNA are that RNA uses ribose, rather than deoxyribose, as its sugar backbone, and RNA replaces the nucleotide base thymine (T) with uracil (U). In a process known as transcription, RNA polymerase synthesizes a complementary RNA (ribonucleic acid) copy of a DNA strand. A complementary copy is not a duplicate, but rather a base-pair inverse of the original. For example, if a DNA base-pair sequence is ATGTCC, the RNA complement will be UACAGG.

DNA nucleotde
DNA polymerase

DNA replication. The DNA strands unwind, and the enzyme DNA polymerase unites nucleotides in each chain according to bases present on the old chain. The new strand then unites with an old strand to form two new double helixes.

Transcription

The bases on a strand of mRNA code for different amino acids, which assemble to form proteins in a process called translation. Translation involves several steps. Different codons, or combinations of three base pairs, correspond to each of the 20 amino acids commonly used in proteins. GUU, for instance, is the three-letter

Translation

Structure of a tRNA

THE GENETIC CODE*

SECOND LETTER

FIRST LETTER	U	C	A	G	THIRD LETTER
U	Phenylalanine	Serine	Tyrosine	Cysteine	**U**
	Phenylalanine	Serine	Tyrosine	Cysteine	**C**
	Leucine	Serine	STOP	STOP	**A**
	Leucine	Serine	STOP	Tryptophan	**G**
C	Leucine	Proline	Histidine	Arginine	**U**
	Leucine	Proline	Histidine	Arginine	**C**
	Leucine	Proline	Glutamine	Arginine	**A**
	Leucine	Proline	Glutamine	Arginine	**G**
A	Isoleucine	Threonine	Asparagine	Serine	**U**
	Isoleucine	Threonine	Asparagine	Serine	**C**
	Isoleucine	Threonine	Lysine	Arginine	**A**
	Methionine (Start)	Threonine	Lysine	Arginine	**G**
G	Valine	Alanine	Aspartate	Glycine	**U**
	Valine	Alanine	Aspartate	Glycine	**C**
	Valine	Alanine	Glutamate	Glycine	**A**
	Valine	Alanine	Glutamate	Glycine	**G**

* The amino acids encoded by mRNA triplets (codons). Although the code depicted above is used by most organisms, subcellular organelles and some ciliate protists show minor variations. The code is also said to be degenerate because more than one triplet may code for a single amino acid.

Codon-Anticodon Pairing

5' end of anticodon	3' end of codon
G	U or C
C	G only
A	U only
U	A or G
I	U, C, or A

code for valine, and UGG is the code for tryptophan. Amino acids are attached to transfer RNA (tRNA) molecules, which "read" the codon and carry the amino acid to the correct position. Ribosomes are involved in joining the amino acids together. Protein synthesis ends when a tRNA reaches a stop codon, such as UGA.

XIV. NATURAL SELECTION

A. Evolution

Evolution is the process by which populations change over time. Charles Darwin's *The Origin of Species*, published in 1859, outlines several key concepts in the study of evolution: fitness, adaptation, and natural selection. An organism's fitness is determined by the ability to produce viable offspring. Fitness is often confused with the ability of an organism to survive in an environment. However, this is not the criterion; a healthy female tiger may be the strongest and fastest in the region, but her fitness is zero if she never mates. On the other hand, a male elephant seal that mates with many females has high fitness. Adaptation is a change in the genetic makeup of a population that increases its fitness. Natural selection is based on the principle that an individual with high fitness is more likely to reproduce successfully than a less fit individual. Natural selection tends to adapt the characteristics of an organism to its environment. For example, in early giraffe populations, natural selection favored individuals with long necks that could reach the leaves of trees. The result over time was a population shift toward individuals with very long necks that were better suited to life in the African savanna.

XV. POPULATION GENETICS

A. Hardy-Weinberg Equilibrium

Natural selection acts on individuals, but evolution acts on populations. Genetically speaking, evolution is defined as the changes in allele frequencies of a population. The Hardy-Weinberg law is a hypothetical model that examines circumstances that cause evolution. In simple terms, if random sexual selection is the only factor affecting allele frequencies, then no evolution will occur—a situation known as Hardy-Weinberg equilibrium. The frequencies for this situation are 80 percent for the dominant allele, and 20 percent for the recessive allele. However, if there are mutations, chance events, or unequal reproductive successes among genotypes in the population, the allele frequencies will not match those for Hardy-Weinberg equilibrium, and evolution will occur. The following example illustrates this principle with regard to scale color in fish.

Equilibrium Allele Frequencies:

AA	Aa	aa
p^2	pq	q^2
.64	.32	.04

Phenotype:

Blue scales	Blue scales	White scales
	A $p = .8$	a $q = .2$
A $p = .8$	$AA = .8 \times .8 = .64$	$Aa = .8 \times .2 = .16$
a $q = .2$	$Aa = .8 \times .2 = .16$	$aa = .2 \times .2 = .04$

Overall: $p^2 + 2pq + q^2 = 1$,

$p = .8$ and $q = .2$

B. Mutations or Random Events

Mutations or random events can, by chance, quickly change the genetic makeup of a small population, a concept called genetic drift. If a nonlethal mutation in an individual greatly increases its fitness, that mutation will be passed on to many offspring. After only a few generations, the new gene will become common in the population. In the same way, a gene can disappear from a population if a random event kills individuals with a certain genotype.

C. Reproductive Isolation

An extreme case of genetic drift is the founder effect, where a small number of individuals branch off the main population and colonize a new habitat. As the "colonists" are reproductively isolated from the larger population, the genetic makeup of their population can change drastically. For example, imagine that a country of people with varying eye color sends a group of homozygous brown-eyed colonizers to a distant island. The new island community will have only brown eyes, representing a dramatic shift in the allele frequency for that population.

When a population becomes reproductively isolated, it evolves into a species. There are several mechanisms that bring about reproductive isolation.

Allopatric Speciation

Allopatric speciation arises from the separation of populations by a geographic barrier, such as a river or a mountain. The barrier prevents gene flow between the populations, and natural selection acts on each population separately. Allopatric speciation, for example, describes the genetic divergence of an animal on an island from the same animal on the mainland (e.g., Darwin's finches of the Galapagos Islands).

Parapatric Speciation

Parapatric speciation occurs when a small part of a larger population branches off in the absence of geographic speciation, in which a small part of a larger population separates itself without the presence of a geographic barrier. This can happen if selective pressures, such as temperature, predation, and food availability on a fringe of a population's range differ from those affecting the larger range.

Sympatric Speciation

In sympatric speciation, a new species originates within a larger population, usually by a genetic mutation. Sympatric speciation occurs frequently in plants, when chromosomal doubling results in unique genotypes that can reproduce only with each other.

XVI. COMMUNITY ECOLOGY AND POPULATION ECOLOGY

A. Communities

Populations of organisms are assembled in nature as a community. For instance, different types of coral, fish, mollusks, arthropods, and microscopic species together form the community of a coral reef. The interactions between these species and within each species in the community are studied in the field of ecology. Ecology seeks to answer such questions as these: Which species will be successful? What factors affect the abundance of a species or group of species? What allows these organisms to coexist?

Succession

Communities are not permanent. In a gradual process called succession, the species composition in an area can change, and one community gives way to another. A grassy meadow, for example, can become overgrown with trees and become a forest community.

Niche

The role that an organism plays in a community is called its niche. An organism's niche first refers to its habitat, that is, where it physically lives in the community. A niche is also defined by the conditions under which an organism can live, and the way in which an organism utilizes the resources in its environment. Temperature range, moisture level, food preference, and feeding time are examples of factors that shape an organism's niche. The competitive exclusion principle states that no two species of organisms can occupy the same niche in the same place and time. For this reason, organisms are likely to exploit different resources and develop varying niches. For instance, different northeastern warbler species consistently forage in different zones of a tree. One species feeds on the bottom seeds, another feeds on the top, and a third feeds in the middle, thereby avoiding competition for the limited resources in a single zone. It is important to note that all the warblers are physically able to feed on seeds from the entire tree. Therefore, they theoretically could exploit greater resources and have a much larger niche than they actually occupy. The notion of the theoretical niche is called the fundamental niche. However, many factors in nature often limit the fundamental niche to a smaller realized niche.

B. Community Interactions

Competition (for food, mates, and territory) is a major force shaping communities.

Competition

There are two types of competition: intraspecific competition, which occurs between individuals of the same species, and interspecific competition, which occurs between species.

Predation—Predator-Prey Oscillations

Predation is another major interaction that shapes communities. Organisms invest heavily in ways to avoid predation, resulting in such characteristics as camouflage, poisons, and protective coverings. An interesting defense against predators is mimicry. In Batesian mimicry, a harmless species resembles a dangerous species; in Mullerian mimicry, two poisonous species look alike.

Predation is also important for controlling the size of prey populations. A classic example of a predator-prey oscillatory relationship occurs between the lynx and the hare. When lynx populations are high, these animals reduce the numbers of hare. Conversely, low numbers of lynx allow hare populations to increase.

Symbiosis

A close association between two different types of organisms in a community is called a symbiotic relationship. Parasitism is a symbiotic relationship wherein one organism benefits and the other is harmed. A lamprey is an example of a parasite, absorbing its nourishment solely from the body fluid of a host shark. In mutualism, both organisms benefit from the interaction. Many corals, for example, benefit from the metabolic products of the single-celled algae called zooxanthellae, which in turn derive essential nutrients from the coral. Commensalism is a relationship in which one organism benefits, while the other is neither helped nor harmed.

C. Ecosystems

All organisms, at every level of the ecosystem, require energy and nutrients to function. In general, organisms are grouped as either producers or consumers. Primary producers, namely plants, are self-feeding (autotrophs), capturing energy from inorganic nutrients. Consumers, namely animals, fungi, and bacteria, cannot make their own food (heterotrophs) and obtain nutrients by eating producers or other heterotrophs.

Some Examples of Ecological Pyramids

The flow of food through an ecosystem is described by simplified diagrams called food webs. Each step in a food web is referred to as a trophic level. Primary producers are the first trophic level, herbivores (animals that feed exclusively on plant material) are the second, and carnivores (animals that feed on other animals) are the third. The 10 percent rule estimates that only 10 percent of energy transfers from a lower trophic level to a higher one. You might ask whether there is a higher trophic level than the carnivores. When carnivores (or organisms on any other level) die, the decomposers (mostly fungi and bacteria) occupy the trophic level that returns the energy to the producers.

Generalized Food Web

The Carbon Cycle

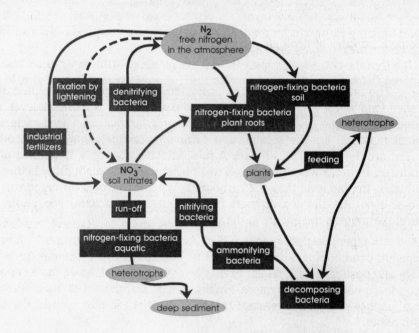

The Nitrogen Cycle

D. Populations

Populations of organisms are highly dynamic. A species in an area can increase dramatically in number when times are good, and crash quickly if times are bad. The study of population dynamics is called population ecology. This field, for instance, predicts for fishermen whether a population of fish will decline or increase on a given coastline.

Several key terms are used by population ecologists. One is carrying capacity (K), the limit to the number of individuals in a species. The limit is based on the concept that a habitat has a finite amount of resources, such as food, water, and space, to support a population. The population, therefore, cannot grow indefinitely. Eventually it will reach the carrying capacity and the numbers of individuals will stabilize.

Different species have different strategies to maximize the growth of their populations. *K*-selected species are those that produce few offspring, invest heavily in parental care, and thus have offspring with a good chance of surviving to reproductive age. Humans are examples of a *K*-selected species. On the other hand, an *r*-selected species has a large number of offspring and provides little parental investment, with the result that only a select few offspring survive to reproduce. Flies and most fish are examples of *r*-selected species. In stable environments there tend to be more *K*-selected species, while in variable environments *r*-selected species are common.

XVII. ANIMAL BEHAVIOR

A. Nature versus Nurture

Behavioral science explores the way in which animals respond to their environment. The expression "Nature versus nurture" names two ways in which scientists have sought to explain the complex causes of behavior. The "nature" view is that many aspects of behavior are inherited. There is an evolutionary basis to these behaviors, and they are hard-wired into the neural circuitry of the organism. An example of a simple genetic behavior is the fixed action pattern (F.A.P.), where a stimulus in the environment consistently triggers a programmed response sequence. A hatchling bird opening its mouth for food, an insect building a nest, and a baby suckling at a mother's breast are all demonstrating F.A.P.'s.

Certain behaviors, however, can be modified with experience through the process of learning. This is the "nurture" view. Habituation is a simple form of learning in which an animal stops reacting to unimportant stimuli. A barnacle tentacle ignoring an indigestible particle is an example of habituation. Imprinting is a type of learning that combines inherited and learned behaviors. It happens during a critical period in an animal's development, when an innate behavior is customized to environmental information. A goose following its mother is displaying an imprinted behavior. If the mother is replaced by a human during the first few hours of life, the goose will follow that person as its "mother" for the rest of its life. Classical conditioning, in which an animal associates one stimulus with another, is another type of learning. An often-cited example of classical conditioning is Pavlov's experiment showing that dogs associate the image of meat with eating. In operant conditioning, an organism learns how to react to a stimulus through negative and positive feedback. For example, if you get sick from eating a certain food, you learn not to eat it anymore. Finally, insight learning takes place when an animal applies previous experience to a new situation; in other words, the animal is "thinking."

B. Social Behavior and Kin Selection

Social behavior is a vital part of life for many species. There are many complex behaviors associated with societies of animals, such as competition for hierarchy, communication, parental investment in offspring, and courtship behavior. Sometimes, an animal will put itself in harm's way in order to benefit the other members of the society. An example is a ground squirrel that gives an alarm call. By giving the call, the individual warns others of danger but puts itself in peril by not immediately running away. This act, called an altruistic behavior, is selected for evolutionarily because it increases the fitness of closely related individuals, a concept called kin selection.

GENERAL CHEMISTRY REVIEW OUTLINE (SNS Q41–Q69)

I. OVERVIEW

    A. A Method of Attack

    B. Problem Solving

    C. Scope of Examination

    D. General Concepts

II. ATOMIC AND MOLECULAR STRUCTURES

    A. Basic Concepts

    B. Electron Configuration, Orbital Types, and Quantum Numbers

        1. Lewis Dot Diagrams

        2. Atomic Theory

        3. Quantum Numbers

            a. Principal Quantum Number (n)

            b. Azimuthal Quantum Number (l)

            c. Magnetic Quantum Number (m_l)

            d. Spin Quantum Number (m_s)

        4. Order of Orbital Sequencing

    C. Molecular Geometry and Bond Types

        1. Molecular Geometry

        2. Bond Types

            a. Ionic

            b. Metallic

            c. Covalent

            d. Molecular

III. PERIODIC PROPERTIES

    A. Reading the Periodic Table

    B. Periodic Trends

        1. Atomic Radius

        2. Ionization Energy

        3. Electronegativity

        4. Electron Affinity

        5. Melting and Boiling Points

    C. Group Characteristics

IV. STOICHIOMETRY

    A. Percent of Composition

        1. Mole and Molar Mass

        2. Empirical Formulas

        3. Molecular Formulas

    B. Types of Reactions and Balancing Equations

        1. Types of Reactions

            a. Combination Reactions

            b. Decomposition Reactions

            c. Single-Replacement Reactions

            d. Double-Replacement Reactions

      e. Combustion Reactions
      f. Oxidation-Reduction Reactions (Half-Reactions)
      g. Neutralization Reactions (Hydrolysis Reactions)

  2. Balancing Equations

      a. Steps in Balancing Coefficients
      b. Calculations from Balanced Equations

V. GASES

A. General Concepts—Standard Temperature and Pressure (STP)
B. Kinetic Molecular Theory of Gases
C. Graham's Law of Effusion
D. Dalton's Law of Partial Pressures
E. Boyle's Law and Charles's Law
F. Ideal Gas Law

  1. Density = Grams per Liter
  2. Molar Mass

VI. LIQUIDS AND SOLIDS

A. Graphical Analysis

  1. Heterogeneous Reactions versus Homogenous Reactions
  2. Energy Changes Accompanying Changes of State

B. Summary of Characteristics of States of Matter
C. Phase Diagrams

VII. SOLUTIONS

A. Basic Definitions
B. Concentration Calculations

  1. Conventional Concentration Units
  2. Mole Fraction

C. Types of Problems

  1. Weight/Weight Calculation
  2. Weight/Volume Calculation
  3. Density Problems
  4. Dilution Problems

D. Colligative Properties

  1. Lowering the Vapor Pressure
  2. Lowering the Freezing Point
  3. Boiling Point Elevation
  4. Osmotic Pressure

VIII. ACIDS AND BASES

A. Basic Information

  1. Brönsted-Lowry's Definition
  2. Arrhenius's Definition
  3. Lewis's Definition

B. pH and pOH

  1. Explanation of Formulas
  2. The pH and pOH Scales

IX. CHEMICAL EQUILIBRIUM

A. Equilibrium Constant

1. Changes in Reactant/Product Concentration
2. Changes in Pressure and Volume
3. Changes in Temperature

B. Acid/Base Calculations
C. Precipitation

1. K_{sp}

X. OXIDATION-REDUCTION REACTIONS

A. Oxidation and Reduction Definitions
B. Determination of Oxidation Numbers
C. Steps in Balancing Redox Reaction Equations
D. Electrochemical Concepts and Calculations

1. Electrolytic Cell
2. Faraday's Law
3. Galvanic Cell

a. Electromotive Force (emf)
b. Standard Electrode Potential (E^o)

XI. THERMODYNAMICS AND THERMOCHEMISTRY

A. Laws of Thermodynamics

1. First Law
2. Second Law
3. Third Law

B. Hess's Law
C. Spontaneity Prediction

1. Gibbs Free Energy
2. Standard Free-Energy Change

XII. CHEMICAL KINETICS

A. Rate Laws
B. Reaction Orders
C. Activation Energy and Enthalpy
D. Half-Life

XIII. NUCLEAR REACTIONS

A. Radioactive Decay
B. Alpha, Beta, and Gamma Decay

I. OVERVIEW

A. A Method of Attack

The general chemistry section is the second part of the Survey of the Natural Sciences. Remember that there will be no formal divisions between the three science sections that comprise the Survey of the Natural Sciences. Question 41 will begin the general chemistry section.

The general chemistry section is not only important in its own right. Because you will need a solid foundation in general chemistry to answer many of the organic chemistry questions, your score in organic chemistry will also be affected by your knowledge of general chemistry. For this reason, it would be prudent to place emphasis on the review of general chemistry prior to your review of organic chemistry.

For the biology section you are required to memorize and understand concepts; the general chemistry section requires that you problem-solve as well. This actually works to your advantage. How so?

B. Problem Solving

With a thorough review of the topics outlined in the scope of examination, you will have seen all of the possible types of questions that can be asked of you. There is virtually no chance that you will be asked to solve a problem that you can't work; understanding the basic concepts will get you far. Armed with the periodic table and a firm grasp of how to solve the common types of problems, you should do well on this section.

This review has been constructed to work through examples step by step, with an explanation of terminology preceding most of the problems presented. Remember that you will be given no formulas on the DAT, and calculators are not permitted. You will have a periodic table that you can display on your screen by clicking on the "Exhibit" button in the lower right-hand corner. Do not forget that the periodic table is there—you will undoubtedly need it to correctly answer several questions! And, most certainly, do not waste time now trying to memorize parts of the table—that time can be utilized in better ways. Limit your review to the major topics, and master them. You should be able to talk out the steps in solving the problems. The ADA will most likely switch the given information around and ask you to solve for a variable that you are not used to or will change the problem in some other fashion.

The following is presented as a guide to attacking the problems on the exam. Although you may not need to follow the guide step by step on easier problems, it should help on difficult problems for which you cannot immediately see the path to the answer.

- *Identify the given facts.* What do you know from the question?
- *Identify what you are solving for or what is being asked.* Look at the answer choices.
- *Sketch a diagram or chart.* If you are asked to balance an equation or calculate the number of moles of a compound, a diagram or chart will help you think through the question.
- *Solve the problem.* The three methods for solving a problem given below are listed in order from most desirable to least desirable.

  1. Knowledge-based approach: You have prior knowledge of what is being asked, and the information you possess leads you to the right solution.
  2. Simplification: This involves breaking a complex problem down into simpler tasks. Then you can see more clearly how to solve these tasks individually and then solve the larger problem.
  3. Backward induction: Here, you look at the answers, and then narrow the choices by eliminating the incorrect or unlikely ones. This method uses trial and error to solve for the answers given.

- *Check the logic.* Does your answer make sense?

If you know the material and follow the problem-solving steps given above, regardless of what is asked you should be able to work the problem out. Think of the general chemistry section as a series of problems that can be solved by using knowledge and logic. If only the biology section were that straightforward!

C. Scope of Examination

The area of chemistry encompasses more than any student could be expected to review, so the folks at the ADA have narrowed the field to a limited number of testable topics, listed below. *The best method of preparation is to achieve a superior level of knowledge of the topics outlined in the scope of the examination.* This review assumes that you have been exposed to the majority of terms and concepts. It is recommended that you refer to a general chemistry textbook to review any areas on which you feel a more thorough review is needed. Checking off the topics as you review them will ensure that you cover all the topics before exam day. The following is the scope of examination as defined by the ADA Department of Testing Services:

- Stoichiometry (percent of composition, empirical formulas from percent of composition; balancing equations; weight/weight, weight/volume, density problems)
- Gases (kinetic molecular theory of gases; Graham's, Dalton's, Boyle's, Charles's and the ideal gas laws)
- Liquids and Solids
- Solutions (colligative properties, concentration calculations)
- Acids and Bases
- Chemical Equilibrium (molecular, acid/base, precipitation, and equilibrium calculations)
- Thermodynamics and Thermochemistry (laws of thermodynamics; Hess's law; spontaneity prediction)
- Chemical Kinetics (rate laws; activation energy; half-life)
- Oxidation-Reduction Reactions (balancing equations; determination of oxidation numbers, electrochemical concepts and calculations)
- Atomic and Molecular Structure (electron configuration, orbital types; Lewis dot diagrams, atomic theories; molecular geometry; bond types; quantum mechanics)
- Periodic Properties (including categories of nonmetals, transition metals, and nontransition metals)
- Nuclear Reactions

D. General Concepts

The following basic concepts are not reviewed in this section because it is assumed that you have knowledge of them. Only a brief mention is given here; refer to a text, if necessary, for further information on these general concepts of chemistry.

- Matter is anything that occupies space and has mass.
- Weight is related to mass and gravitational force, weight can vary, but mass does not. Inertia is resistance to a change in direction.
- Density is mass divided by volume ($D = M/V$).
- Matter exists in three states: solid, liquid, and gas.
- Solids have definite size and shape.
- Liquids have size but not shape.
- Gases have neither shape nor size.
- If a substance consists of just one type of atom, it is an element.
- Combinations of elements in definite groupings are compounds.
- Mixtures can vary in composition.
- Energy exists in many forms and is either kinetic or potential.
- Reactions can be classified as exothermic ($\Delta H < 0$) or endothermic ($\Delta H > 0$), according to the equation $\Delta H = H_{products} - H_{reactants}$.

- Heat is measured by three common temperature scales: Celsius, Fahrenheit, and Kelvin. (See the appendix for formulas and relationships.)
- The International System (Système International, SI) of units is used in chemistry. (Common SI units are listed in the appendix.)
- Exponential notation is used in chemistry. Remember that exponents of 10 are added in multiplication and subtracted in division.
- The factor-label method of conversion is used to convert from one form of dimensional analysis to another. (In this commonly used system, units are crossed out in most chemical calculations.)
- Precision is concerned with the reliability or reproducibility of a measurement.
- Accuracy is concerned with the closeness of a measurement to an accepted value.
- Uncertainty is related to significant figures. (You need to know which digits are significant in a given measurement.)

II. ATOMIC AND MOLECULAR STRUCTURES

A. Basic Concepts

The *atom* is the smallest representative particle of an element. The atom is composed of smaller subunits:

- *proton:* a positively charged subatomic particle found in the nucleus
- *neutron:* an electrically neutral subatomic particle found in the nucleus and having approximately the same mass as the proton
- *electron:* a negatively charged subatomic particle found *outside* the nucleus; its mass is $\dfrac{1}{1836}$ the mass of a proton

Each principal energy level within an atom contains one or more sublevels. (Note that in the older terminology, the terms *shell* and *subshell* were used; the newer terminology has replaced *shell* with *principal energy level* and *subshell* with *sublevel*.)

The *valence principal energy level* refers to the electron population of the outer principal energy level. This number is important because these electrons come into contact with other atoms when forming compounds. In the periodic table the elements in each column have the same number of valence electrons.

Representation of valence electrons as dots around the atomic symbol.

B. Electron Configuration, Orbital Types, and Quantum Numbers

The term *electron configuration* refers to the arrangement of electrons in an atom. In the most stable configuration of an atom the electrons are in their lowest possible energy state (ground state). As mentioned before, electrons are located in orbitals outside the nucleus and are in states of rapid motion.

1. Lewis Dot Diagrams

A Lewis dot diagram shows an element surrounded by a series of dots, which represent the valence electrons of the element.

Elements normally represented with Lewis electron-dot symbols.

Counting Electrons
Around Cl Atoms

Counting Electrons
Around P Atom

Diagram illustrating how to count electrons around each atom by drawing a circle that includes all nonbonding electrons and all bonding electrons for that atom.

The *octet rule* states that atoms lose, gain, or share electrons until they are surrounded by eight valence electrons. The *noble gases* (except helium) have eight valence electrons and are therefore quite stable.

2. Atomic Theory

John Dalton (1766–1844) was responsible for explaining the *law of conservation of mass* and the *law of definite proportions,* and he created the atomic theory. His postulates were as follows:

- Matter is made up of small particles known as atoms.
- All atoms of a given element are identical.
- A chemical compound is composed of elements that are present in a definite, fixed numerical ratio.
- A compound is formed when atoms of more than one element combine.
- Atoms of different elements have different properties.
- In chemical reactions, atoms merely reshuffle from one combination to another; the atoms themselves do not change.

The *law of constant composition* states that the elemental composition of a pure compound is always the same. The *law of conservation of mass* (law of conservation of matter) states that matter is neither created nor destroyed in chemical reactions. The *law of multiple proportions* states that, when two elements combine to form more than one compound, in each case the masses of the elements that combine are ratios of small whole numbers.

Each atomic orbital has no more than two electrons of opposite spin.

3. Quantum Numbers

a. Principal Quantum Number (n)

The principal quantum number tells us an electron's *energy level*. It is related to the average distance of the electron from the nucleus. The number n can have any positive integer value (1, 2, 3...). The larger the value of n:

- the farther the distance between the nucleus and the electron,
- the larger the average energy of the levels belonging to the shell,
- the less the difference in energy between adjacent shells: the difference between $n = 5$ and $n = 6$ is less than that between $n = 2$ and $n = 3$.

Note: The maximum number of electrons in energy level n is expressed as $2n^2$.

b. Azimuthal Quantum Number (l)

The azimuthal quantum number tells us the *angular momentum magnitude*. Each shell is made up of one or more subshells, designated as l. The number of subshells for a shell is equal to the value of n. The value of l may be 0 to $n - 1$.

Example:

If a shell has three subshells, what are the l values?

If the subshell n is 3, the l values are 0, 1, and 2. We associate letters with l values as follows: $0 = s$, $1 = p$, $2 = d$.

c. Magnetic Quantum Number (m_l)

This number tells us the *angular momentum orientation*. It is the orientation of an orbital in space. The values for m_l are all integers from -1 to $+1$.

PRINCIPAL QUANTUM NUMBER, n (SHELL)	ANGULAR MOMENTUM QUANTUM NUMBER, l (SUBSHELL)	SUBSHELL LABEL	MAGNETIC QUANTUM NUMBER (m_l)	NUMBER OF ORBITALS IN SUBSHELL
1	0	$1s$	0	1
2	0	$2s$	0	1
	1	$2p$	$-1, 0, +1$	3
3	0	$3s$	0	1
	1	$3p$	$-1, 0, +1$	3
	2	$3d$	$-2, -1, 0, +1, +2$	5
4	0	$4s$	0	1
	1	$4p$	$-1, 0, +1$	3
	2	$4d$	$-2, -1, 0, +1, +2$	5
	3	$4f$	$-3, -2, -1, 0, +1, +2, +3$	7

d. Spin Quantum Number (m_s)

This number tells us the *electron spin direction*. Its values are $\pm\dfrac{1}{2}$. The significance of the spin is explained by the Pauli exclusion principle, which states that in a given atom no two electrons can have exactly the same quantum numbers. Each orbital can be filled by only two electrons, and the electrons can spin in only two directions: $+$spin and $-$spin.

ELEMENT	n	l	m_l	m_s
H	1	0	0	$\pm\dfrac{1}{2}$
He	2	0	0	$\pm\dfrac{1}{2}$
Li	2	0	0	$\pm\dfrac{1}{2}$
Be	2	0	0	$\pm\dfrac{1}{2}$
B	2	1	−1	$\pm\dfrac{1}{2}$
C	2	1	0	$\pm\dfrac{1}{2}$
N	2	1	+1	$\pm\dfrac{1}{2}$
O	2	1	−1	$\pm\dfrac{1}{2}$
F	2	1	0	$\pm\dfrac{1}{2}$
Ne	2	1	+1	$\pm\dfrac{1}{2}$
Na	3	0	0	$\pm\dfrac{1}{2}$
Mg	3	0	0	$\pm\dfrac{1}{2}$
Al	3	1	−1	$\pm\dfrac{1}{2}$
Si	3	1	0	$\pm\dfrac{1}{2}$
P	3	1	+1	$\pm\dfrac{1}{2}$
S	3	1	−1	$\pm\dfrac{1}{2}$
Cl	3	1	0	$\pm\dfrac{1}{2}$
Ar	3	1	+1	$\pm\dfrac{1}{2}$
K	4	0	0	$\pm\dfrac{1}{2}$
Ca	4	0	0	$\pm\dfrac{1}{2}$

Example:
Which of the following quantum numbers are possible, and which are not possible, according to the rules for assigning quantum numbers?

1. $1, 0, 0, \dfrac{1}{2}$ Possible

2. $3, 2, 2, -\dfrac{1}{2}$ Possible

3. $3, 1, 2, -\dfrac{1}{2}$ Not possible

4. $1, 3, 0, \dfrac{1}{2}$ Not possible

5. $2, 0, 1, -\dfrac{1}{2}$ Not possible

6. $5, 0, 0, \dfrac{1}{2}$ Possible

4. Order of Orbital Sequencing
Electrons fill sublevels starting with the lowest energy level first, then the next higher energy level, and so on, following the order below:

$1s\ 2s\ 2p\ 3s\ 3p\ 4s\ 3d\ 4p\ 5s\ 4d\ 5p\ 6s\ 4f\ 5d\ 6p\ 7s\ 5f\ 6d$

This sequence is much easier to remember if you understand the logic. The following figure illustrates that, if you start at the upper left and read the periodic table as you would text, the filling sequence makes sense. The maximum number of electrons in the *s* sublevel is 2 (one orbital); the *p* sublevel can hold 6 (three orbitals); the *d* holds 10 (five orbitals); and the *f* holds 14 (seven orbitals).

Periodic table divided to show the regions where *s*, *p*, *d*, and *f* electrons are the highest energy electrons in each atom.

Often chemists use an abbreviated version to simplify the electronic configuration. Inner electrons are represented by a noble gas, and valence electrons are written in electronic configuration. For example:

$$Fe = 1s^2 2s^2 2p^6 3s^2 3p^6 4s^2 3d^6$$

$$Fe = [Ar]: 4s^2 3d^6$$

When writing an electron configuration, keep *Hund's rule* in mind. This rule states that, for degenerate orbitals, the lowest energy is achieved when the number of electrons with the same spin is maximized. An orbital diagram is used to demonstrate this concept.

Orbital diagrams for the first 10 elements, showing only the valence electrons.

Example:

Write the orbital diagrams for hydrogen, helium, and nitrogen.

H has 1 electron in the ground state and is depicted as $\uparrow$ ($1s^1$).

He has 2 electrons with opposite spins and is shown as $\uparrow\downarrow$ ($1s^2$).

N has 7 electrons and is shown as $\uparrow\downarrow$ $\uparrow\downarrow$ $\uparrow$ $\uparrow$ $\uparrow$ ($1s^2 2s^2 2p^3$).
$\quad\quad 1s \quad 2s \quad 2p$

A very common type of question asks you to write the electron configuration of a given element. An element such as scandium (Sc) would probably be chosen to test your awareness to go from $4s^2$ to $3d^1$. If you understand the sequencing of the periodic table, you will be able to write the electron configuration of any element.

C. Molecular Geometry and Bond Types

1. Molecular Geometry

Molecular geometry is the shape of the molecule that can be predicted by using the Lewis dot diagram. The *valence-shell electron-pair repulsion (VSEPR) theory* states that the geometry of the electrons around an atom will be an arrangement such that the electron pairs are as far away from each other as possible.

NOTATION	SHAPE	ANGLE(S)
AX	Linear	180°
AX_2	Linear	180°
AX_3	Trigonal planar	120°
AX_4	Tetrahedral	109.5°
AX_5	Trigonal bipyramidal	120°, 90°
AX_6	Octahedral	90°

The above table includes basic shapes of substances without nonbonding pairs. *Derived structures* of the basic structures have nonbonding pairs and are variations of the basic shapes. Nonbonding pairs take up slightly more space than do atoms. The trigonal planar structure, AX_3, is *bent* with a nonbonding electron pair in place of an atom. This and other derived structures are listed in the table below.

BASIC STRUCTURE	DERIVED STRUCTURE	SHAPE	ANGLE(S)
AX	AE	Single atom	None
AX_2	AXE	Linear diatomic	180°
AX_3	AX_2E	Bent	120°
AX_4	AX_3E	Triangular pyramidal	109.5°
AX_4	AX_2E_2	Bent	109.5°
AX_5	AX_4E	Seesaw	120°, 90°
AX_5	AX_3E_2	T-shaped	90°
AX_5	AX_2E_3	Linear	180°
AX_6	AX_5E	Square pyramidal	90°
AX_6	AX_4E_2	Square planar	90°

Commonly asked questions on the DAT refer to the following shapes:

- Bent (H_2O, SO_2)
- Linear (CO_2, $BeCl_2$)
- Trigonal pyramidal (NH_3)
- Trigonal planar (BF_3, BH_3)
- Tetrahedral (CH_4, CCl_4)

2. Bond Types
A chemical bond results from the concurrent sharing of electrons to two nuclei.

TYPE OF BOND	EXAMPLE	CHARACTERISTICS
a. Ionic	Nacl	Solids *Atoms held together via electrostatic forces called ionic bonds* • transfer of electrons from metals to non-metals • hard, brittle • high melting points • poor conductors of electricity
b. Metallic	Na, Fe	Solids *Metallic bonds (positively charged ions in sea of electrons)* • variable hardness • variable melting points • good conductors of electricity • ductile and malleable with high deformity
c. Covalent	Diamond	Solids, Liquids, Gases *covalent bonds* • poor conductors of electricity and heat *polar covalent bonds* • unequal sharing of bonding electron pair • electronegativity difference of 0.4–0.7 • dipole moment *non-polar covalent bonds* • equal sharing of bonding electron pair • same electronegativity • diatomic molecules (H_2, Cl_2, O_2)
d. Molecular	CO_2	*van der Waals forces (London dispersion)* *hydrogen bonds* • low melting points • poor conductors of electricity • high boiling points

III. PERIODIC PROPERTIES

A. Reading the Periodic Table

In the periodic table the elements are listed by increasing *atomic number*, from 1 to 115. In this example, the *atomic number* is above the symbol, and the atomic mass is below.

| 11 |
| **Na** |
| 22.98976 |

The atomic number indicates the total number of protons, which also equals the total number of electrons in a neutral atom.

The mass number is *number of neutrons + number of protons*, or *atomic number + number of neutrons*. This works out because electrons have practically no mass, and protons and neutrons have masses of about 1. Atomic numbers will always be whole numbers, and mass numbers will have several digits past the decimal point.

Isotopes are atoms with the same number of protons, but different numbers of neutrons. Therefore, isotopes have the same atomic number but different atomic masses. The term *isoelectric* refers to the fact that, when an atom loses or gains an electron, it becomes equivalent, in number of electrons, to the atom corresponding to its new charge.

Example:
1. Cl^- is isoelectric to Ar.
2. Si^{2-} is isoelectric to S.

The elements are organized in the periodic table in periods (rows) and groups (columns). As mentioned previously, atoms in the same column have the same valence orbitals and are more similar to each other than atoms in the same row. Each row corresponds to the principal quantum number.

Common form of the periodic table, showing groups of related elements.

B. Periodic Trends

1. Atomic Radius
Atomic radii increase on the periodic table as you move down and to the left. Within a group, the radius increases downward because each period has an additional outer principal energy level of electrons and is larger than the preceding principal energy level. The radius decreases as you move to the right of a row because the additional protons in the nucleus create a stronger positive charge that is able to draw electrons to the nucleus. With a stronger nucleus acting on electrons at the same distance, the electrons are drawn closer and a smaller radius results.

Keep in mind that, as an example, Mg^{2+} has a smaller radius than Mg because of loss of electrons. There is less electron-electron repulsion, and the electrons move closer to the nucleus. *Cations are always smaller* than neutral atoms of the same element, whereas *anions are always larger.*

2. Ionization Energy
Ionization energy is the energy that is needed to remove an electron from an atom. Remember that helium has the highest ionization energy; *ionization energy increases on the periodic table as you move up and to the right.*

3. Electronegativity

Electronegativity is a measure of the ability of an atom to acquire an additional electron. *Electronegativity increases as you move up and to the right* on the periodic table. Remember that fluorine has the highest electronegativity.

H 2.1																	
Li 1.0	Be 1.5											B 2.0	C 2.5	N 3.1	O 3.5	F 4.0	
Na 1.0	Mg 1.3											Al 1.5	Si 1.8	P 2.1	S 2.4	Cl 2.9	
K 0.8	Ca 1.1	Sc 1.2	Ti 1.3	V 1.5	Cr 1.6	Mn 1.6	Fe 1.7	Co 1.7	Ni 1.8	Cu 1.8	Zn 1.7	Ga 1.8	Ge 2.0	As 2.2	Se 2.5	Br 2.8	
Rb 0.8	Sr 1.0	Y 1.1	Zr 1.2	Nb 1.3	Mo 1.3	Tc 1.4	Ru 1.4	Rh 1.5	Pd 1.4	Ag 1.4	Cd 1.5	In 1.5	Sn 1.7	Sb 1.8	Te 2.0	I 2.5	
Cs 0.7	Ba 0.9	La 1.1	Hf 1.2	Ta 1.4	W 1.4	Re 1.5	Os 1.5	Ir 1.6	Pt 1.5	Au 1.4	Hg 1.5	Tl 1.5	Pb 1.6	Bi 1.7	Po 1.8	At 2.2	
Fr 0.7	Ra 0.9	Ac 1.0															

Periodic table showing the electronegativities of the elements.

4. Electron Affinity

Electron affinity is the energy required to add an electron to an atom. Fluorine has the highest electron affinity. Electron affinity increases on the periodic table as you move up and to the right. This concept is closely related to electronegativity.

5. Melting and Boiling Points

Melting and boiling points tend to decrease from the top to the bottom of a group for metals. Nonmetals show an increase from top to bottom.

C. Group Characteristics

Group IA (Alkali metals)

- Metallic character increases as you go down the group.
- React easily with nonmetals (one electron in outer principal energy level).

Group IIA (Alkaline earth metals)

- Two electrons in outer principal energy level.

Groups IIIB–VIIIA and IB–IIB (Transitional elements)

- Most have metallic character.
- Good electrical conductors.
- Various oxidation states.

Transitional elements have unusual characteristics. If you are questioned about a characteristic that is unfamiliar, the element involved is most likely transitional.

Group VIIA (Halogens)

- Seven electrons in outer shell.
- Fluorine has highest electronegativity.

Group 0 (Noble gases)

- Nonreactive because of full outermost principal energy level.
- Have no electronegativity.

IV. STOICHIOMETRY

The term *stoichiometry* refers to the quantitative relationships among compounds in a chemical reaction. Knowing these relationships among reactants and products enables chemists to produce the desired amount of products with just the right amount of reactants. Stoichiometry involves the factor-label (or the "crossing-out-units") method of conversion. It is important to form the habit of writing the units because they are as important as the numbers that are associated with them. Showing units will also help you see what you have been given and what you are looking for in a problem. Be sure to cancel the units as you work out stoichiometry problems.

A. Percent of Composition

It is important to understand the *law of constant composition*. The elemental composition of a pure compound is always the same. For example:

- ^{12}C has 12.00 atomic mass units per atom.
- 12 amu ^{12}C has 6.02×10^{23} atoms.

Avogadro's number $= 6.02 \times 10^{23} = 1$ mole.

1. Mole and Molar Mass

A *mole* (mol) is the amount of any substance that contains as many units as the number of atoms in 12 grams of ^{12}C. It is the central unit of measurement in chemistry.

The percentage of a given element in a compound is given by the following formula:

$$\text{Percent of element} = \frac{(\text{atoms of element}) \, (\text{atomic mass})}{\text{formula mass of compound}} \times 100$$

Examples:

1. What percentage of oxygen is present in $KClO_3$?

$$\% \, O = \frac{(3) \, (16 \, g)}{122.6 \, g} \times 100 = 39.2\%$$

2. Given a 60-gram sample of $KClO_3$, how many grams of oxygen are present?

$$(0.392)(60) = 23.520 \, g$$

2. Empirical Formulas

An *empirical formula* gives the simplest whole-number ratio of elements in a particular compound. You may be asked to find the empirical formula from a given percent composition.

Example:

The percent composition of a compound is as follows: 12.1% C, 16.2% O, and 71.7% Cl. What is the empirical formula of this compound?

1. Assume that there are 100 g of sample. Therefore, there are 12.1 g of C, 16.2 g of O, and 71.7 g of Cl.

2. Convert grams to moles for each element. Obtain the molar masses (g/mol) of the elements from the periodic table.

moles C $= (12.1 \, g) \times (1 \, \text{mol C}/12.0 \, g) = 1.01 \, \text{mol C}$
moles O $= (16.2 \, g) \times (1 \, \text{mol O}/16.0 \, g) = 1.01 \, \text{mol O}$
moles Cl $= (71.7 \, g) \times (1 \, \text{mol Cl}/35.5 \, g) = 2.02 \, \text{mol Cl}$

3. Divide by the smallest number of moles calculated (1.01 mol O) to get a ratio. The ratio of C:O:Cl is 1:1:2. Therefore, the empirical formula is $COCl_2$.

3. Molecular Formulas

The *molecular formula* gives the actual number of atoms of each element in a particular compound.

You may be asked to find the molecular formula from the empirical formula. The molecular formula of the molecule will be a multiple of the ratio found in determining the empirical formula. In the example above, the empirical formula for $COCl_2$ had the ratio 1:1:2, so the ratio of the molecular formula must be

1	×	1:1:2	=	1:1:2 or $COCl_2$
2	×	1:1:2	=	2:2:4 or $C_2O_2Cl_4$
3	×	1:1:2	=	3:3:6 or $C_3O_3Cl_6$
4	×	1:1:2	=	4:4:8 or $C_4O_4Cl_8$

The molecular mass must be supplied in the question to determine which formula is correct.

Example:

Given the empirical formula $COCl_2$, what is the molecular formula if the mass of the compound is 294 grams?

The mass of $COCl_2$ is about 99 grams; $\frac{294}{99}$ = approximately 3. Therefore, 3 times the empirical formula gives the molecular formula $C_3O_3Cl_6$.

B. Types of Reactions and Balancing Equations

1. Types of Reactions

There are often questions on the DAT asking you to identify a given reaction as to type. There are four major types of reactions: combination, decomposition, single-replacement, and double-replacement. Three other common reactions are included here as well. To understand why reactions take place, you need first to understand several basic concepts: *heat of formation, solubility, entropy, enthalpy,* and *limiting reactants*.

a. Combination Reactions

Combination reactions involve the formation of one product by two or more substrates. These reactions are also called synthesis reactions. If the heat of formation is negative, the reaction proceeds spontaneously and is exothermic. A reaction will occur spontaneously to achieve a lower energy state. With large negative values of heat the reaction proceeds rapidly, whereas with small negative values the reaction proceeds at a barely noticeable rate. In the following reaction, 1 mole of zinc and 1 mole of sulfur combine to form 1 mole of zinc sulfide:

$$Zn + S \rightarrow ZnS \ (\Delta H = -48.5 \text{ kcal})$$

b. Decomposition Reactions

Decomposition reactions involve the formation of two or more products by one substrate. A very high positive value for the heat of formation indicates that a reaction will decompose explosively. Conversely, a very high negative value for the heat of formation indicates that the reaction is highly exothermic and will be difficult to decompose. In the following example, a low negative value for the heat of formation results in the decomposition of 2 moles of mercuric oxide:

$$2HgO \rightarrow 2Hg + O_2 \quad (\Delta H = -21.7 \text{ kcal/mol})$$

c. Single-Replacement Reactions

In a single-replacement reaction a single element reacts with a compound to produce a different element and a new compound:

$$2AgNO_3 + Zn \rightarrow 2Ag + Zn(NO_3)_2$$

In this single-replacement reaction the element zinc replaces silver, producing a new single element and a new compound.

d. Double-Replacement Reactions

Double-replacement reactions involve two compounds. The cations for each compound switch places.

$$MgSO_4 + BaCl_2 \rightarrow MgCl_2 + BaSO_4$$

In this reaction the two cations replaced each other, thus the term *double-replacement reaction.*

e. Combustion Reactions

Combustion reactions start by combining an organic (carbon-containing) substance with oxygen and then continue to form carbon dioxide and water:

$$C_5H_{12} + 8O_2 \rightarrow 5CO_2 + 6H_2O$$

If the original organic compound contains an element other than carbon, hydrogen, and oxygen, these elements must be in their elemental states in the product.

f. Oxidation-Reduction Reactions (Half-Reactions)

Oxidation-reduction reactions involve the transfer of electrons by a compound or an ion. If electrons are on the right (product) side, an oxidation reaction has occurred. If the electrons are on the left side, a reduction reaction occurred. These reactions are usually broken down into two half-reactions to help keep track of the electrons.

$$Fe^{2+} \rightarrow Fe^{3+} + e^-$$ oxidation half-reaction
$$I_2 + 2e^- \rightarrow 2I^-$$ reduction half-reaction

As long as the electrons cancel, the half-reactions can be combined to form a complete oxidation-reduction reaction.

$$I_2 + 2Fe^{2+} \rightarrow 2Fe^{3+} + 2I^-$$

g. Neutralization Reactions (Hydrolysis Reactions)

This is a form of a double-replacement reaction using an acid and a base to form salt and water. It is also referred to as a neutralization reaction because the acid and base are neutralized.

$$HCl + NaOH \rightarrow NaCl + H_2O$$

2. Balancing Equations

Since atoms are neither created nor destroyed in any reaction, equal numbers of atoms of each element must be maintained on both sides of the equation.

Remember: *Subscripts are never changed when balancing equations. Coefficients in front of a compound are changed.* Therefore, the amount, not the identity, of a substance changes. Balancing equations is done largely by trial and error. The process is best accomplished by balancing the most complex molecule first.

a. Steps in Balancing Coefficients

Example:
Balance the following equation:

$$C_4H_{10} \text{ (l)} + O_2 \text{ (g)} \rightarrow CO_2 \text{ (g)} + H_2O \text{ (l)}$$

First, balance the carbons:

$$C_4H_{10} + O_2 \rightarrow 4CO_2 + H_2O$$

Next the hydrogens:

$$C_4H_{10} + O_2 \rightarrow 4CO_2 + 5H_2O$$

Then the oxygens:

$$C_4H_{10} + \frac{13}{2}O_2 \rightarrow 4CO_2 + 5H_2O$$

Equations can contain only whole numbers, so multiply everything by 2:

$$2C_4H_{10} + 13O_2 \rightarrow 8CO_2 + 10H_2O$$

Look over the equation to make sure everything checks out. The coefficients indicate the numbers of molecules and the numbers of moles involved in the reaction.

$2C_4H_{10}$	+	$13O_2$	$\rightarrow$	$8CO_2$	+	$10H_2O$
2 molecules		13 molecules		8 molecules		10 molecules
$2(6.02 \times 10^{23}$ molecules)		$13(6.02 \times 10^{23}$ molecules)		$8(6.02 \times 10^{23}$ molecules)		$10(6.02 \times 10^{23}$ molecules)
2 mol		13 mol		8 mol		10 mol

b. Calculations from Balanced Equations

A common type of problem that may be asked requires calculations from your balanced equation. Use the above reaction to solve the following problem.

Example:
In the above combustion reaction, if 10 grams of C_4H_{10} is the amount of reactant, how many grams of H_2O are produced?

The sequence of steps is as follows:

1. Grams of reactant: 10 g $2C_4H_{10}$ *multiplied by...*

2. Moles of reactant: $\dfrac{1 \text{ mol } C_4H_{10}}{58 \text{ g } C_4H_{10}}$ (58 g is calculated from summation of atomic weights) *multiplied by...*

3. Moles of product: $\dfrac{10 \text{ mol } H_2O}{2 \text{ mol } C_4H_{10}}$ *multiplied by...*

$\dfrac{18 \text{ g } H_2O}{1 \text{ mol } H_2O}$ *gives...*

4. Grams of product: 15.5 g H_2O.

Other related problems are *weight/weight problems, weight/volume problems,* and *density problems.* These types of problems involve solute/solution reactions, and are discussed in Section VII, Solutions.

V. GASES

A. General Concepts—Standard Temperature and Pressure (STP)

When dealing with gases, we consider them to be in a hypothetical "ideal" state. We assume that they have nonexistent intermolecular forces and occupy no volume. Volumes of gases change extensively with changes in pressure and temperature. Gases as a whole have distinct properties, making them unique from solids and liquids.

- Gases expand to fill their containers (gas volume = volume of container); volumes of solids and liquids are not determined by container.
- Gases are quite compressible under high pressure (pressure = force/area); solids and liquids are not as compressible.
- Gases form homogenous mixtures with each other regardless of their identities; with liquids this is not always the case.

Standard temperature and pressure (STP) of the gas laws:

- Temperature = 0.0°C (273.15 K)
- Pressure = 1 atmosphere
- Volume of 1 mole of any gas at STP = 22.4 liters

All gases show similar physical characteristics and behaviors. To understand the gas laws, it is important to understand the kinetic molecular theory of gases.

B. Kinetic Molecular Theory of Gases

The *kinetic molecular theory of gases* may be summarized as follows:

- Attractive and repulsive forces between gas molecules are negligible.
- The volume of all the molecules of the gas is negligible compared to the volume in which the gas is contained.
- Collisions between gas molecules are elastic; henceforth there is no gain or loss of energy.
- Gas molecules collide with each other and the walls of their container in a random, continuous motion.

The average kinetic energy of gas particles is proportional to their absolute temperature and is the same for all gases at a given temperature.

C. Graham's Law of Effusion

Effusion is the flow of gas from one compartment to another through a small opening. Rates of effusion can be compared by keeping the temperature and pressure the same. *Graham's law* states that the rates of effusion are inversely proportional to the square roots of the densities of the gases:

$$\frac{\text{Rate of effusion of gas A}}{\text{Rate of effusion of gas B}} = \sqrt{\frac{\text{Density of B}}{\text{Density of A}}} = \sqrt{\frac{\text{Mm of B}}{\text{Mm of A}}}$$

where Mm is equal to molecular mass.

Lightweight gases effuse and diffuse more rapidly than gases of larger molecular weight.

D. Dalton's Law of Partial Pressures

Dalton's law states that the total pressure of a mixture of gases is equal to the sum of the individual pressures exerted by all the gases.

$$P_{total} = P_1 + P_2 + P_3 + \ldots$$

This relationship allows us to write the following equation:

$$P_{total} = \frac{RT}{V}(n_1 + n_2 + n_3 + \ldots)$$

where $R = 0.0821$ L-atm/K-mol, T = Kelvin temperature, and n = number of moles.

Example:
What pressure, in atmospheres, is exerted by a mixture of 3.00 grams of H_2 and 8.00 grams of N_2 at 273 K in a 10.0-liter vessel?

$$n_{H_2} = 3.00 \text{ g } H_2 \times \frac{1 \text{ mol } H_2}{2.02 \text{ g } H_2} = 1.49 \text{ mol } H_2$$

$$n_{N_2} = 8.00 \text{ g } N_2 \times \frac{1 \text{ mol } N_2}{28.0 \text{ g } N_2} = 0.286 \text{ mol } N_2$$

Now that we have the numbers of moles, we can move on.

$$P_{total} = \frac{RT}{V}(n_1 + n_2 + n_3 + \ldots)$$

$$= \frac{(0.0821 \text{ L-atm/K-mol})(273 \text{ K})}{10.0 \text{ L}} \times (1.49 \text{ mol} + 0.286 \text{ mol})$$

$$= 3.98 \text{ atm}$$

Another simplified formula that may come in handy is

$$P_{partial} = P_{total} \times \text{mole fraction}$$

E. Boyle's Law and Charles's Law

With *Boyle's law*, pressure and volume are inversely proportional to one another and temperature is constant; therefore, ignore the denominator in the combined gas law formula given below. With *Charles's law*, volume and absolute temperature are directly proportional and pressure is constant; therefore, ignore P in the numerator of the formula:

$$\frac{P_1 V_1}{T_1} = \frac{P_2 V_2}{T_2}$$

There are no direct questions on the DAT on the combined gas law; but if you can remember the relationships it states, you will find it easier to memorize Boyle's and Charles's laws.

F. Ideal Gas Law

The *ideal gas law* combines the principles of Boyle's law, Charles's law, and Avagadro's principle:

$$PV = nRT$$

The ideal gas law assumes that each gas occupies the entire volume of the vessel with its own partial pressure. We can use this relationship to find the density and molar mass of the gas.

1. Density = Grams per Liter

- Obtain the number of grams from n(grams/molecular weight).
- Obtain the number of liters by solving the ideal gas law equation for V.

2. Molar Mass

- Divide the weight by the volume.
- Multiply this number (grams/liter) by 22.4 liters/mole.

VI. LIQUIDS AND SOLIDS

A. Graphical Analysis

Typical heating curve, bringing a sample from the solid state on the left to the gaseous state on the right.

On the above figure, M.P. = melting point and B.P. = boiling point.

$A \rightarrow B$ = specific heat (amount of heat needed to raise the temperature of 1 g of substance 1°C) of a solid (cal/g°C)

$B \rightarrow C$ = heat of fusion (cal/g°C); melting (reverse is freezing = crystallization)

$C \rightarrow D$ = specific heat of a liquid (cal/g°C)

$D \rightarrow E$ = heat of vaporization (kcal/mol); liquid $\rightarrow$ gas (reverse is condensation)

$E \rightarrow F$ = specific heat of a gas (cal/g°C)

Sublimation is the phase change from solid to gas without passing through the liquid phase.

1. Heterogeneous Reactions versus Homogeneous Reactions
Homogeneous reactions occur in one phase (Example: solid only). Heterogeneous reactions occur in two or more phases (Example: solid and liquid).

2. Energy Changes Accompanying Changes of State
The calorie (cal) is a unit of thermal energy. One calorie is equal to 4.184 joules (J). The joule is the SI unit for quantity of heat.

Example:
Calculate the calories necessary to change 50 grams of ice at –10°C to steam at 130°C.

Necessary constants:

Specific heat of ice = 0.49 cal/g°C ΔH_{fusion} = 1.44 kcal/mol

Specific heat of water = 1.00 cal/g°C $\Delta H_{vaporization}$ = 9.72 kcal/mol

Specific heat of steam = 0.48 cal/g°C

Approach this problem by breaking down the process into simple steps:

1. Change ice (solid) at –10°C to ice (solid) at 0°C.
   Calories = grams × specific heat × temperature change
   = 50 g × 0.49 cal/g°C × 10°C
   = 245 cal

2. Change ice (solid) at 0°C to water (liquid) at 0°C.
   Calories = moles × ΔH_{fusion} × 1,000 cal/kcal
   = 50 g × 1 mol/18 g × 1.44 kcal/mol × 1,000 cal/kcal
   = 4,000 cal

3. Change water (liquid) at 0°C to water (liquid) at 100°C.
   Calories = 50 g × 1.00 cal/g°C × 100°C = 5,000 cal

4. Change water (liquid) at 100°C to steam (gas) at 100°C.
   Calories = 50 g × 1 mol/18 g × 9.72 kcal/mol × 1,000 cal/kcal
   = 27,000 cal

5. Change steam (gas) at 100°C to steam (gas) at 130°C.
   Calories = 50 g × 0.48 cal/g°C × 30°C = 720 cal

Finally, calculate the total calories.

6. 245 cal + 4,000 cal + 5,000 cal + 27,000 cal + 720 cal = 36,965 cal
   36,965 cal × 1 kcal/1,000 cal = 37 kcal

B. Summary of Characteristics of States of Matter

In the following table, the states of matter are listed in decreasing order according to the four characteristics of density, expandability, diffusibility, and compressibility (e.g., solids are the most dense, whereas gases are the least dense).

DENSITY	EXPANDABILITY	DIFFUSIBILITY	COMPRESSIBILITY
1. Solids	Gases	Gases	Gases
2. Liquids	Liquids	Liquids	Liquids
3. Gases	Solids	Solids	Solids

C. Phase Diagrams

Another popular series of questions on the DAT involves phase diagrams. A phase diagram is a graphical way to show the different states of matter under which equilibrium exists. Defining the areas on the graph has been the route the DAT has taken to test knowledge on this section.

The *critical point* is the point where the vapor pressure curve ends. Beyond this point the gas and liquid phases are indistinguishable. The *triple point* is the point where all three curves intersect. At this point all three phases are in equilibrium.

A typical phase diagram of the pressure-temperature regions where gas, liquid, and solid phases exist. Each line represents an equilibrium between two phases, and the triple point indicates the pressure and temperature at which all three phases are in equilibrium.

VII. SOLUTIONS

A. Basic Definitions

Solute:	substance that is dissolved in a solution.
Solvent:	dissolving medium of a solution; usually the component present in greater amount.
Electrolyte:	solute that produces ions in solution (conducts electric current).
Non-electrolyte:	substance that does not ionize in water, thereby resulting in a nonconducting solution.
Saturated solution:	solution that has the maximum amount of solute that can be dissolved in the solvent at the particular temperature.
Unsaturated solution:	solution that has more capacity for solute to be dissolved.
Supersaturated solution:	solution containing more solute than a saturated solution.
Solvation:	clustering of solvent molecules around a solute particle.
Hydration:	water is the solvent that clusters around solute.
Miscible:	capable of mixing in all proportions.

B. Concentration Calculations

1. Conventional Concentration Units

- Molarity (M) — The number of moles of solute per liter of solution
- Molality (m) — The number of moles of solute per kilogram of solvent
- Normality (N) — The number of equivalents of solute per liter of solution (1 equivalent of reagent A will react with 1 equivalent of reagent B as in acid-base and oxidation-reduction reactions)

Example:
What is the normality of 2.5 M H_2SO_4?

2 H ions $\times$ 2.5 M = 5.0 N

2. Mole Fraction

The mole fraction is the ratio of the number of moles of a particular component to the total number of moles in a solution.

Example:

A solution contains 3.0 moles of water and 2.0 moles of methanol. What is the mole fraction of water?

3.0 mol/(3.0 mol + 2.0 mol) = 0.60

C. Types of Problems

1. Weight/Weight Calculation

These types of problems deal with the *weight fraction*.

$$\text{Weight fraction} = \frac{\text{grams of component}}{\text{total grams of solution}}$$

Multiplying the answer by 100 gives the *weight percent*.

2. Weight/Volume Calculation

To find the weight/volume percent, use the following formula:

$$\text{Weight/volume percent} = \frac{\text{weight of solute (g)}}{\text{volume of solution (mL)}} \times 100$$

3. Density Problems

Density, as you know, is equal to mass/volume. This value can be used to help calculate the weight percent. Density acts as a conversion factor to go from milliliters to grams in the denominator.

Example:

Solution X has a molarity of 1.433 M and a density of 1.012 grams per milliliter. Find the weight percent.

1.433 M = 1.099 mol X/1,000 mL solution

1.12g/ml = 1.012 g solution/1.000 mL solution

If each milliliter has a mass of 1.012 g, then 1000 mL must have a mass of 1,012 g. Now you can use this information to find the weight percent.

4. Dilution Problems

If a solution is diluted or concentrated, the number of moles *does not change*, but the volume of solution and the concentration *do change*. The formula is as follows:

$$M_1 \times V_1 = M_2 \times V_2$$

D. Colligative Properties

The colligative properties of the solvent depend on the *concentration* of solute particles present, not on the kind of solute particles. Typical problems involve vapor pressure lowering, freezing point lowering, boiling point elevation, and osmotic pressure.

1. Lowering the Vapor Pressure

If a solute (A) is added to a pure solvent (B), the vapor pressure above the solvent decreases. The more particles dissolved in a solvent, the lower the vapor pressure. Raoult's law governs this relationship.

$$\Delta \text{ vapor pressure} = (\text{mole fraction}) \times \text{vapor pressure of pure solvent}$$

$$\text{mole fraction} = \text{moles of solute/moles of solute + moles of solvent)}$$

2. Lowering the Freezing Point

The more particles of solute added to a solution, the greater the reduction of temperature needed to allow the molecules to orient themselves in a crystalline structure.

$$\Delta \text{ freezing point depression} = K_f \times \text{molality}$$

where K_f is a constant for the solvent ($1.86°C/m^{-1}$ for water).

3. Boiling Point Elevation

Boiling occurs when the vapor pressure is equal to the external pressure on the surface. Since adding solutes lowers the vapor pressure, a higher temperature is needed to raise the vapor pressure and cause the solution to boil.

$$\Delta_{\text{boiling point}} = K_b \times \text{molality}$$

where K_b is a constant depending on solvent.

4. Osmotic Pressure

Solvent moves across a semipermeable membrane if the solute concentrations on the two sides of the membrane are not the same (i.e., are either hypotonic or hypertonic), *not* isotonic.

$$\text{Osmotic pressure} = \text{molarity of solution} \times R \times T$$

where R is a constant and T is the temperature in kelvins.

Start of Osmotic Pressure Experiment   End of Osmotic Pressure Experiment

Start of an osmotic pressure experiment with equal pressures acting on both compartments. At the end of the experiment the pressure developed is the osmotic pressure.

VIII. ACIDS AND BASES

A. Basic Information

An *acidic solution* is an aqueous solution that has a pH less than 7. It contains more H^+ ions than OH^- ions. A *basic solution* is an aqueous solution than has a pH greater than 7. It contains more OH^- ions than H^+ ions. Brönsted-Lowry, Arrhenius, and Lewis have provided different definitions of the same concept. Be sure that you can see that all three describe the same concept.

1. Brönsted-Lowry's Definition

An *acid* is a substance that donates a proton (H^+) to another substance. A *base* is a substance that accepts a proton (H^+) from another substance.

In a solution, when an acid donates a proton, the acid becomes a substance that can now accept a proton. This is the concept behind conjugate acid-base pairs.

$$AH \quad + \quad B \quad \leftrightarrow \quad BH^+ \quad + \quad A^-$$

| acid | base | conjugate acid | conjugate base |

A conjugate acid forms when a proton is added to a base. A conjugate base forms when a proton is lost from an acid. The stronger the acid, the weaker the conjugate base; the opposite is true for a strong acid. This concept applies also to bases.

2. Arrhenius's Definition

An *acid* is a substance that, in the presence of an aqueous solution, donates a H^+ to that solution. A *base* is a substance that, in the presence of an aqueous solution, produces OH^-. The amount of dissociation defines the strength of the acid or base. A substance that dissociates completely is considered to be a strong acid or base (large K_a or K_b), and one that dissociates partially is considered to be weak (small K_a or K_b).

$$AH \xrightarrow{H_2O} A^- + H^+$$

$$K_a = \frac{[A][H]}{[HA]}$$

3. Lewis's Definition

An *acid* is a substance that accepts a pair of electrons. A *base* is a substance that donates a pair of electrons.

| Lewis acid | Lewis base | Lewis acid-base compound |

The term *amphoteric* (*amphiprotic*) refers to a substance that can function as an acid or a base, depending on its environment.

B. pH and pOH

1. Explanation of Formulas

pH (potential for Hydrogen) measures the hydrogen ion concentration $[H^+]$. The formula is as follows:

$$pH = -\log [H^+] = \log \frac{1}{[H^+]}$$

pOH measures the hydroxide ion concentration. Here is the formula:

$$pOH = -\log [OH^-] = \log \frac{1}{[OH^-]}$$

The equilibrium-constant expression for the autoionization of water is as follows:

$$K[H_2O] = K_w = [H^+][OH^-] = 1.0 \times 10^{-14}$$

2. The pH and pOH Scales

pH   1   2   3   4   5   6   7   8   9   10   11   12   13   14

Strong acid ←————————————— neutral ————————————→ Strong base

pOH   14   13   12   11   10   9   8   7   6   5   4   3   2   1

IX. CHEMICAL EQUILIBRIUM

A. Equilibrium Constant

At equilibrium, the rate of the forward reaction equals that of the reverse reaction. Rate will be discussed more fully in Section XIII, Chemical Kinetics, but it is helpful to give this equation here:

$$\text{Rate} = k[A]^x [B]^y$$

We write this equation for both the forward and reverse reactions of a particular reaction at equilibrium. By setting them equal to each other and solving for k, we get the equilibrium constant.

Example:
What is the equation for the equilibrium constant of the following reaction?

$$2[A] + [B] \longleftrightarrow 3[C] + 2[D]$$

$$\text{Rate (forward)} = k[A]^2 [B]; \text{Rate (reverse)} = k[C]^3 [D]^2$$

$$k_{forward} [A]^2 [B] = k_{reverse}[C]^3 [D]^2$$

$$K_{eq} = \frac{[C]^3 [D]^2}{[A]^2 [B]}$$

Note: Pure solids and liquids are not in the equilibrium constant expression.

To determine the direction of the reaction (i.e., if products or reactants are favored in the given reaction), you must find the value of Q_c, the reaction quotient. This value, Q_c, is found with the same method as k_c. Rather than using the concentrations at equilibrium, Q_c utilizes the experimental set of concentrations.

By comparing Q_c to k_c, we can tell whether the given reaction will favor the formation of products or reactants, or whether the reaction is at equilibrium.

$Q_c = K_{eq}$ The reaction is at equilibrium.

$Q_c > K_{eq}$ The reaction favors the reactants.

$Q_c < K_{eq}$ The reaction favors the products.

$$aA + bB \longleftrightarrow cC + dD$$

$$Q_c = \frac{[C]^c [D]^d}{[A]^a [B]^b}$$

Example:

$$A + B \longleftrightarrow 2C$$

Given: $K_{eq} = 62$ at 500°C; $[A] = 7.69 \times 10^{-2}$; $[B] = 3.45 \times 10^{-4}$; $[C] = 5.21 \times 10^{-3}$ at 500°C.

Is this equation at equilibrium or will a reaction take place to reach equilibrium? If a reaction takes place to reach equilibrium, will it favor the formation of products or reactants?

1. Write the reaction quotient, Q_c:

$$Q_c = \frac{[C]^2}{[A][B]}$$

2. Substitute concentrations given in the question:

$$Q_c = \frac{(5.21 \times 10^{-3})^2}{(7.69 \times 10^{-2})(3.45 \times 10^{-4})} = 1.02$$

$$Q_c = 1.02 \text{ at } 500°C$$

$$k_{eq} = 62 \text{ at } 500°C$$

$Q_c < k_{eq}$, therefore a reaction will take place in order to reach equilibrium. It will favor the formation of products as it moves in a forward direction.

If a reaction is at equilibrium, any change in stress to the system will cause the reaction to move to the left or right to counterbalance that alteration. In these problems, either the reactants or the products will be favored. The following examples illustrate how changes in concentration, pressure/volume, and temperature will affect a reaction at equilibrium.

1. Changes in Reactant/Product Concentration

Increasing the concentration of a substance causes the reaction to use that substance, making more of the substances on the other side of the equation. Increasing concentration causes a shift to the other side.

2. Changes in Pressure and Volume

Increasing the pressure of a system at equilibrium will cause a shift to the side that reduces pressure. An increase in volume has the same effect as a decrease in pressure.

Example:

What will occur with an increase in pressure in the following reaction at equilibrium?

$$N_2 \text{ (g)} + 3H_2 \text{ (g)} \leftrightarrow 2NH_3 \text{ (g)}$$

There are 2 moles of gas on the right side of the equation and 4 moles on the left. An increase in pressure favors the formation of more NH_3. The reaction favors the side with fewer gas molecules.

3. Changes in Temperature

We treat heat as a product in an exothermic reaction, and as a reactant in an endothermic reaction.

Example:

Add heat to the following endothermic reaction:

$$\text{Reactants} \longleftrightarrow \text{products}$$

When heat is added, the reaction will try to normalize by shifting to the right:

$$\text{Reactants} + \text{HEAT} \longleftrightarrow \text{products}$$

B. Acid/Base Calculations

Some acid/base calculations have already been addressed (pH, K_a, etc.) in other sections. Neutralization, buffers, and titration must be reviewed as well.

The formula for *neutralization* is

$$\text{Volume}_{acid} \times \text{Normality}_{acid} = \text{Volume}_{base} \times \text{Normality}_{base}$$

A *buffer* is a solution that undergoes a limited change in pH upon addition of a small amount of acid or base. *Buffering capacity* refers to the amount of acid or base the buffer can neutralize before the pH begins to change to an appreciable degree.

The *Henderson-Hasselbach equation* is used to estimate the pH of a buffer.

$$pH = pK_a + \log \frac{[\text{base}]}{[\text{acid}]}$$

Note that when:

$$[\text{base}] = [\text{acid}], pH = pK_a$$

Titration is a method used to determine the pH of an unknown solution. A *standard solution* of known concentration is mixed with the unknown solution. The *equivalence point* is reached when the numbers of equivalents of the standard and unknown solutions are equal in the titration procedure. The *end point* is the point in the titration when the indicator changes color, showing that enough standard solution has been added to terminate the reaction. A *titration curve* is a graph of pH as a function of the volume of standard solution added.

C. Precipitation

1. K_{sp}

The *solubility product constant* (K_{sp}) is equal to the product of the molar concentrations of ions in a saturated solution, each raised to a power equal to its coefficient in the balanced equation.

Dissolution: A_xB_y (s) $\longleftrightarrow$ xA^{y+} (aq) + yB^{x-} (aq)

Solubility product constant, $K_{sp} = [A^{y+}]^x \times [B^{x-}]^y$

Often a reaction is written out and you are asked to formulate the expression for the K_{sp}; or the solubility data are given, and you are asked to find the K_{sp}.

Example:
The molar solubility in water of $Pb(IO_3)_2$ is 4.0×10^{-5} mole per liter. What is the value of K_{sp}?

$$Pb(IO_3)_2 \text{ (s)} \longleftrightarrow Pb^{2+} \text{ (aq)} + 2IO_3^- \text{ (aq)}$$

$$K_{sp} = [Pb^{2+}] [IO_3^-]^2$$

Upon dissolution:

$$1 \text{ mol } [Pb^{2+}] \rightarrow 4.0 \times 10^{-5} \text{ mol/L}$$

$$2 \text{ mol } [IO_3^-] \rightarrow 4.0 \times 10^{-5} \text{ mol/L} \times 2$$

$$K_{sp} = (4.0 \times 10^{-5}) (8.0 \times 10^{-5})^2$$

$$= 2.6 \times 10^{-13}$$

The *ion product* is the product of the concentrations of the dissolved ions, each raised to its stoichiometric coefficient.

Ion product < K_{sp}:	Unsaturated	No precipitate will form.
Ion product = K_{sp}:	Saturated	No precipitate will form.
Ion product > K_{sp}:	Unsaturated	Precipitation occurs.

X. OXIDATION-REDUCTION REACTIONS

A. Oxidation and Reduction Definitions

Oxidation is the loss of an electron by a substance. *Reduction* is the gain of an electron by a substance. An easy mnemonic to remember is *"LEO the lion says GER"* (lose e^- → oxidation; gain e^- → reduction). These two processes occur simultaneously in oxidation-reduction (redox) reactions, thereby conserving the original number of electrons. An *oxidizing agent* is *reduced* and causes the other atom to be oxidized. A *reducing agent* is *oxidized* and causes the other atom to be reduced.

B. Determination of Oxidation Numbers

Oxidation numbers are used to keep track of the changes that take place in a redox reaction. The rules for assigning numbers are as follows:

- A free element (Na, H_2, P_4, N_2) has the oxidation number 0.
- The oxidation number of any monatomic ion (an ion of only one atom) is equal to the charge on the ion ($Na+ = +1$; $Al^{3+} = +3$).
- The oxidation number of oxygen is –2 except in peroxides, where it is –1 (peroxides = H_2O_2; Na_2O_2).
- The oxidation number of hydrogen is +1 except when it occurs after a metal ion, when it is –1.
- The oxidation number of fluorine is –1.
- The oxidation numbers of Group IA elements are +1.
- The oxidation numbers of Group IIA elements are +2.
- The sum of all the oxidation numbers in a compound is 0, except for polyatomic ions, where the sum is equal to the charge of the ion.

C. Steps in Balancing Redox Reaction Equations

- Determine what substances are undergoing oxidation and what substances are undergoing reduction.
- Write the half-reaction for each process.
- Balance each half-reaction equation.
  Acidic solution: Use H_2O and H^+.
  Basic solution: Use H_2O and OH^-.
- Balance charges, using electrons.
- Multiply one or both half-reactions by a whole-number factor to get the electrons lost to equal the electrons gained.
- Add the two balanced half-reactions

Example:
Balance the following equation, which involves an acidic solution:

$$Cr_2O_7^{2-} (aq) + Cl^- (aq) \rightarrow Cr^{3+} (aq) + Cl_2 (g)$$

Steps 1 and 2:

$$Cr_2O_7^{2-} (aq) \rightarrow Cr^{3+} (aq) \qquad Cl^- (aq) \rightarrow Cl_2 (g)$$

Step 3:
Since this is an acidic solution, use H_2O and H^+ to balance the half-reaction equations:

$$14 H^+ (aq) + Cr_2O_7^{2-} (aq) \rightarrow 2Cr^{3+} (aq) + 7 H_2O (l)$$

and

$$2Cl^- (aq) \rightarrow Cl_2 (g)$$

Step 4:

Equalize the total charge on both sides.

$$6e + 14\,H^+\,(aq) + Cr_2O_7{}^{2-}\,(aq) \rightarrow 2Cr^{3+}\,(aq) + 7\,H_2O\,(l)$$

and

$$2Cl^-\,(aq) \rightarrow Cl_2\,(g) + 2e^-$$

Step 5:

Multiply the second half-reaction equation by 3 to equalize the electrons on both sides.

$$6Cl^-\,(aq) \rightarrow 3Cl_2(g) + 6e^-$$

Step 6:

Finally, add the two balanced half-reactions.

$$14\,H^+\,(aq) + Cr_2O_7{}^{2-}\,(aq) + 6\,Cl^- \rightarrow 2Cr^{3+}\,(aq) + 7\,H_2O\,(l) + 3Cl_2\,(g)$$

D. Electrochemical Concepts and Calculations

1. Electrolytic Cell

An electrolytic cell has nonspontaneous reactions that are driven by an outside source of electrical energy (electrolysis). The oxidation-reduction reactions occur in the electrodes. The *positive electrode* (*anode*) is where *oxidation* takes place. The *negative electrode* (*cathode*) is where *reduction* takes place.

An electrolytic cell can be used to decompose molten sodium chloride:

$$2NaCl\,(l) \rightarrow 2Na\,(l) + Cl_2\,(g)$$

Setup of an electrolytic cell.

2. Faraday's Law

Faraday's law states that the amount of oxidation-reduction reaction occurring in an electrolytic cell is proportional to the amount of current passing through. It relates the number of electrons to the amount of electric charge. The coulomb (C) is the unit of electric charge.

$$96{,}485\,C = 1\text{ mole electrons} = 1\text{ faraday (F)}$$

3. Galvanic Cell

A galvanic cell that produces an electric current as a spontaneous reaction occurring between the electrolytes of the cell, for example, a battery. The two half-cells must be separated from each other but connected by a salt bridge, which allows ions to be exchanged.

The galvanic cell.

a. Electromotive Force (emf)

Electromotive force (emf) is the driving force that pushes the electrons through the circuit. It is the potential difference between the electrodes of the cell.

b. Standard Electrode Potential ($E°$)

The value $E°$ is the emf measured under standard conditions, thus allowing a comparison between half-cell reactions. The standard conditions are as follows:

- The temperature is 25°C.
- The concentration of each ion is 1 M.
- The partial pressure of each gas in the reaction is 1 atmosphere.
- Metals are in their pure states.

When $E°$ values are compared, the *higher number is oxidized*, and the *lower number is reduced.*

$$\text{Emf of cell} = E_{\text{oxidation}} + E_{\text{reduction}}$$

Note: The half-cell potential for a reduction reaction is equal in magnitude but opposite in sign to the half-cell potential for an oxidation reaction.

A positive emf value indicates a spontaneous reaction, while a negative one indicates a nonspontaneous reaction.

XI. THERMODYNAMICS AND THERMOCHEMISTRY

A. Laws of Thermodynamics

1. First Law

The total energy of a system and its surroundings is conserved. Energy is neither created nor destroyed.

Change in internal energy (ΔE) = heat added (q) + work done on system (w)

2. Second Law

In any spontaneous process the entropy of the universe increases. Processes that are spontaneous in one direction are not spontaneous in the reverse direction. *Entropy* (*S*) is a measure of the randomness of a system.

3. Third Law

The entropy of a pure crystalline substance at absolute zero (0.0 K or –273°C) is zero.

B. Hess's Law

Hess's law states that, whether a reaction occurs in one step or in a series of steps, the change in enthalpy is an additive property. Change in enthalpy (ΔH) refers to the thermal energy gained or lost when a change takes place under constant pressure.

Example:

Using the given information, predict the ΔH for the reaction $SO_2 \rightarrow SO_3 + \frac{1}{2} O_2$

$$S + \frac{3}{2} O_2 \rightarrow SO_3 \quad \Delta H = -54.31 \text{ kcal/mol}$$

$$S + O_2 \rightarrow SO_2 \quad \Delta H = -32.92 \text{ kcal/mol}$$

Solve this problem by reversing the second equation. Change the sign of ΔH, and then subtract the terms on each side of the equation to get the final equation.

$$
\begin{array}{lll}
S + \frac{3}{2} O_2 & \rightarrow SO_3 & \Delta H = -54.31 \text{ kcal/mol} \\
SO_2 & \rightarrow S + O_2 & \Delta H = -32.92 \text{ kcal/mol} \\
\hline
SO_2 & \rightarrow SO_3 + \frac{1}{2} O_2 & \Delta H = -21.39 \text{ kcal/mol}
\end{array}
$$

C. Spontaneity Prediction

1. Gibbs Free Energy

Gibbs free energy (*G*) is a thermodynamic state function that combines enthalpy and entropy. For a change occurring at a constant temperature and pressure, the formula is

$$\Delta G = \Delta H - T \Delta S$$

Entropy (*S*) is a measure of the randomness of a system. *Enthalpy* (*H*) is a measure of the amount of heat. If ΔG is negative, the reaction is spontaneous and forward. If ΔG is zero, the reaction is at equilibrium. If ΔG is positive, the reaction is nonspontaneous, but the reverse reaction is spontaneous.

2. Standard Free-Energy Change

The standard free-energy change for a reaction equals the sum of the standard free-energy values per mole of each product, each multiplied by the corresponding coefficient in the balanced equation, minus the corresponding sum for the reactants.

$$\Delta G° = \sum n \Delta G°_f \text{ (products)} - \sum m \Delta G°_f \text{ (reactants)}$$

Example:

$$N_2 \ (g) \ + \ 3H_2 \ (g) \rightarrow 2 \ NH_3 \ (g)$$

For $N_2(g)$: $\Delta G^\circ_f = 0.0$
For $H_2(g)$: $\Delta G^\circ_f = 0.0$
For $NH_3(g)$: $\Delta G^\circ_f = -16.66$ kJ/mol

Set up the equation and plug in the numbers:

$$\Delta G = 2\Delta G^\circ_f \ (NH_3) - [3\Delta G^\circ_f \ (H_2) + \Delta G^\circ_f \ (N_2)]$$

$$\Delta G = -33.32 \text{ kJ}$$

XII. CHEMICAL KINETICS

A. Rate Laws

The rate of a reaction is the change in concentrations of the reactants divided by the time. The rate law for almost all reactions, $aA + bB \rightarrow cC + dD$, has a rate proportional to $[A]^a \ [B]^b$.

$$\text{Rate} = k \ [A]^a \ [B]^b$$

Example:
Find the rate law from the given information:

TRIAL	$[A]_{INITIAL}$ (M)	$[B]_{INITIAL}$ (M)	INITIAL RATE (M/S)
1	0.100	0.100	2.0×10^{-5}
2	0.100	0.200	4.0×10^{-5}
3	0.200	0.200	16.0×10^{-5}

Look for the trials in which the concentrations are the same (i.e., trials 1 and 2). In trial 2, the concentration of B doubles while the concentration of A stays the same, and the rate increases by 2.

Trial 1 rate: $k \ [A]^x \ [B]^y = k(1.00)^x \ (1.00)^y$

Trial 2 rate: $k \ (1.00)^x \ (2.00)^y$

Now, divide rate 2 by rate 1:

$$\frac{\text{Rate 2}}{\text{Rate 1}} = \frac{4.0 \times 10^{-5}}{2.0 \times 10^{-5}} = \frac{\cancel{k} \ \cancel{(1.00)^x} \ (2.00)^y}{\cancel{k} \ \cancel{(1.00)^x} \ (1.00)^y} = (2.00)^y$$

$$2 = (2.00)^y$$

$$y = 2$$

Make the same comparison between trials 2 and 3, and find $x = 2$.
The overall *reaction order* is the sum of the two orders ($2 + 2 = 4$).

To find the rate law, solve for k using the data from any of the trials and the values for x and y:

$$\text{Rate} = k \ [A]^x \ [B]^y \rightarrow k = \frac{\text{rate}}{[A]^x \ [B]^y}$$

$$k = \frac{2.0 \times 10^{-5} \text{ M/s}}{(1)^2 \ (1)^2}$$

Rate law $= 2.0 \times 10^{-5} \text{ M}^{-2} \text{ s}^{-1} \ [A]^2 \ [B]^2$

B. Reaction Orders

- *Zero-order reactions* have a constant rate, and they occur independently of the concentrations of the reactants.
- *First-order reactions* have a rate $\propto [A]^x$, where $x = 1$. The rate is therefore proportional to the concentration of one reactant.
- *Second-order reactions* have a rate $\propto [A]^1[B]^1$, or a rate $\propto [A]^2$.

Note: Third-order and higher order reactions are also feasible, as well as mixed-order reactions (fractional order).

Chemical reactions are usually accelerated by

- increasing the concentrations of reactants,
- increasing the temperature of reaction,
- increasing the surface area of reaction,
- the presence of a catalyst.

A *homogenous catalyst* is a catalyst that is in the same state as the reactants. A *heterogeneous catalyst* is in a different phase than the reactants.

C. Activation Energy and Enthalpy

Reaction profiles illustrating the activation energy of reverse reactions and the fact that ΔH of the reverse reaction is opposite in sign to ΔH of the forward reaction.

In this reaction profile E_a is the activation energy of the reaction. It is the difference in potential energy between the activated complex and the reactants and represents the energy of collision necessary to drive this reaction. The activation energy can be reduced by the addition of a catalyst. The catalyst works by increasing the frequency of collisions in the forward reaction (E_a) and similarly in the reverse reaction ($E_{a \text{ reverse}}$). $E_{a \text{ reverse}}$, the activation energy of the reverse reaction, is the difference between the potential energy of the transition state and the products.

ΔH represents the change in enthalpy. Enthalpy is equal to the potential energy of the products minus the potential energy of the reactants. If this number is negative, the reaction is exothermic (heat is released). If this number is positive, the reaction is endothermic (heat is absorbed).

The *transition state* (activated complex) is the arrangement of reactant and product molecules at the point of maximum energy in the rate-determining step of a reaction.

Collision theory states that reactant molecules must possess the correct orientation and enough energy to combine and form an activated complex.

D. Half-Life

The half-life ($t_{1/2}$) is the length of time required for the concentration of a reactant to decrease to one-half of the original amount.

For a first-order reaction:

$$t_{1/2} = \frac{0.693}{k}$$

For a second-order reaction:

$$t_{1/2} = \frac{1}{k\,[X]}$$

In these formulas, k = rate constant of reaction and X = initial concentration.

Here is an example of the most common type of question asked in this category: Given x grams, use the equation

$$\frac{x}{2^n} = \text{remaining amount}$$

where n = number of half-lives and x = number of grams.

This equation gives the final product remaining.

XIII. NUCLEAR REACTIONS

A. Radioactive Decay

Radioactivity occurs as a result of an unstable nucleus that spontaneously emits energy and/or small subatomic particles. Radioactive isotopes emit subatomic particles including the electron (beta particle), neutron, helium nucleus (alpha particle), and positron. As a result, the nuclear mass and/or nuclear charge changes, forming a radioisotope.

In the past, the questions for this section have taken one of two forms. You may be required to fill in the missing element, or simply identify the type of radioactive decay.

B. Alpha, Beta, and Gamma Decay

TYPE OF DECAY	CHARGE	RADIATION	PENETRATING POWER
Alpha	+2	4_2He	1
Beta	−1	Electrons	100
Gamma	0	High-energy photons	1,000

Alpha decay is a form of radioactivity that involves the emission of helium nuclei, termed alpha (α) particles, $^{4}_{2}\text{He}$:

$$^{222}_{86}\text{Rn} \quad \rightarrow \quad ^{218}_{84}\text{Po} \quad + \quad ^{4}_{2}\text{He}$$

or

$$^{222}_{86}\text{Rn} \quad \rightarrow \quad ^{218}_{84}\text{Po} \quad + \quad \alpha$$

Beta decay involves the emission of electrons. Beta particles (β) have no mass and have a charge of −1, indicated as $^{0}_{-1}\text{e}$.

$$^{14}_{6}\text{C} \quad \rightarrow \quad ^{14}_{7}\text{N} \quad + \quad ^{0}_{-1}\text{e}$$

or

$$^{14}_{6}\text{C} \quad \rightarrow \quad ^{14}_{7}\text{N} \quad + \quad \beta$$

Neutrons are emitted in nuclear reactions ($_0^1 n$):

$$_{49}^{21}Sc \rightarrow \ _{50}^{20}Ca \ + \ _0^1 n \ + \ _{-1}^0 e$$

Positrons are the positive equivalents of beta particles. Positrons have no mass and a +1 charge.

$$_6^{11}C \rightarrow \ _5^{11}B \ + \ _{+1}^0 \beta$$

Reactions involving positrons may also involve *electron capture,* a process whereby an electron combines with a proton to form a neutron:

$$_6^{11}C \ + \ _{-1}^0 \beta \rightarrow \ _5^{11}B$$

Gamma rays are emitted when decay occurs, leaving the nucleus with excess energy. The loss of this excess energy is called gamma radiation. No change of charge or mass occurs with gamma radiation. *X rays* are similar to gamma rays; neither is incorporated into written equations, nor does either change the identity of the isotope.

ORGANIC CHEMISTRY REVIEW OUTLINE (SNS Q71-100)

I. OVERVIEW

    A. A Method of Attack
    B. The Visual Thought Process
    C. Organic Models
    D. Scope of Examination
    E. General Concepts

II. BONDING

    A. Three Types of Bonds

        1. Ionic
        2. Covalent
        3. Hydrogen

    B. Orbitals

        1. Atomic Orbitals
        2. Molecular Orbitals

            a. Sigma Bond
            b. Pi Bond

        3. Hybrid Orbitals

            a. sp^3
            b. sp^2
            c. sp

    C. Bond Rotation and Energy; Newman Projections

        1. Rotation and Energy
        2. Newman Projections

            a. Ethane
            b. Butane

        3. Energy Diagrams

    D. Other Related Concepts

        1. Ring Strain
        2. Cyclohexane
        3. Bond Cleavage

III. NOMENCLATURE

    A. IUPAC Rules
    B. General Molecular Formulas

        1. Alkanes

            a. Alkyl Substituents
            b. Rings

        2. Alkenes

   a. Cis and Trans Isomers
   b. *E* and *Z* Isomers
   c. Dienes and Trienes

  3. Alkynes

 C. Naming Benzene Compounds

  1. Monosubstitution
  2. Disubstitution
  3. Trisubstitution and Other Substitutions

 D. Alcohols: Primary (1°), Secondary (2°), Tertiary (3°)
 E. Ethers
 F. Carbonyl Compounds

  1. Aldehydes
  2. Ketones
  3. Carboxylic Acids
  4. Esters

 G. Amines and Amides

IV. STEREOCHEMISTRY

 A. General Information

  1. Importance: The Thalidomide Example
  2. Stereoisomers
  3. Chirality/Chiral Centers
  4. Optical Activity

 B. Fischer Diagrams

  1. Concepts
  2. Relevance to Carbohydrates
  3. Rule of 2^n

 C. Absolute Configuration

V. AROMATICITY

 A. General Information

  1. Conjugation
  2. Resonance and Delocalization

 B. Rules for Determining Aromaticity
 C. Electrophilic Aromatic Substitution (EAS)

  1. General Concepts and Mechanism
  2. Types, Reagents, and Products

 D. Effects of Substituents on Electrophilic Aromatic Substitution

  1. General Concepts
  2. Activators and Deactivators

VI. CHEMICAL AND PHYSICAL PROPERTIES OF MOLECULES

 A. General Concepts

  1. Polarity
  2. Solubility

B. Alkanes, Alkenes, and Alkynes

    1. Alkanes
    2. Alkenes and Alkynes

C. Alcohols, Ethers, and the Carbonyl Compounds

    1. Alcohols
    2. Ethers
    3. Aldehydes
    4. Ketones
    5. Carboxylic Acids

D. Carbohydrates, Lipids, and Amines

    1. Carbohydrates
    2. Lipids
    3. Amines

E. Optically Active Stereoisomers

VII. ACID-BASE CHEMISTRY

A. General Information

    1. Relevance to Understanding Reactions
    2. Review of Definitions

        a. Brönsted-Lowry Acid and Base
        b. Lewis Acid and Base

    3. Strength and Stability of Acids and Bases

B. Resonance

    1. Terms and Concepts
    2. Rules for Drawing Resonance Forms
    3. Effects of Resonance on Acidity

C. Inductive Effects and Electronegativity

VIII. MECHANISMS AND REACTIONS OF THE MAJOR FUNCTIONAL GROUPS

A. General Information

    1. A Brief Review
    2. Structure and Stability of Radicals

B. Alkane Reactions

    1. Free-Radical Halogenation of Alkanes
    2. Nucleophilic Substitution and Elimination

        a. The Basics
        b. S_N1
        c. S_N2
        d. $E1$
        e. $E2$

C. Alkene and Alkyne Reactions

    1. Markovnikov's Rule—HX Addition
    2. Anti-Markovnikov Reactions—Radical Halogenation

D. Reactions of Oxygen-Containing Molecules

  1. Alcohols

    a. Oxidation to Aldehydes

    b. Dehydration to Alkenes

    c. Formation of Esters from Alcohols and Carboxylic Acids

  2. Aldehydes and Ketones

    a. Reactions with Grignard Reagents

    b. Reactions with Alcohols

    c. Oxidation

    d. Aldol Condensation

    e. Keto-Enol Tautomerism

  3. Carboxylic Acids

    a. Nucleophilic Substitution Reaction

    b. Esterification

    c. Formation of Anhydrides

E. Reactions of Carbohydrates and Amines

  1. Carbohydrates

  2. Amines

IX. SYNTHESIS

A. General Information

B. Alkanes—Wurtz Reaction

C. Alkenes and Alkynes

  1. Alkenes

    a. Dehydrohalogenation

    b. Dehydration

    c. Dehalogenation

  2. Alkynes

    a. Dehydrohalogenation

    b. Dehalogenation

D. Alcohols, Aldehydes, and Ketones

  1. Alcohols

    a. Hydration of Alkenes

    b. Grignard Reagents

    c. Reduction of Adehydes and Ketones

  2. Aldehydes

    a. Mild Oxidation of a 1° Alcohol

    b. Oxidation of a Diol

  3. Ketones

    a. Mild Oxidation of a 2° Alcohol

    b. Ozonolysis

    c. Decarboxylation of Carboxylic Acids

E. Carboxylic Acids, Esters, and Ethers

I. OVERVIEW

A. A Method of Attack

The organic chemistry section is the third and last part of the Survey of the Natural Sciences. There will be only 30 questions on which to demonstrate your knowledge of organic chemistry. Students should realize that the American Dental Association does not expect dental school applicants to have a full mastery of the subject matter. Thankfully, the ADA realizes that practicing dentists do not need a Ph.D. in organic chemistry. However, *a solid foundation in the major concepts is expected. The goal of this review is to thoroughly cover the concepts that are outlined in the ADA's scope of examination.*

    The approach you choose for your review of organic chemistry is important. This review should be different from your reviews of both biology and general chemistry. The biology review called for extensive memorization, and the general chemistry review emphasized analytic problem solving skills. *The organic chemistry review demands both.* The best method of studying organic chemistry is to *visualize* and *conceptualize* the interactions of the molecules involved and to understand why certain reactions occur. Too many students attempt to learn organic chemistry through memorization alone. Finding similarities and trends among reactions is much more useful than memorizing individual reactions. Taking the time to think through the concepts presented is vital to a successful outcome on the actual exam. Each topic included in the ADA scope of exam can be tested through an infinite number of questions, and the student who can apply general principles to a wide range of problems will be the most successful.

B. The Visual Thought Process

It has been stressed that the best method of preparation is to fully visualize the topic discussed. But how do you implement this method into your review for the DAT? The following example may be helpful. In the review of the chemical and physical properties of alkanes, the following statement is made: "Alkanes are *nonpolar hydrocarbons that are insoluble in water.*" You should visualize hydrogens in hybridized *sp³* tetrahedral bonding and the carbon backbone and should realize that, because of the symmetry, no dipole is created. This explains why alkanes are *nonpolar hydrocarbons.* In addition, the structure of water should come to mind. You will recall that the H_2O molecule is in a bent formation with two lone pairs of electrons, creating a dipole. By realizing that polar and nonpolar molecules are not soluble with one another, you can see that the claim that alkanes are *insoluble in water* can be justified.

The visual thought process also identifies what information is known and what is not. For example, if you, the diligent student, were able to visualize the hydrocarbon configuration but could not link it to the solubility in water, you would refer to Section VI.A.2 on solubility and then make the link between polarity and solubility. It takes time to adopt this thought process, which is slow and tedious, but we believe that *it is the most efficient and effective method of learning organic chemistry.*

C. Organic Models

Model sets are an excellent aid in this visual type of learning. Since, however, model sets are not allowed in the actual exam, *they should only be used initially to understand the concepts presented.* The organic chemistry section intentionally tests the student's ability to visualize in three dimensions. The only way to improve this ability is through practice.

D. Scope of Examination

It is important to keep in mind that the goal of your review of organic chemistry is to score well on this section of the DAT. *Mastering the fundamental concepts outlined in the scope of examination is the best method of preparation for the DAT.* Following is the scope of examination, as defined by the ADA Department of Testing Services:

- Bonding (atomic orbitals, molecular orbitals, hybridization, Lewis structures, bond angles, bond lengths)
- Mechanisms (energetics, structure and stability of intermediates: S_N1, S_N2, elimination, addition, free-radical substitution mechanisms)
- Chemical and Physical Properties of Molecules (stability, solubility, polarity, inter- and intramolecular forces: separation techniques)
- Organic Analysis (introductory IR and 1H NMR spectroscopy, simple chemical tests)
- Stereochemistry (conformational analysis, optical activity, chirality, chiral centers, places of symmetry, enantiomers, diasteriomers, meso compounds)
- Nomenclature (IUPAC rules for identification of functional groups in molecules)
- Reactions of the Major Functional Groups (prediction of reaction products and important mechanistic generalities)
- Acid-Base Chemistry (resonance effects, inductive effects, prediction of products and equilibria)
- Aromaticity (concepts of aromaticity, electrophilic aromatic substitution)
- Synthesis (identification of the product of, or the reagents used in, a simple sequence of reactions)

A one-year introductory course covering the major concepts of organic chemistry is required by most dental schools. This review assumes that you have been exposed to the majority of terms and concepts. It is recommended that you refer to an organic chemistry textbook to review areas for which you feel additional study is needed.

Check off each topic on the outline as you review the material. Doing so will ensure that, by the end of your review, you have covered all the topics outlined in the ADA's scope of examination.

E. General Concepts

Organic chemistry assumes a fundamental knowledge of general chemistry. *Review general chemistry before beginning this section.* Organic chemistry is the study of carbon-containing molecules. *Electrophiles* are electron loving (are themselves electron deficient), and *nucleophiles* are nucleus loving (are themselves electron rich). Bonds form between the two. Nature prefers lower states of energy, which are more stable. High-energy bonds are more reactive and less stable; low-energy bonds are less reactive and more stable. *Electronegativity* is the ability of an atom to attract electrons. Electronegativity increases on the periodic chart upward and to the right. The number of *valence electrons* determines the number of bonds an atom will form. *Atomic orbitals* are theoretic regions around the nucleus that have a high probability of containing electrons.

|||||||····   into the plane of paper

▶   out of the plane of paper

Valency, you recall, determines the number of bonds formed by an atom. Carbon has four electrons in its outer shell and forms four bonds to obtain an octet. Be sure to review *Lewis structures* and the *octet rule* in Section II of general chemistry.

II. BONDING

Understanding electronegativity, the octet rule, valency, and trends of the periodic table is essential to understanding bonding. Refer to the general chemistry section for a review of these concepts if you have not done so already.

A. Three Types of Bonds

1. Ionic
Ionic bonds form between atoms with different electronegativities. An atom with a high electron affinity will take electrons from an atom with a low ionization potential. Ionic bonds are strong bonds that have great intermolecular forces, resulting in high melting and boiling points.

2. Covalent
In ionic bonding, electrons are transferred from atom to atom. The atoms of covalent bonds, however, have similar electronegativities and therefore share electrons. Covalent bonds are found in diatomic molecules and in most organic compounds. A difference in electronegativity of atoms in a covalently bonded molecule creates a polar covalent bond. In fact, most covalent bonds are polar, and the molecule creates a dipole. This simply means that the atom in the bond with less

electronegativity takes on a slightly positive charge (+), and the atom with greater electronegativity takes on a slightly negative charge (−). Understanding this concept is key to understanding why organic reactions occur as they do.

3. Hydrogen

Hydrogen bonds form a weak dipole interaction between a hydrogen atom and a negatively charged atom. Hydrogen bonding determines most of the physical properties of organic molecules.

1.   2.   3.   4.

No Net Dipole   No Net Dipole   Net Dipole   Net Dipole

B. Orbitals

1. Atomic Orbitals

Atomic orbitals are theoretic areas around the nucleus where electrons of a given energy level can be found. These orbitals are often referred to *as electron clouds*. An *s* orbital takes on a *spherical cloud*, whereas a *p* orbital is more elongated and resembles a *dumbbell-shaped cloud*.

s p_y

2. Molecular Orbitals

The sharing of electrons in covalent bonds results in an overlap of two of the atomic orbitals, forming two *molecular orbitals*. One of these will be of *higher energy* and *antibonding*, while the other will be of *lower energy* and *bonding*. Electrons fill the bonding, lower energy level first.

a. Sigma Bond

End-on-end overlap of orbitals forms a sigma (σ) bond. The bonding of four hydrogen atoms to a carbon atom results in four sigma bonds. A sigma bond allows the two bonded atoms to *freely rotate*.

Methane with 4 σ bonds

b. Pi Bond

The pi (π) bond is formed from the *parallel overlap of p orbitals*. These parallel overlaps are above and below the plane of the sigma bond. *Pi bonds do not permit rotation.*

Single bonds are sigma bonds, double bonds contain one sigma and one pi bond, and triple bonds contain one sigma and two pi bonds.

π bonds

3. Hybrid Orbitals

Hybridization of atomic orbitals occurs to achieve lower energy states and results in shapes more conducive to overlapping when atomic orbitals become molecular orbitals. This overlapping creates stronger bonds. It is important to remember that nature does not like high-energy states and that chemical reactions occur primarily to obtain lower energy states. Therefore, while paradoxical, the stronger the bond the less energy in the system. Strong bonds and low energy create very stable systems.

Hybridization is the result of nature's creating a system to reduce the energy in the bond and thus achieve a more stable system. This desire to achieve stability results in a change of electron configuration. In the hybridization of carbon (6 electrons, electron configuration of $1s^2\ 2s^2\ 2p^2$), an electron from the $2s$ orbital moves into the vacant $2p_z$ orbital. Then each of the three $2p$ orbitals and the one $2s$ orbital has one electron. The mixing of these four orbitals (that is, the hybridization) results in four identical hybrids that are one part s and three parts p.

p_x p_y p_z $p_{x,\,y,\,z}$

a. sp³

The sp^3 hybrid orbital consists of one s (spherical) and three p (dumbbell-shaped) orbitals that are mixed to form four new sp^3 orbitals. These four orbitals are arranged in a *tetrahedral* conformation, which maximizes the distance between the electron clouds. The angle between clouds created by sp^3 hybridization is 109.5°.

sp^3

b. sp²

The *sp²* hybrid consists of one *s* orbital and two *p* orbitals that mix to form three *sp²* orbitals. The fourth *p* orbital remains unhybridized. This planar conformation creates an angle of 120° between the orbitals. The three *sp²* orbitals lie on the same plane, and the unhybridized dumbbell-shaped *p* orbital is perpendicular to this plane (the *p* orbital is 90° from the plane of the three *sp²* orbitals).

sp^2

c. sp

When one *s* and one *p* orbital form a hybrid, two *sp* orbitals are created and two *p* orbitals remain unhybridized. The two *sp* orbitals are 180° apart (linear), and the two unhybridized orbitals are perpendicular to each other and to the *sp* orbitals. The *lengths* and *strengths* of these hybridized orbitals are *inversely related*, with the *sp* bond being the shorter and stronger.

Two unhybridized *p* orbitals

COMPARISON OF sp, sp², AND sp³ ORBITALS

	sp³	*sp²*	*sp*
Conformation	Tetrahedral	Planar	Linear
Angle (°)	109.5	120*	180†
Number of orbitals	4	4	4
Hybridized	4	3	2
Unhybridized	0	1	2

*sp² orbitals are 90° from the unhybridized *p* orbital.

†*sp* orbitals are 90° from the two unhybridized *p* orbitals.

TYPE	STRENGTH	LENGTH	SIGMA	PI	FREE ROTATION
sp³	Weak	Long	1	0	Yes
sp²	⇓	⇓	1	1	No
sp	Strong	Short	1	2	No

C. Bond Rotation and Energy; Newman Projections

1. Rotation and Energy

The free rotation about a single bond creates a variety of arrangements of atomic structures, some more energetically desirable than others. For example, an ethane molecule has two carbons, each having three hydrogens and one sp^3 bond between the carbons. The ethane molecule can be illustrated with the dotted-line wedge, the sawhorse, or the *Newman projection*.

Dotted-Line
Wedge

Sawhorse

Newman Projection

2. Newman Projections

Newman projections are used to illustrate the energetically favorable and unfavorable positionings of atoms.

a. Ethane

The Newman projection of ethane helps to visualize the positioning of the hydrogens on the carbons. The projection is drawn looking down the axis of the carbon-carbon bond. In the case of ethane, the closer the hydrogens are to one another, the greater the energy and the less stable the molecule. The *anti* is the most favorable positioning, followed by the *gauche*. The *eclipsed* is the least favorable positioning. Rotating the back carbon 60° will change the positioning from anti to gauche, and with another turn the positioning goes from gauche to eclipsed. In ethane, the gauche and anti positionings are identical (sometimes referred to as *staggered*); however, with the addition of more carbons the anti position is indeed more energetically favorable.

Eclipsed

Gauche

Staggered
or
Anti

b. Butane

The Newman projection of butane shows a slightly more complicated situation. In this projection, the axis that is rotated is between the second and third carbons. Rotating the third carbon (out of view) illustrates the various positions possible. The eclipsed position of two methyl groups is more energetically unfavorable than is an eclipsed conformation of hydrogen and methyl.

CH₃   CH₃   CH₃   CH₃

CH₃   CH₃

                                                                    CH₃

Eclipsed   Gauche   Anti

3. Energy Diagrams

As a rule of thumb, *a molecule attains the lowest possible energy by maximizing the distance between its atoms.* In most energetically unfavorable positions the larger groups are eclipsed, and in the most energetically favorable position the larger groups are anti to each other. The relative energy states of molecules are represented by energy diagrams.

Below is the *energy diagram* for butane.

1. Anti
2. CH₃—H Eclipsed
3. CH₃—CH₃ Gauche
4. CH₃—CH₃ Eclipsed
5. CH₃—CH₃ Gauche
6. CH₃—H Eclipsed
7. Anti

D. Other Related Concepts

1. Ring Strain

The most *ring strain* is found in cyclopropane. This molecule gives off a great amount of energy when the ring is broken because of its extreme divergence from the desired bond angle. Of all the cycloalkanes, the six-membered ring *cyclohexane* has the least strain created from bond angles stretching from their desired angle. The molecule benzene, discussed in Section III.C, has no ring strain.

2. Cyclohexane

Cyclohexane is a molecule that appears in two conformations, the *chair* and the *boat*. The molecule undergoes *ring flip*, switching between boat and chair conformations, to maximize the distance between substitutents. The chair conformation has *six axial* hydrogens (vertically oriented) and *six equatorial* hydrogens (horizontally oriented). Hydrogens in the same position (equatorial or axial) on adjacent carbons are trans to one another. Hydrogens in the axial position are cis to hydrogens in the equatorial position on adjacent carbons. For further explanation of cis and trans, see page 159. The following illustration may help to clarify the positioning of hydrogens on the chair configuration of cyclohexane. Also, if an organic model set is available, building the cyclohexane and then inverting the ring between the chair and boat conformations will help to visualize this transformation.

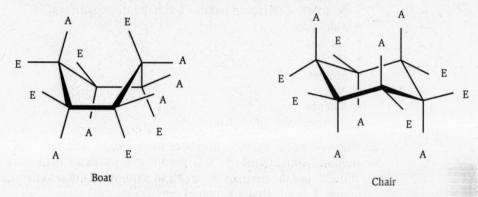

Boat   Chair

3. Bond Cleavage

In *heterolytic cleavage* (*heterolytic* means *"different breaking"*) both electrons are taken by one of the atoms in a molecule. This results in charged products. A simple example of heterolytic cleavage is the dissolution of water. In *homolytic cleavage* (*homolytic* means *"similar breaking"*) each atom takes one electron. No charge results from homolytic cleavage; however, *radicals* are formed that are extremely reactive. This topic will be further discussed in Section VIII on reactions.

III. NOMENCLATURE

A. IUPAC Rules

1. Determine the longest continuous chain of carbon atoms and use this as the parent name. When a functional group is present, use the longest chain that includes the functional group. Drop the *-e* from the alkane name, and add the suffix of the corresponding functional group.

FUNCTIONAL GROUP(S)	SUFFIX	GENERALIZED STRUCTURAL FORMULA	EXAMPLE
Alkane	-ane	R–H	pentane
Alkene	-ene	R=H	pentene
Alkyne	-yne	R H	pentyne
Alcohol	-ol	R–OH	pentanol
Aldehyde	-al	$\overset{\text{O}}{\overset{\|}{\text{R–C–H}}}$	pentanal
Ketone	-one	$\overset{\text{O}}{\overset{\|}{\text{R–C–R}}}$	pentanone
Carboxylic acid	-oic	$\overset{\text{O}}{\overset{\|}{\text{R–C–OH}}}$	pentanoic acid

2. Locate the substituent(s) present, and number the longest chain including the substituent in such a way that the substituent receives *the lowest possible number*. Functional groups take on the parent name. If more than one functional group exists, the groups are *prioritized*; the one with greatest priority takes on the parent name, and the others are treated as substituents. Functional groups are listed in order of *decreasing priority* as follows:

- Carboxylic acids and their derivatives [esters (-oate), amides, nitriles (-nitrile), -C(N), acid halides (-yl halide), anhydrides]
- Aldehydes
- Ketones
- Alcohols
- Amines
- Alkynes
- Alkenes
- Halogens and alkyl groups

3. Use dashes to separate numbers from words, and commas to separate numbers from numbers. If a group appears more than once as a substituent, use the prefixes *di-*, *tri-*, and *tetra-* in addition to the numbers (example: 2,2-dimethyl-3-heptene).

$$CH_3$$
$$|$$
$$C - C - C = C - C - C - C$$
$$|$$
$$CH_3$$

4. Name substitutents alphabetically when two or more exist (example: 2-ethyl-3-methylheptane). The prefixes *iso-*, *sec-*, *tert-*, and *neo-* are *included* in alphabetizing, but, *di-*, *tri-*, and *tetra-* are *excluded*.

5. For cylic compounds use the prefix *cyclo-*.

Examples of IUPAC nomenclature:

1. 3-Methylpentane

$$CH_3 - CH_2 - CH - CH_2 - CH_3$$
$$|$$
$$CH_3$$

2. 3-Bromo-2-chloropentane

$$CH_3 - CH_2 - CH - CH - CH_3$$
$$|\quad|$$
$$Br\quad Cl$$

3. 2-Heptene

4. Cyclohexene

5. Butanal

$$CH_3 - CH_2 - CH_2 - \overset{\overset{\displaystyle O}{\|}}{C} - H$$

6. Butanoic acid

$$CH_3 - CH_2 - CH_2 - \overset{\overset{\displaystyle O}{\|}}{C} - OH$$

7. 3,3-Dimethyl-5-ethyl-6-propylnonane

$$CH_3 - \overset{\overset{\displaystyle CH_3}{|}}{\underset{\underset{\displaystyle CH_2 - CH_3}{|}}{C}} - CH_2 - \overset{\overset{\displaystyle CH_2 - CH_3}{|}}{\underset{\underset{\displaystyle CH_2 - CH_2 - CH_3}{|}}{CH}} - CH - CH_2 - CH_2 - CH_3$$

NUMBER OF CARBON ATOMS	PREFIX	NAME	MOLECULAR FORMULA
1	meth-	methane	CH_4
2	eth-	ethane	C_2H_6
3	prop-	propane	C_3H_8
4	but-	butane	C_4H_{10}
5	pent-	pentane	C_5H_{12}
6	hex-	hexane	C_6H_{14}
7	hept-	heptane	C_7H_{16}
8	oct-	octane	C_8H_{18}
9	non-	nonane	C_9H_{20}
10	dec-	decane	$C_{10}H_{22}$

B. General Molecular Formulas

1. Alkanes

The general formula for alkanes is C_nH_{2n+2}. This means that, for any given number of carbon atoms, there are 2 more than twice that number of hydrogen atoms. The names of alkanes have the suffix -*ane*.

a. Alkyl Substituents

Alkyl substituents are named by adding -*yl* to the prefix (methane becomes methyl). *Iso-*, *sec-*, *tert-*, and *neo-* are prefixes used to further describe the structure of the alkyl substituent. Some common alkyl substituents are listed below.

NUMBER OF CARBON ATOMS	NAME	STRUCTURAL FORMULA
1	methyl-	CH_3-
2	ethyl-	CH_3-CH_2-
3	propyl-	$CH_3-CH_2-CH_2-$
3	isopropyl-	$CH_3-\underset{\underset{\displaystyle}{\|}}{CH}-CH_3$
4	butyl-	$CH_3-CH_2-CH_2CH_2-$
4	*sec*-butyl-	$CH_3-CH_2-\underset{\underset{\displaystyle CH_3}{\|}}{CH}$

(continued)

NUMBER OF CARBON ATOMS	NAME	STRUCTURAL FORMULA
4	isobutyl-	CH_3 \\ $CH-CH_2-$ / CH_3
4	*tert*-butyl-	CH_3 | CH_3-C- | CH_3
5	pentyl-	$CH_3-CH_2-CH_2-CH_2-CH_2-$
5	*sec*-pentyl-	$CH_3-CH_2-CH_2-CH-$ | CH_3
5	isopentyl-	$CH_3-CH-CH_2-CH_2-$ | CH_3
5	*tert*-pentyl-	CH_3 | CH_3-CH_2-C- | CH_3
5	neopentyl-	CH_3 | CH_3-C-CH_2- | CH_3

b. Rings

Carbon chains that form a ring have the same general molecular formula as alkenes, C_nH_{2n}. Two hydrogens are lost from the bond that forms the ring.

Cyclohexane

$C_6 H_{12}$

2. Alkenes

The general formula for alkenes is C_nH_{2n}. Alkenes have a *double bond* between two adjacent carbon atoms and therefore have *two fewer hydrogen atoms than alkanes*. The names of alkenes have the suffix *-ene*.

a. Cis and Trans Isomers

The terms *cis-* and *trans-* refer to the substituents of planar molecules that are not free to rotate because of pi bonds. These terms are used to identify the isomers. Cis alkenes have the larger substituents on the same side of the double bond, and trans alkenes have the larger substituents on opposite sides.

b. E and Z Isomers

IUPAC uses *E/Z* terminology to describe the placement of substituents on planar molecules. This nomenclature is another method of describing cis/trans isomers. *E* refers to opposite sides, or trans. *Z*, refers to the same side ("Zame side"), or cis.

$$H \diagdown \qquad \diagup H$$
$$C = C$$
$$CH_3CH_2 \diagup \qquad \diagdown CH_2CH_3$$

$$H \diagdown \qquad \diagup CH_2CH_3$$
$$C = C$$
$$CH_3CH_2 \diagup \qquad \diagdown H$$

cis-3-Hexane   *trans*-3-Hexane

c. Dienes and Trienes

Alkenes that have two double bonds are dienes, and alkenes that have three bonds are trienes. If the double bonds are separated by a single bond, the structure is referred to as *conjugated*.

or

3. Alkynes

The general formula for alkynes is C_nH_{2n-2}. Alkynes have a *triple bond* between two adjacent carbon atoms and therefore have *four fewer hydrogen atoms than alkanes*. The names of alkynes have the suffix *-yne*.

C. Naming Benzene Compounds

Without substituents, the fully conjugated six-carbon ring, with three double bonds, is called a *benzene* molecule (1,3,5-cyclohexatriene). Benzene is quite unique because of its overlapping *p* orbitals, and will be discussed at length in Section V on aromaticity. The prefixes *phenyl-* and *benzyl-* are often used when a benzene ring appears in a molecule as a substituent, rather than as the functional group.

Benzene   Phenyl   Benzyl

1. Monosubstitution

The following are common monosubstituted benzene rings.

| Toluene | Phenol | Aniline | Benzoic Acid | Benzaldehyde |

2. Disubstitution

Substituents are listed alphabetically in such a way that they receive the lowest number. The prefixes *ortho-*, *para-*, and *meta-* are used to describe disubstituted benzene rings.

Ortho-
(1,2-disubstitution)

Meta-
(1,3-disubstitution)

Para-
(1,4-disubstitution)

3. Trisubstitution and Other Substitutions

Benzene rings that have more than two substituents cannot be described in terms of *ortho-*, *meta-*, *para-*. For these, the substituents are listed alphabetically in such a way that they receive the lowest possible number.

2,3-Dichlorophenol

1,3-Dibromo-5-chlorobenzene

3-Bromo-4-chloro-analine

D. Alcohols: Primary (1°), Secondary (2°), Tertiary (3°)

Alcohols are named by adding the suffix *-ol*. For multiple *hydroxy groups* (−OH groups), the prefixes *di-*, *tri-*, etc., are added (diols and triols).

According to the number of carbon atoms bonded to the carbon with the hydroxy group, alcohols are often referred to as primary (1°), secondary (2°), or tertiary (3°).

1°   2°   3°

E. Ethers

Ethers are named using two different methods. Simple molecules are usually named by listing the alkyl groups in order of increasing size and then adding the word *ether*. More complex molecules are usually named by following the "alkyl-*oxy*alkane" format, giving the larger group the parent name and adding the suffix *-oxy* to the smaller group.

ethyl butyl ether   or   ethoxybutane

F. Carbonyl Compounds

In naming compounds with carbonyl groups (C = O), the Greek letters α, β, and γ are used to describe the relative positions of the carbon atoms attached to the carbonyl carbon.

carbonyl carbon

1. Aldehydes

Identify the longest chain containing the aldehyde group, and number the chain starting at the carbonyl carbon. Add the suffix *-al*.

2. Ketones

Identify the longest carbon chain containing the carbonyl carbon. Number the chain so that the carbonyl carbon gets the lowest possible number. Add the suffix *-one*.

3. Carboxylic Acids

Identify the longest chain containing the COOH group. Number the chain starting at the carbonyl carbon. Add the suffix *-oic* and "acid."

4. Esters

Ester nomenclature is similar to ether nomenclature in that the functional group divides the molecule into two parts that are individually named. The section of the molecule bonded to the oxygen is referred to as the alcohol portion and is the first part of the name. The part that is bonded to the carbonyl carbon is referred to as the carboxylic acid portion and is the second part of the name.

2, 3-Dimethylbutanal   2-Methylbutyl-3-methylbutanoate

3-Pentanone

G. Amines and Amides

There are two ways of naming amines. When the amino group appears in a molecule as a branched side chain, it is given a number that identifies its position and the prefix *amino-*. Otherwise, the alkyl substituent is given the suffix *-amine.*

2-Aminobutane

Triethylamine

Special attention should be given to the naming of amides; this nomenclature is quite different. The base name is the longest carbon chain containing the amide, with the numbering starting at the carbonyl carbon. An N- is used to indicate each group bound to the nitrogen. (*Note*: Nitrogen forms a maximum of three bonds.)

3-Hydroxy-N-methylbutanamide

IV. STEREOCHEMISTRY

A. General Information

The spatial relationships of atoms within a molecule can determine how the molecule as a whole reacts. Two molecules with the same number and type of atoms may have completely different properties, and therefore are truly different molecules. Some molecules, on the other hand, may be so similar in structure and properties that only certain tests can differentiate them.

1. Importance: The Thalidomide Example

The infamous example that illustrates the importance of stereochemistry is a drug called thalidomide that was prescribed in the 1960s to alleviate morning sickness. A mixture of *both* stereoisomers was administered to pregnant women. Later it became tragically evident that, while one stereoisomer in the mixture relieved morning nausea, the other caused severe birth defects.

2. Stereoisomers

For two molecules to be considered stereoisomers, they must have identical atoms and connectivity. Stereoisomers differ in the spatial configuration of their atoms. Stereoisomers are either *enantiomers* or *diastereomers*. Enantiomers are *nonsuperimposable mirror images of each other* (i.e., like a pair of gloves or a left and a right ear). Their difference lies in the orientation of atoms at one carbon. Diastereomers *are not mirror images of each other*. They differ in the orientation of atoms at two or more carbons.

3. Chirality/Chiral Centers

An *sp*³ carbon atom with four different substituents is asymmetric and has the property of *chirality*. This carbon is called the *chiral center* in an enantiomer. If a plane of symmetry can be drawn, the molecule is *achiral*.

4. Optical Activity

Light waves normally exist in all planes, but if the light waves are filtered through a polarizer, only those oscillating in one plane pass through. This light is *plane-polarized light*. *Optically active compounds* will rotate this light *counterclockwise/levorotary*, or *clockwise/dextrorotary*. Enantiomers rotate light in equal amounts and in opposite directions. If equal amounts of two enantiomers are present (a *racemic mixture*), the *rotation will be zero*. *Meso compounds* have an internal plane of symmetry, are not optically active, and, in relation to optically active compounds, are diastereomers. No meso compounds are enantiomers.

A.   Plane-polarized light

B.   Rotation

or

L⁻   D⁺

C.   Meso example

CH₃

H ——— Cl

H ——— Cl   internal
                   plane of
                   light

CH₃

B. Fischer Diagrams

1. Concepts

Often it is necessary to distinguish stereoisomers from each other. To illustrate the methods of doing so, we must first review *Fischer diagrams*. In a Fisher diagram, the vertical *y*-axis is representative of bonds going into the plane of the paper, and the horizontal *x*-axis is representative of bonds coming out of the plane of the paper.

2. Relevance to Carbohydrates

The molecule *glyceraldehyde* is the standard of reference for the D/L naming system of other carbohydrate molecules. (*Note*: This is not the same system as the use of D/L descriptors to identify the direction of rotation of plane-polarized light.) Glyceraldehyde has two enantiomers, D-*glyceraldehyde* and L-*glyceraldehyde*, on which this system is based. With the carbonyl carbon placed at the top of a Fischer diagram, the orientation of the hydroxy group on the bottom carbon determines the designation: D-(hydroxy on the right) or L-(hydroxy on the left). D and L describe enantiomers, whereas diastereomers are given different names. An *anomer* is a diastereomer that has a different configuration at the first carbon (designated as alpha or beta). An *epimer* is a diastereomer that has a different configuration at the second carbon.

Therefore: A/B and C/D are enantiomers;
A/C, A/D, B/C, B/D are diastereomers

3. Rule of 2^n

There is a quick method for finding the number of possible stereoisomers. First find the number of chiral centers (n); then use the following formula to find the number of possible diastereomers that exist for that molecule: number of diastereomers = 2^n.

$n = 3$, $2^3 = 8$

8 diastereomers

3 chiral carbons

C. Absolute Configuration

To identify stereoisomers other than carbohydrates, it is necessary to assign an *absolute configuration* using the *R/S* system. The first step is to number the four different groups on the chiral carbon as 1, 2, 3, and 4 according to priority, 1 being the highest priority and 4 the lowest. The rules for assigning absolute configuration follow:

1. The atom directly bonded to the chiral carbon usually determines the priority of the group—*the higher the atomic number of this atom, the greater the priority of the group.*
2. If double or triple bonds exist, the atoms so bonded are considered to be doubled or tripled in atomic number.

The lowest priority group, usually hydrogen, is placed in the back, using a rotated Fischer projection—called the steering wheel approach. If the sequence is 1, 2, 3 *clockwise*, the molecule is designated as *R*; if *counterclockwise*, as *S*.

V. AROMATICITY

A. General Information

Before discussing the rules of aromaticity, it is necessary to state what these molecules have in common: *conjugation, resonance*, and *delocalization*.

1. Conjugation

A molecule that has double bonds separated by single bonds is *conjugated*, causing a linking of adjacent *p* orbitals. These *p* orbitals form two electron clouds: one above and one below the axis of the carbon-carbon bonding.

2. Resonance and Delocalization

The linking of the *p* orbitals to form clouds of electrons is due to *resonance*. Besides being conjugated, the molecule must be in a planar configuration so that the *p* orbitals line up. The effect of resonance is a cloud of *delocalized* electrons, *yielding a very stable molecule*. As discussed in Section II on bonding, each *p* orbital has one electron. When six *p* orbitals are aligned, with three conjugated pi bonds, the six electrons completely fill the lower energy bonding molecular orbital. This is a very favorable energetic situation. The molecule can be in a chain configuration or a ring configuration.

B. Rules for Determining Aromaticity

When the fully conjugated planar molecule, with overlapping p orbitals, is present in a ring, the term *aromatic* is applied. Benzene is the most commonly found aromatic, but many others exist that do not resemble benzene. The following three questions provide a guide to establishing whether or not a molecule is aromatic:

1. Are the atoms in a ring configuration (cyclic geometry)?
2. Are $4n + 2$ pi electrons present, where $n = 0, 1, 2, 3, 4$, etc. (Huckel's rule)?
3. Does each member of the ring have an sp^2 or sp hybridized configuration?

If all three conditions are true for the molecule, it is aromatic. The following molecules are common aromatics.

These molecules are *not* aromatic:

Note: Because aromatics are so unique, reactions specific to these compounds will be discussed in this section rather than in Section VIII on the general reactions and mechanisms of major groups.

C. Electrophilic Aromatic Substitution (EAS)

1. General Concepts and Mechanism

It should be obvious that aromatic molecules are perfect targets for electrophiles. The molecule is electron rich, and the electron cloud is quite accessible. The electrophile draws an electron from the ring forming, a resonance-stabilized *carbocation* (a positively charged carbon molecule). To reestablish aromaticity, the nonaromatic intermediate is deprotonated; that is, it loses the hydrogen bound to the carbon that accepted the electrophile. The loss of the proton causes the extra electron maintained in the system to eliminate the carbocation.

The electrophilic aromatic substitution (EAS) can be illustrated as follows:

2. Types, Reagents, and Products

Knowledge of the reagents used in the various types of EAS reaction can assist in quickly predicting the products.

TYPE OF EAS	REAGENT	PRODUCT
Friedel-Crafts acylation	CH_3COCl / $AlCl_3$	$CH_3C=O$
Halogenation	X_2 / FeX_3	$-X$ (Cl, Br)
Nitration	HNO_3 / H_2SO_4	$-NO_2$
Alkylation	RX / AlX_3	$-R$ (1°)
Sulfonation	SO_3 / H_2SO_4	$-SO_3H$

D. Effects of Substituents on Electrophilic Aromatic Substitution

1. General Concepts

When EAS occurs with a substituted benzene ring, the characteristics of the ring in reactions are changed. These benzene substituents, classified as activators/electron-donating groups or deactivators/electron-withdrawing groups, will polarize the electron clouds and therefore alter the orientation (ortho/para or meta) and speed at which groups will add through EAS. *It is the substituent(s) on the benzene ring that determine the orientation and rate of reaction of the incoming group.* Because of their importance, these substituents are classified so that the products of the reaction can be predicted.

2. Activators and Deactivators

The activators and deactivators are listed in a prioritized method according to the strength with which they affect incoming groups. This is important when there is more than one substituent already on the benzene ring and one substituent directs ortho/para orientation and the other directs meta. Halogens are an exception to the rule that ortho/para directors are activators and meta directors are deactivators. This anomaly is due to the strong electronegativity of halogens.

ACTIVATORS:	DEACTIVATORS:
1. are electron-*donating* groups,	1. are electron-*withdrawing* groups,
2. *increase* the rate of reaction,	2. *decrease* the rate of reaction,
3. are *ortho, para* directors.	3. are *meta* directors.

CLASSIFICATION	EXAMPLES	PRIORITY
Ortho/para activators	$-NH_2$, $-OH$, $-NHR$, $-OCH_3$, $-C_6H_5$ (−Ph), $-CH_3$	High
Ortho/para deactivators	Halogens (−F, −Cl, −Br, −I)	Medium
Meta deactivators	NO_2, $-COOH$, $-CN$, $-NH_3+$, $-SO_3$, $-CHO$	Low

Example: bromination of phenol

VI. CHEMICAL AND PHYSICAL PROPERTIES OF MOLECULES

A. General Concepts

1. Polarity

The *polarity* of a molecule determines in part how the molecule will react with other molecules. Polarity is due to the geometric configuration of the molecule, often a result of hybridization. The physical properties common to a species are a result of intermolecular interactions determined mostly by the net polarity of the molecule.

No Net Dipole

Net Dipole

2. Solubility

Solubility is a measure of how readily a compound will dissolve in another compound. The *solvent* is generally added to the *solute*. The important concept to remember is that *polar compounds solvate polar compounds* and *nonpolar compounds solvate nonpolar compounds*.

B. Alkanes, Alkenes, and Alkynes

1. Alkanes

Alkanes are *nonpolar hydrocarbons* that are *insoluble in water*. Their melting and boiling points are relatively low. The *higher the molecular weight* (the greater the number of carbons), the *higher the boiling point*. The interaction of the electrons with each other, due to what are called *van der Waals* forces, causes this increase in boiling point. If two alkanes have the same formula weight (differing only in connectivity of atoms), the one that has more extensive branching has the lower boiling point because the branching prevents the molecules from being packed together as tightly as occurs in a straight chain. This results in weaker intermolecular forces and therefore a lower boiling point. Branching often has the reverse effect on the melting point. Usually the melting point increases because of an increase in symmetry, which aids in the formation of crystal lattices.

Alkanes with 1–4 carbons are gases; alkanes with 5–17 carbons are liquids; alkanes with 18 or more carbons are solids. *Combustion* of alkanes due to oxidation yields water and CO_2 and is an *exothermic* reaction.

2. Alkenes and Alkynes

The melting points and boiling points of alkenes and alkynes increase with an increase in molecular weight. In general, alkenes and alkynes have physical properties similar to those of alkanes. However, the presence of the double bond in alkenes creates cis/trans isomerization, as previously discussed. This can affect the net polarity of the molecule and therefore affect intermolecular interactions.

C. Alcohols, Ethers, and the Carbonyl Compounds

1. Alcohols

Alcohols have higher boiling points than alkanes because of the hydrogen bonding of the hydroxy group. The lone pairs of electrons on the oxygen are free to bond to neighboring hydroxy hydrogens. As the carbon chain grows in length, the polarizing effect of the hydroxy group diminishes and the molecule acts as a non-polar molecule. Alcohols that have five or fewer carbons exhibit a net dipole and are water soluble. Alcohols react with acids, which protonate the oxygen, creating a positive charge that reacts with a nucleophile.

2. Ethers

Ethers cannot form intermolecular hydrogen bonds as alcohols do because, in place of the hydroxy hydrogen, ethers have an alkyl group. Therefore, in comparison to alcohols of similar weight, ethers have lower melting and boiling points. An increase in the carbon chain length increases the melting point and boiling point because of van der Waals forces. Solubility in water decreases with increasing carbon chain length. Ethers react with acids, which protonate the oxygen, creating a positive charge that reacts with a nucleophile.

3. Aldehydes

All carbonyl compounds have higher boiling points than comparable alkanes because the polarity of the carbonyl group creates strong intermolecular forces. Aldehydes have melting and boiling points higher than those of ketones, but lower than those of carboxylic acids.

4. Ketones

Ketones have low boiling and melting points because they lack the hydrogen that the other carbonyl compounds use to hydrogen-bond to adjacent molecules. The boiling and melting points of ketones are lower than those of comparable alcohols.

5. Carboxylic Acids

Because of extensive hydrogen bonding, carboxylic acids have higher melting and boiling points than aldehydes and ketones. Also, as a result of their very strong polarity, these acids have higher melting and boiling points than alcohols. Resonance at the carbonyl group creates an electrophilic carbon and a nucleophilic oxygen.

D. Carbohydrates, Lipids, and Amines

Carbohydrates, lipids, and amines are referred to as the organic molecules of biological importance. These are the molecules that make up our living tissues and biological chemicals, and their reactions are vital to life-sustaining processes.

1. Carbohydrates

The oxidation of carbohydrates, which are polyhydroxylated molecules comprised of aldehydes and ketones, is responsible for the metabolism of stored energy and the formation of ATP. *Mutarotation* (change from axial to equilibrial positions) is responsible for the equilibration of the alpha and beta forms of the cyclical molecule. Optical rotation occurs because of mutarotation.

2. Lipids

Lipids include a variety of compounds some of which are phospholipids, waxes, and fatty acids. A lipid is a nonpolar molecule with a carboxyl head and a long hydrocarbon tail (the polarity created by the carboxyl is overshadowed by the large number of nonpolar hydrocarbons). If the chain contains double bonds, it is either unsaturated (contains one double bond) or polysaturated (contains more than one double bond). Fats are the primary energy-storage molecules. The large number of carbon-hydrogen bonds, which release energy when metabolized, explains why fats provide twice as much energy per gram as do carbohydrates and proteins.

Micelles are spherical bodies comprised of many fatty acid soap molecules. The carboxylate groups are hydrophilic and polar; these ends point outward. The hydrophobic and nonpolar hydrocarbon ends point inward. Micelles are soluble in water because the nonpolar ends are shielded. A micelle can trap a nonpolar molecule (i.e., grease, fats, dirt) by engulfing it into the nonpolar internal region while remaining solvated in the polar medium.

3. Amines

Amines are nitrogen-containing compounds derived from ammonia. The lone pair of electrons on the nitrogen affects many properties of amines. As expected, the electrons are involved in hydrogen bonding, giving amines high melting and boiling points. The electrons enable the amine to react as a nucleophile, and its effects on basicity are discussed in Section VIII.E.

E. Optically Active Stereoisomers

All optically active stereoisomers have the same physical properties with the exception of the rotation of plane-polarized light. In other words, enantiomers show the same IR and NMR spectroscopic results (discussed in Sections X.C and X.D) and have the same boiling points, melting points, and solubility.

VII. ACID-BASE CHEMISTRY

A. General Information

1. Relevance to Understanding Reactions

A thorough review of acid-base chemistry could very well be the best approach in preparing for the organic chemistry section of the DAT. In most reactions, the acidity or basicity of the reactants determines the products. The ability to predict the way in which a compound will react with another compound is a necessary tool for success on test day. In addition, resonance and inductive effects, two favorites of the ADA Department of Testing Services, are covered in this section as related topics. You will find it very difficult to grasp the information presented in Sections VIII and IX on mechanisms, reactions, and synthesis if you have not mastered the fundamentals of acid-base chemistry. *Therefore, be sure to spend adequate time and effort in reviewing this section—there is a high probability that this investment will equate to a better score on the DAT.*

2. Review of Definitions
a. Brönsted-Lowry Acid and Base

A Brönsted-Lowry *acid* can *donate a proton*. A Brönsted-Lowry *base* can *accept a proton*. Under the Brönsted-Lowry definitions, acids and bases equilibrate into conjugate acids and conjugate bases. The conjugate base of an acid is usually a molecule that has given off a proton and has taken on a negative charge, therefore becoming a Brönsted-Lowry base. The conjugate acid of a base is usually a molecule that has taken on a proton, becoming positively charged and likewise a Brönsted-Lowry acid.

Brönsted-Lowry reactions involve two acids and two bases in equilibrium, as is easily seen with the addition of an acid to water. The *dissociation equilibrium* must shift to the right for an acid to be characterized as strong. The following equation illustrates that strong acids exist on the right side of the equilibrium. In calculating the K_a, this increases the value of the numerator, and therefore strong acids have large K_a values.

$HA + H_2O \leftrightarrow H_3O^+ + A^-$
acid + base $\leftrightarrow$ conjugate acid + conjugate base

or

Conjugate acid + conjugate base $\leftrightarrow$ acid + base

$$K_a = \frac{[H_3O^+] \ [A^-]}{[HA]}$$

b. Lewis Acid and Base

A Lewis *acid* is *an electron pair acceptor*. A Lewis *base* is *an electron pair donor*. Whenever a lone pair of electrons exists in a Lewis dot structure, the molecule is a base. Whenever a vacant *p* orbital exists, the molecule is an acid. When dealing with ions, remember that cations are acids and anions are bases.

Base—analine   Acid—carboxylic acid

3. Strength and Stability of Acids and Bases

Remember: The more stable a conjugate base, the stronger the acid. The more stable a conjugate acid, the stronger the base.

Therefore, the stronger the conjugate base, the weaker the acid, and the stronger the conjugate acid, the weaker the base. To evaluate the strength of an acid or a base, it is necessary to evaluate the stability of its conjugate. Resonance, inductive effects, and electronegativity will affect the stability of the conjugate.

B. Resonance

1. Terms and Concepts

To understand resonance and to be able to draw resonance forms, it is necessary to understand that *electrons are not static*. Electrons are constantly moving from one atom to the next. Learning what will cause the electrons to leave an atom is crucial. When electrons move around within the atomic framework of a molecule, this phenomenon is referred to as *resonance*. Pictorial representations of the positions that electrons may have are called *resonance forms*. A combination of these resonance forms is a representative structure called a *resonance hybrid*.

Resonance increases the stability of a molecule. The more stable an individual resonance form is, the greater its contribution to the resonance hybrid. As discussed in Section V on aromaticity, delocalization of electrons can occur with adjacent p orbitals connected by pi bonds. In the case of benzene, it was shown that through delocalization the electrons were spread over the cyclical structure, forming what were described as electron clouds above and below the ring. It was also mentioned that all aromatic compounds are extremely stable molecules.

2. Rules for Drawing Resonance Forms

It is important to be able to draw resonance structures quickly. The following rules should help in understanding which electrons move where and why:

- Atoms do not move; only electrons move.
- A molecule that has a charge does not lose the charge unless there is interaction with another molecule.
- The total number of electrons does not change.
- The Lewis structures of molecules must remain accurate when electrons move.
- Electrons will move toward a positive charge.
- Negative charges prefer to be on electronegative atoms.
- A resonance form with a greater number of covalent bonds is more stable than one with fewer covalent bonds.
- A resonance form that has fewer charges is more stable than one with a greater number of charges.
- A resonance form with complete octets is more stable than one that lacks complete octets.

3. Effects of Resonance on Acidity

One method of determining the strength of an acid is to evaluate the resonance of the conjugate base.

Remember: Resonance increases stability, and strong acids have stable conjugate bases.

A.

$$Cl-CH_2-\overset{\overset{O}{\|}}{C}-OH \quad \xrightarrow{-H^+} \quad Cl-CH_2-\overset{\overset{O}{\|}}{C}-O^- \quad \longleftrightarrow \quad Cl-CH_2-\overset{\overset{O^-}{|}}{C}=O$$

Hybrid

$$Cl-CH_2-\overset{\overset{O}{\|}}{C}-O$$

B.

Hybrid

C. Inductive Effects and Electronegativity

When the electron density of a molecule shifts toward the more electronegative atom, a partially positive charge is created. This charge can help stabilize the conjugate base of an acid that is deprotonated. When the electronegative atom bonds to a hydrogen atom in the acid (HF or HBr), the effect increases the stabilization of the conjugate. When, however, there are atoms between the electronegative atom and the hydrogen (Cl-CH$_2$-COOH or Cl-CH$_2$-CH$_2$-OH), the *effect is termed inductive*.

The shift of electron density is simply polarization due to a highly electronegative atom. The farther the hydrogen is from the electronegative element, the less the effect.

$$Cl - CH_2 - \overset{\overset{\displaystyle O}{\|}}{C} - OH$$

$$\delta^- \quad \overleftarrow{\quad +\quad} \quad \delta^+$$

VIII. MECHANISMS AND REACTIONS OF THE MAJOR FUNCTIONAL GROUPS

A. General Information

1. A Brief Review

A very brief reminder of some concepts from Section XII on kinetics of the general chemistry chapter is included in this section. *You should review the relevant topics of general chemistry before reviewing this section.*

A reaction that gives off heat is *exothermic*, and one that absorbs heat is *endothermic* (a change in *enthalpy* occurs). Some reactions do not proceed directly from reactants to products; these reactions create *intermediates* in *transition states*. The difference between the energy levels of the reactants and the intermediates is the *activation energy*. *Catalysts* (enzymes) lower the activation energy. Gibbs free-energy diagrams graphically illustrate these concepts.

2. Structure and Stability of Radicals

Very often the intermediates in reactions are radicals, and an assessment of their stability is necessary in order to predict the products. The determinants for stability discussed in Section VII hold true for determining the stability of radicals as well. In general, the more substituted the alkyl radical, the more stable it becomes. The following diagram indicates, in order of stability, the radicals most frequently encountered.

$$3° \qquad\qquad 2° \qquad\qquad 1°$$

B. Alkane Reactions

1. Free-Radical Halogenation of Alkanes

This reaction involves three steps: initiation, propagation, and termination. *Initiation* is the formation of a halogen radical. These initial halogen radicals are formed by heat or light in an *endothermic* process, requiring much energy. *Propagation* is a chain reaction in which a product and another halogen radical are formed. In this homolytic cleavage, the halogen radical bonds with hydrogen, creating HX and an alkyl radical. The radical produced in the propagation step splits a nearby X_2 molecule, and the reaction continues until the reactant is fully exhausted or all the radicals bind in the termination step. The *termination* step, which involves two halogen radicals coming together to form a bond, is exothermic and creates a lower, more stable, and therefore more desirable energy state. The general reaction sequence is as follows:

1. Initiation

$$X_2 \xrightarrow[\Delta]{hv} X - X \longrightarrow 2X^{\bullet}$$

2. Propagation

$$X^{\bullet} \quad H - H_2 C - R \longrightarrow R - \overset{\bullet}{C}H_2 + HX$$

$$R - \overset{\bullet}{C}H_2 \quad X - X \longrightarrow R - CXH_2 + X^{\bullet}$$

3. Termination

$$2 \; R - \overset{\bullet}{C}H_2 \longrightarrow RCH_2CH_2R$$

$$R - \overset{\bullet}{C}H_2 + X^{\bullet} \longrightarrow R - CXH_2$$

$$2X^{\bullet} \longrightarrow X_2$$

2. Nucleophilic Substitution and Elimination
a. The Basics

Four types of reactions, described in subsections b–e below, occur when electron-rich and electron-deficient compounds come into contact. The first two reactions result in substitution on alkanes, whereas the second two result in elimination and therefore the formation of alkenes. Substitution and elimination have characteristic trends that help in determining which type of reaction will occur. Rate-determining steps, first- and second-order rates, and steric considerations are evaluated for each reaction. A rate-determining step is the step in a reaction that requires the most activation energy. First-order rates of reaction are determined by the concentration of one reactant. Second-order reaction rates are determined by the concentrations of two of the reactants. (*Note*: Zero-order-rate reactions occur regardless of the concentrations of the reactants.)

b. $S_N 1$

This is a *two-step, unimolecular, first-order reaction*. The first step involves the formation of a carbocation intermediate by the dissociation of a leaving group. The second step, as logic predicts, involves an attack by a nucleophile (any carbocation is an obvious target for a nucleophile). This nucleophile becomes the substituted part. $S_N 1$ reactions are first order: they depend only on the concentration of the substrate. The stability of the carbocation determines its reactivity. If a more stable carbocation can be formed in this transition state, formation will occur through a process called *carbocation rearrangement*. It is important to note, when reviewing the mechanism of the $S_N 1$ reaction, that the carbocation can be attacked by the nucleophile from either side, causing a *racemic mixture* (two stereoisomers are produced). This reaction prefers bulky electrophiles (3° < 2° < 1°) and favors *aprotic solvents*—free of protons for hydrogen bonding.

c. $S_N 2$

This is a *one-step, bimolecular, second-order reaction* in which the nucleophile attacks the bond of the electronegative leaving group and there is *no formation of a carbocation*. Just as the leaving group dissociates, the incoming nucleophile bonds. This one-step reaction has *no rate-determining step*.

One of the easiest ways to determine whether a reactant favors the $S_N 1$ or $S_N 2$ reaction is to evaluate the bulk of the reactant. *Inversion of configuration occurs* with S_N2. The *steric hindrance* of large groups physically prevents both the leaving group and the nucleophile from reacting in one step. Therefore, *only primary and secondary carbons will react via S_N2. Tertiary carbons will react only go by S_N1.* The S_N2 reaction favors *protic solvents*—protons readily available for hydrogen bonding.

d. E1

This is a *two-step, unimolecular, first-order reaction* similar to the S_N1 reaction. E1's first step is the dissociation of the leaving group, forming the carbocation. Rather than adding a nucleophile in the next step, however, the compound loses a proton to the nucleophile (strong base). The most *substituted double bond forms, trans preferably*. The rate-determining step is the formation of the carbocation. The E1 rate is determined by the concentration of the substrate.

e. E2

This is a *one-step, bimolecular, second-order reaction* similar to the S_N2. The E2 is a more effective elimination reaction than the E1. The term antiperiplanar, used to describe the position of the proton in reference to the leaving group, refers to the proton's being on the partially positive end. Because of steric hindrances E2 reactions do not occur with bulky groups. No rearrangement occurs. The rate is determined by the concentrations of both the nucleophile/base and the substrate.

Here is a comparison of the characteristics of nucleophilic substitution and elimination reactions:

S_N1 vs. E1:   E1 favors higher temperatures.

S_N2 vs. S_N1: S_N1's are typically more polar and protic, and have increased substitution, weak nucleophiles, and a low concentration of nucleophiles.

S_N2 vs. E2:   E2 favors bulky bases with increased branching and heat.

E1 vs. E2:   E2 favors a stronger base and a higher concentration of the base.

C. Alkene and Alkyne Reactions

The electrons in the pi bonds of alkenes and alkynes are responsible for the reactions with other compounds. Generally, these two types of substances react as electron-rich compounds.

1. Markovnikov's Rule—HX Addition

Markovnikov's rule states that the electrophilic addition of a hydrogen to a double bond will occur at the carbon that has the greatest number of hydrogens. Stability of the carbocation intermediate dictates the placement of substituents in this addition reaction.

$$CH_3 - CH_2 - CH = CH_2 \longrightarrow CH_3 - CH_2 - CH^{+}- CH_3 \longrightarrow CH_3\,CH_2\,CHCH_3$$
$$\mid$$
$$Cl$$

HCl addition   Major product

2. Anti-Markovnikov Reactions—Radical Halogenation

The result of an anti-Markovnikov reaction is that a nucleophile attaches itself to the lesser substituted carbon. The hydrogen bonds to the carbon with fewer hydrogens in an anti-Markovnikov reaction.

D. Reactions of Oxygen-Containing Molecules

In the presence of acids, the hydroxy group is replaced in a substitution reaction or removed in an elimination reaction.

1. Alcohols
a. Oxidation to Aldehydes

With a weak oxidizing agent, such as pyridinium chlorochromate (PCC), a primary alcohol can be oxidized to an aldehyde. With further oxidation the alcohol will continue to react until it forms a carboxylic acid.

PCC as Oxidizing Agent

b. Dehydration to Alkenes

Dehydration is one method of creating alkenes. The hydroxy group and a hydrogen leave in an elimination reaction, producing water and an alkene.

$$H_3C - CH_2OH \xrightarrow[\text{H}_2\text{SO}_4]{\text{Heat}} H_2C = CH_2 + H_2O$$

c. Formation of Esters from Alcohols and Carboxylic Acids

In the most common method of creating an ester, the alcohol hydroxyl group and the proton from the acid leave and the alkyl group from the alcohol bonds to the resonance-stabilized deprotonated carbonyl group on the acid. The hydroxyl group from the alcohol and the proton from the acid combine to form water, leaving behind an ester.

$$R — COOH + R' — OH \underset{\longleftarrow}{\overset{H^+}{\longrightarrow}} R — \overset{\overset{\displaystyle O}{\|}}{C} — OR' + H_2O$$

2. Aldehydes and Ketones

Aldehydes and ketones are subject to nucleophilic attack.

a. Reactions with Grignard Reagents

When Grignard reagents and other nucleophiles come in contact with alde- hydes and ketones, addition reactions occur. These reactions result in the forma- tion of a number of alcohols. Grignards are alkylmagnesium halides with the general formula RMgX.

$$R — \overset{\overset{\displaystyle O}{\|}}{C} — R' + R'' MgBr \longrightarrow R — \underset{\underset{\displaystyle R''}{|}}{\overset{\overset{\displaystyle OMgBr}{|}}{C}} — R' \overset{H_2O}{\longrightarrow} R — \underset{\underset{\displaystyle R''}{|}}{\overset{\overset{\displaystyle OH}{|}}{C}} — R'$$

$$R — CHO + R'MgBr \longrightarrow R — \overset{\overset{\displaystyle OMgBr}{|}}{CH} — R' \overset{H_2O}{\longrightarrow} R — \underset{\underset{\displaystyle OH}{|}}{CH} — R'$$

$$HCHO + RMgBr \longrightarrow R — CH_2 — OMgBr \overset{H_2O}{\longrightarrow} R — CH_2OH$$

b. Reactions with Alcohols

When the electrophilic carbon is attacked by an alcohol, the aldehyde or ke- tone undergoes a nucleophilic addition reaction and adds to the carbonyl group. When one alcohol reacts, the result is either the formation of a hemiacetal from an aldehyde or the formation of a hemiketal from a ketone. When a second molecule reacts, the hemiacetal and hemiketal form the acetal and ketal, respectively.

1.
$$R — CHO + R' — OH \overset{H^+}{\longrightarrow} R — \underset{\underset{\displaystyle H}{|}}{\overset{\overset{\displaystyle OH}{|}}{C}} — OR' \quad \text{Hemiacetal}$$

2.
$$R — \underset{\underset{\displaystyle H}{|}}{\overset{\overset{\displaystyle OH}{|}}{C}} — OR' \underset{H^+}{\overset{R'OH}{\longrightarrow}} R — \underset{\underset{\displaystyle H}{|}}{\overset{\overset{\displaystyle OR'}{|}}{C}} — OR' \quad \text{Acetal}$$

3.
$$R — \overset{\overset{\displaystyle O}{\|}}{C} — R' + R''OH \overset{H^+}{\longrightarrow} R — \underset{\underset{\displaystyle OR''}{|}}{\overset{\overset{\displaystyle OH}{|}}{C}} — R' \quad \text{Hemiketal}$$

4.

$$R - \underset{\underset{OR''}{|}}{\overset{\overset{OH}{|}}{C}} - R' \xrightarrow{R''OH, H^+} R - \underset{\underset{OR''}{|}}{\overset{\overset{OR'}{|}}{C}} - R' \qquad \text{Ketal}$$

c. Oxidation

The oxidation of aldehydes involves two common reagents, Tollen's and Benedict's. Note that the oxidation of alcohols with Tollen's reagent is often referred to as the silver mirror test. Since, whenever there is oxidation there is reduction (and vice versa), Tollen's reagent forms silver metal from the reduction of a silver salt *only in the presence of an aldehyde*.

Tollen's reagent

$$RCHO + Ag(NH_3)_2 \xrightarrow{OH^-} R\overset{\overset{O}{\|}}{C}O^- + Ag^+$$

Benedict's reagent

$$RCHO + Cu^{2+} \xrightarrow{OH^-} R\overset{\overset{O}{\|}}{C}O^- + Cu_2OH$$

d. Aldol Condensation

When an aldehyde and a ketone come together in the presence of a dilute acid or base, the two molecules combine. The products are either hydroxyaldehydes or hydroxyketones.

e. Keto-Enol Tautomerism

Any carbonyl compound with an alpha hydrogen is subject to interconversion between keto and enol forms. (*Note*: the term *enol* refers to a compound that contains a double bond and an alcohol.) The conversion is referred to as tautomerism. The keto form is more stable.

Base catalyzed

Acid or base will give the same product.

Acid catalyzed

3. Carboxylic Acids

Carboxylic acids are acidic because of the stability of the carboxylate ion, the conjugate base.

> **Remember: When more halides are bonded to the acid, the electron density is shifted away from the carbonyl group, facilitating deprotonation; halides make acids stronger.**

a. Nucleophilic Substitution Reaction

Whereas aldehydes and ketones prefer nucleophilic addition reactions, carboxylic acids prefer nucleophilic substitution reactions. The general reaction is as follows:

$$X = Cl^-, Br^-, {}^-OR, {}^-NH_2$$

b. Esterification

The reaction of a carboxylic acid with an alcohol results in an ester and water.

$$RCOOH + R'OH \underset{}{\overset{H^+}{\rightleftharpoons}} R - \overset{\overset{\displaystyle O}{\|}}{C} - OR + H_2O$$

c. Formation of Anhydrides

The reaction of two carboxylic acids creates a special type of molecule referred to as an *anhydride*.

$$2\ RCOOH \longrightarrow R - \overset{\overset{\displaystyle O}{\|}}{C} - O - \overset{\overset{\displaystyle O}{\|}}{C} - R + H_2O$$

E. Reactions of Carbohydrates and Amines

1. Carbohydrates

There are three reactions to note for carbohydrates: glycoside formation, ether formation, and ester formation. Glycosides are nonreducing sugars (i.e., negative Tollen's silver mirror test). They are acetals that do not undergo mutorotation. The formation of ethers and esters is discussed in Section IX on synthesis.

2. Amines

The lone pair of electrons in an amine make this compound act as a nucleophile. Ammonia and primary amines are the best nucleophiles; in more substituted amines the electrons are not able to react with incoming electrophiles because of steric hindrances. Amines react with electrophiles and carbonyls to form *imines* and *amides*, respectively.

1.

2.

IX. SYNTHESIS

A. General Information

In subsections B–E, methods of synthesis are given for various types of organic compounds. Note that there are multiple methods of creating compounds. Some methods yield higher percentages of the desired product, while other methods may work only under special conditions. It is important to learn what reagent will convert one species to another. Familiarity with the basic types of synthesis reactions is far more important than memorization of all of the mechanisms of formation.

B. Alkanes—Wurtz Reaction

The Wurtz reaction, in which the two alkyl groups from the alkyl bromides are joined and sodium bromide is formed as a side product, is used to make longer chains of hydrocarbons.

$$2RBr + 2Na \rightarrow RR + 2NaBr$$

C. Alkenes and Alkynes

1. Alkenes

The substitution of the alkane starting material dictates which method is used to create the pi bond present in alkenes. All three methods involve elimination reactions.

a. Dehydrohalogenation

Dehydrohalogenation involves the removal of hydrogen and a halogen from an alkane with a halogen substituent. Here is an example:

$$CH_3CH_2Br + KOH \longrightarrow CH_2 = CH_2 + H_2O + KBR$$

b. Dehydration

In dehydration, a hydroxy and a hydrogen are removed, forming an alkene and water. The starting material is an alcohol. See Section VIII.D.1.b on the dehydration of alcohols to alkenes.

c. Dehalogenation

Dehalogenation occurs when adjacent carbons of an alkane are substituted with halogens. Here is an example:

$$BrCH_2CH_2Br + Zn \longrightarrow CH_2 = CH_2 + ZnBr_2$$

2. Alkynes

a. Dehydrohalogenation

The dehydrohalogenation process is basically similar to that for the formation of alkenes. The difference is that there is more KOH to remove the alkene hydrogens forming the second pi bond of the alkyne.

b. Dehalogenation

The dehalogenation process is basically similar to that for the formation of alkenes. The difference is that the alkane starting material has two halogens on each of the adjacent carbons, permitting the formation of two pi bonds.

D. Alcohols, Aldehydes, and Ketones

1. Alcohols

a. Hydration of Alkenes

The hydration of alkenes follows Markovnikov's rule:

b. Grignard Reagents

The formation of alcohols using magnesium bromide in the presence of anhydride and ether follows:

1.

$$RMgBr + HCHO \xrightarrow[\text{Ether}]{\text{Anhydride}} RCH_2OMgBr \xrightarrow{H^+} RCH_2OH$$

2.

$$RMgBr + R'CHO \xrightarrow[\text{Ether}]{\text{Anhydride}} \underset{\underset{H}{|}}{\overset{\overset{R'}{|}}{RC}} - OMgBr \xrightarrow{H^+} \underset{\underset{H}{|}}{\overset{\overset{R'}{|}}{RC}} - OH$$

3.

$$RMgBr + R' - \overset{\overset{R''}{|}}{C} = O \xrightarrow[\text{Ether}]{\text{Anhydride}} R' - \underset{\underset{R}{|}}{\overset{\overset{R''}{|}}{C}} - OMgBr \xrightarrow{H^+} R' - \underset{\underset{R}{|}}{\overset{\overset{R''}{|}}{C}} - OH$$

c. Reduction of Aldehydes and Ketones

Formation of an alcohol is easily accomplished by the reduction of carbonyl compounds by $LiAlH_4$ or $NaBH_4$. Ketones reduce to secondary alcohols and aldehydes, and carboxylic acid derivatives reduce to primary alcohols. Some milder reducing agents can reduce carboxylic acid derivatives to aldehydes, but not to alcohols.

2. Aldehydes

a. Mild Oxidation of a 1° Alcohol

This oxidation reaction proceeds as follows:

$$RCH_2OH \xrightarrow{Cu, \Delta} R - CHO$$

b. Oxidation of a Diol

The formation of two aldehydes results from the splitting of a diol, a molecule with two hydroxy groups.

$$R - \underset{\underset{}{\overset{\overset{OH}{|}}{CH}}} - \underset{}{\overset{\overset{OH}{|}}{CH}} - R \xrightarrow{HIO_4} R - CHO + R' - CHO$$

3. Ketones

a. Mild Oxidation of a 2° Alcohol

This oxidation reaction proceeds as follows:

b. Ozonolysis

The starting material for ozonolysis can be linear or cyclic. Depending on the substitution of the double bond, an aldehyde or ketone is formed.

Formation of ketone or aldehyde

c. Decarboxylation of Carboxylic Acids

The decarboxylation reaction proceeds as follows:

E. Carboxylic Acids, Esters, and Ethers

1. Carboxylic Acids

a. Oxidation of Alkenes

This oxidation reaction proceeds as follows:

b. Grignard Reagent with Carbon Dioxide

The two-step formation of a carboxylic acid using carbon dioxide and Grignard reagents proceeds as follows:

c. Oxidation of 1° Alcohols

This oxidation reaction proceeds as follows:

d. Saponification of Esters

This saponification reaction proceeds as follows:

$$R - \overset{\overset{\displaystyle O}{\|}}{C} - O - R' \ + \ NAOH \ \rightleftharpoons \ R'OH + R - \overset{\overset{\displaystyle O}{\|}}{C} - ONa \ \xrightarrow{H^+} \ R - COOH$$

2. Esters—Acid and Alcohol

See Section VIII.D.1 on the reactions of alcohols.

3.Ethers

a. Williamson Ether Synthesis

In Williamson ether synthesis, the reaction between an alcohol and a strong base results in an alkoxide that reacts via an S_N2 process to form an ether.

b. Dehydration

The result of the dehydration of two alcohols is the formation of an ether:

$$2CH_3 - CH_2OH \ \xrightarrow{H_2SO_4, \ \Delta} \ CH_3 - CH_2 - O - CH_2 - CH_3$$

X. ORGANIC ANALYSIS

A. General Concepts

All too often the desired product of a chemical reaction is accompanied by unde-sirable secondary products. The following section discusses tests to determine what organic substances are present and how to separate them to produce a pure yield of the desired product.

B. Some Simple Chemical Tests

When compounds have different solubilities, *extraction* can be used to separate them. Often the compounds are chemically altered to create a species soluble in aqueous solution.

> **Remember: Aqueous acids extract organic bases,**
> **and aqueous bases extract organic acids.**

Distillation is used to separate compounds with different boiling points. When two compounds in a liquid mixture are heated, the one with the lower boil-ing point will vaporize first, leaving behind the higher boiling point compound, which will also vaporize once its boiling point is reached. The vapors can be con-densed and collected, yielding two pure compounds.

Crystallization is a type of purification involving the heating of a solid in a solution until the solvent evaporates. The crystallization of a precipitate follows as the supersaturated solution cools.

Chromatography is the separation of the components of a mixture based on differences in solubility and polarity. Chromatography involves the distribution of solutes between a moving phase and a stationary phase. There are four types of chromatography.

1. *Thin-layer chromatography (TLC)* incorporates a thin layer of stationary phase (typically silicia gel) on a flat surface, usually a glass or plastic plate. The distances traveled by the components of the mixture because of capillary action permit the identification of these components on the basis of characteristic polarity.

2. *Column chromatography* can be thought of as inverted TLC. Rather than traveling across a plate because of capillary action, in column chromatography the mixture runs down a column. The mobile phase can be altered, changing its affinity for the polarity of a solvent.

3. *Gas chromatography* requires the evaporation of a mixture. The vapors are passed through inert gas, the mobile phase, and through a column with the stationary phase.

4. *High-performance liquid chromatography* is done at high pressure with liquids as the mobile phase. The degree of absorbency of ultraviolight light indicates the flow rate of a compound.

Chromatography is a very useful method of identification and separation in the laboratory.

C. Infrared (IR) Spectroscopy

1. Concept of Oscillation Frequencies

The bonds of a molecule can be stretched and bent. The frequency of bond vibrations can be used to identify unknown specimens. Atoms slow the vibrations according to their mass. Each functional group has a range of oscillation frequencies that is determined by the numbers and types of bonds and atoms. When infrared electromagnetic energy passes through a molecule, the molecule will vibrate or absorb the energy, if the natural frequency of the molecule equals the energy, according to this formula:

$$E = h(c/\lambda)$$

Then, since $c/\lambda = v$,

$$E = hv$$

2. Common IR Spectrums

You should memorize the absorbencies of the major functional groups. The units are reciprocal centimeters (cm^{-1}).

FUNCTIONAL GROUP	IR ABSORBANCE (cm^{-1})
–CH	2850–2960
=CH	3020–3100
≡C–H	3300
–C=C–	1650–1670
–C≡C–	2100–2260
Aromatics	1500–1600

FUNCTIONAL GROUP	IR ABSORBANCE (cm⁻¹)
$-C\equiv N$	2210–2260
–O–H	3400–3640, broad
–N–H	3310–3500, broad
C=O	
Aldehyde	1690–1740
Ketone	1680–1750
Esters	1735–1750
Amides	1630–1690
C–O; Ethers and esters	1080–1300

D. Nuclear Magnetic Resonance (NMR) Spectroscopy

1. NMR and the Concept of Chemical Shift Values

Electrons spin, and this spin creates a magnetic field. If a molecule is placed in a magnetic field, some of the protons spinning in the same direction will align with the applied field, whereas others will spin in a direction that creates a field that opposes the applied field. The direction can be changed if a proton spinning against the field absorbs the electromagnetic radiation. At this point, an NMR tracing signal, referred to as a chemical shift value, can be observed.

It is important to note that the *number* of signals describes the number of different protons. The *position* of the signals describes the environment of the proton. The *intensity* of the signals indicates how many of each kind of proton exist. The *splitting* of a signal describes the proton's environment in relation to other protons and is further discussed in the next section.

Here is an example of an NMR tracing.

A table of chemical shift values is given in Section X.D.4.

2. Spin-Spin Splitting

The effect of adjacent and neighboring hydrogens on adjacent carbons is explained in spin-spin splitting. The direction of spin of the nearby proton creates a magnetic field that will oppose or align with that of a given proton. The number of different ways in which the spins can occur determines the number of signal splits that will result. A lone proton signal will be split into four signals, a quartet (one signal is a singlet; two signals, a doublet; three signals, a triplet), if three protons are adjacent. This situation is explained by illustrating the possible spins.

Also, note that like protons will not split each other. Like protons must be chemically and magnetically equivalent. Only one signal results from equivalent protons.

3. Shielding and Deshielding

The electrons create a magnetic field. If this field reduces the strength of the applied field, the proton is shielded; if it enhances the applied field, the proton is deshielded. Shielding creates an upfield shift, to the right, and deshielding creates a downfield shift, to the left.

4. Chemical Shift Values

You should memorize the following chemical shift values of the major functional groups.

FUNCTIONAL GROUP	NMR CHEMICAL SHIFT (δ)
$R-CH_3$	0.8–1.0
$R-CH_2-R$	1.2–1.4
$Ph-CH_3$	2.2–2.5
$R-CH_2-Cl$	3.6–3.8
$R-CH_2-Br$	3.4–3.6
$R-CH_2-I$	3.1–3.3
$R-O-CH_3$	3.3–3.9
$R-CO-CH_3$	2.1–2.6
RCHO	9.5–9.6
Ph–H	6.0–9.5
$RC{\equiv}CH$	2.5–3.1
$R_2C{=}CHR$	5.2–5.7

References: Survey of the Natural Sciences Review

Alcamo, I. Edward. *Anatomy and Physiology the Easy Way*. Hauppauge, NY: Barron's Educational Series, Inc., 1996.

Bresnick, Stephen. *Columbia Review High Yield Organic Chemistry*. Baltimore, MD: Williams and Wilkins, 1996.

Campbell, Neil A. *Biology*, 4th Edition. Menlo Park, CA: The Benjamin-Cummings Publishing Company, Inc., 1987.

Jespersen, Neil. *How to Prepare for the AP Examination: Chemistry*. Hauppauge, NY: Barron's Educational Series, Inc., 1995.

Mascetta, Joseph A. *Chemistry the Easy Way*, 3rd Edition. Hauppauge, NY: Barron's Educational Series, Inc., 1997.

Rudin, Norah. *Dictionary of Modern Biology*. Hauppauge, NY: Barron's Educational Series, Inc., 1997.

Seibel, Hugo R. *How to Prepare for the MCAT*, 8th Edition. Hauppauge, NY: Barron's Educational Series, Inc., 1997.

PERCEPTUAL ABILITY TEST REVIEW

OUTLINE

I. OVERVIEW

A. What Is the Perceptual Ability Test?

The Perceptual Ability Test (PAT) is perhaps the most unusual component of the DAT. It is a measure of your ability to perceive and consider two- and three-dimensional forms and is probably unlike any other type of test you have taken. The test is composed of six parts that appear in the following order: aperture passing, orthographic projection, angle discrimination, paper folding, cubes, and form development.

B. Details of the Test

The PAT is administered second, directly following the Survey of Natural Sciences. There is a total of 90 items on the PAT, divided evenly among the six parts (15 questions each). Although there are 90 questions, only 75 of them are scored. The remaining 15 are experimental questions that are scattered randomly throughout the PAT sections. You will *not* be able to identify these experimental questions. You are given 60 minutes to complete the 90 questions.

    The six parts of the PAT are arranged in sections of 15 questions. However, even though the sections are discrete, they are administered as a unit with no time breaks between them. This means that you have the freedom to skip ahead to a particular section first, if you wish, and later return to address the skipped sections. Within the 60-minute time frame, you may address the PAT as you wish.

C. Taking the Test

Considering the allotted time and the number of test items, you have an average of 40 seconds to complete each question and an average of 10 minutes to complete each section. As you will come to discover through practice, some questions are quite time consuming, while others have answers that seem readily apparent.

    There is no right number of seconds or minutes to spend on each question and section. Perhaps the best rule to follow is that you should progress through the test to completion at a productive pace. If you find yourself spending too much time on a difficult item and thus failing to maintain your established pace, you should leave that question and later, time permitting, return to it. As you take the practice tests in this book, you should time yourself on at least one of the two tests. It might be useful to complete one test at a comfortable pace, but record precisely how long you spent on each perceptual ability section. This will give you an index of the relative time it took you to complete each group of questions.

D. Perceptual Ability? I Just Want to Become a Dentist

In examining the utility of the PAT, the American Dental Association ran a study to assess the correlation between performance on this test and preclinical performance in laboratory settings that require a high degree of manual dexterity. The result is not surprising—performance on the PAT and preclinical performance in laboratory settings are indeed significantly correlated. The study and the practice of dentistry demand the ability to conceive of objects spatially. A strong performance on the PAT reflects the sort of mental agility useful in the profession.

Additionally, it should be mentioned that, in light of the correlation between PAT scores and performance in dental school, Admissions Committees hold the PAT score in high regard. These committees examine with particular care two scores that reflect performance on the DAT: (1) total academic and (2) perceptual ability. Arguably, since several individual scores are figured into the total academic score, the perceptual ability score is the single most important score on the DAT.

E. How Can I Improve My Perceptual Ability?

You will quickly come to learn that perceptual ability (as it is measured by the PAT) isn't something that you either *have* or *don't have*. It is a quality that can be nurtured, developed, and enhanced through training. The following review is a comprehensive preparation guide that addresses the details of what to expect on the test and provides explanatory figures and practice exercises.

The components that you need to perfect are: visual perception and visualization and mental imagery. Even if you have perfect vision, you will find that discipline and practice are needed in order to perceive minuscule details. (If you suspect that you don't have very good vision, now is a good time to invest in a pair of glasses.)

The ability to make use of visualization and mental imagery also improves with practice. As you are preparing for the PAT, continue to challenge yourself with mental imagery tasks even after you close this book. Imagine, for example, how the room you are sitting in would be oriented if the entire unit (the room and all its contents) were rotated and flipped. Try to identify the new positionings of various objects in the room. Exercises like this one will help keep your *mind's eye* active throughout the day.

There are also several creative activities, such as origami, that rely on the same skills you will be refining for the PAT. Origami, the Japanese art of paper folding, is a discipline that requires a lot of structure and precision. The intricate origami folds transform a flat piece of paper into a multidimensional form. Involvement in origami will expand your ability to recognize how flat paper can take on a multitude of forms. This activity is most applicable to the part of the PAT called "form development" but will also contribute to your preparation for the paper-folding questions.

Be creative in choosing supplementary activities for your additional practice. By stacking sugar cubes or children's building blocks, you can create cube formations like those illustrated in this book (see Cubes, Section VI) or can create your own. This offers further practice for the painted-surface-counting questions in the cube section of the PAT. Additionally, by using dice, you can practice imagining the location of the surface dots after repositioning each die. This will contribute to enhanced performance on aperture passing and form development questions.

Preparing for the PAT can actually be quite enjoyable. The following preparation review offers clear, easy to understand approaches to each part of the PAT. In each section of the review are highly useful descriptions of the nature of the test questions and appropriate practice exercises. While the additional activities suggested above will help you to generally improve your perceptual abilities, the exercises in each review section are designed to "target train" your perception, visualization and mental imagery, and logical reasoning skills as they apply specifically to the questions on the DAT.

II. APERTURE PASSING

A. Introduction

The first section of the Perceptual Ability Test is aperture passing. Here you will be presented with an image of a three-dimensional object and the outlines of five different apertures. Your task is to identify the aperture (or opening) that could accommodate the insertion of the solid object.

An aperture is much like a keyhole. It is an opening through which an object can pass. An aperture-passing item as it appears on the DAT is governed by a number of rules, which are outlined below.

- Although the object is presented in a particular position, it may be turned in any direction prior to insertion.
- Once the object has been started through the opening, it may not be rotated, turned, or twisted in any way.
- Both the aperture and the object are drawn to the same scale.
- There are no irregular or surprising shapes in any portion of the object that are not in clear view as is presented in the three-dimensional rendering.
- The correct aperture is always the exact shape of the object's silhouette.
- In each group of apertures, there is only one aperture that can be used to pass the solid object.

A thorough understanding of these parameters will further enhance your ability to make use of strategy. Perhaps more so than on any other section of the Perceptual Ability Test, the questions on aperture passing exploit your understanding of the rules.

Each rule stated above has a number of consequences that can help you locate the correct answer quickly. Also, when in doubt, application of the rules will help you to eliminate one or more incorrect answer choices, thus improving your chances of selecting the correct response.

B. The Rules, Their Consequences, and Your Strategy

Although the object is presented in a particular position, it may be turned in any direction prior to insertion. Usually the three-dimensional form will need to be turned or oriented in a position different from the initial presentation. The aperture-passing questions are largely a test of your ability to mentally maneuver obscure forms and to identify appropriate corresponding silhouettes. For this reason, you should assume that most times a degree of maneuvering is required. You may need to imagine either turning the object to align a particular side, or rotating the object horizontally or vertically in order to accommodate the orientation of the aperture.

Each object has six distinct sides: top, bottom, left, right, front, and rear. This first rule implies that the object may be inserted into the aperture top first, bottom first, or any of the sides first. You need not consider any angular insertions that deviate from a distinct side or top entry. Below is an example of an aperture-passing question. The object is pictured at the left.

Before examining the possible apertures, choices A–E, it is important that you identify the significance of each line in the three-dimensional drawing. The subtleties of the lines are often overlooked. Also, the aperture shapes can bias your viewing, causing you to overlook the intricate detail of the object. You set yourself up for failure if you examine the apertures before thoroughly understanding the drawing.

The subtleties that you should look for in the drawing are reflected in the following questions:

- Are the outermost surfaces of the object (front, rear, top, bottom, and left and right sides) flat, or are there slopes or protrusions?
- From which direction are protrusions noticeable and unnoticeable?
- Are there any holes or recesses in the form? Where are they?
- Are there any stairlike edges? Are the stairs of equal height?

The second rule states that, *once the object has been started through the opening, it may not be rotated, turned, or twisted in any way.* Although there are six sides to choose from as the entry side, in actuality you need to consider only three sides. Remember that, not only must a side be able to enter the aperture, but also the entire form must be able to follow through. Thus, you need consider only three possibilities: a top/bottom entry and the two different side entries (see figures below).

| Entry 1: top/bottom | Entry 2: side/side | Entry 3: side/side |

After you are familiar with the form of the object, you should begin to identify what each of the three silhouettes looks like. A silhouette is an outline of a form that contours the outermost edge. Keep in mind that a silhouette is a contour on a single plane that does not reveal any information about the object's depth. Although the depth of the object is not indicated on a silhouette, all of the points of the object (including the ones that recede into space) will take part in the formation of the silhouette if they extend beyond the image created from the surface being considered. In the following illustration, each of the three silhouettes corresponds to one of the images presented above:

Since, as the third rule states, *both the aperture and the object are drawn to the same scale,* you need to rely heavily on precise comparison between the projected silhouette and the aperture opening. The aperture must accommodate the size of the silhouette. A perfect but smaller silhouette would not allow the three-dimensional shape to be inserted. Hence, it is possible for the aperture to be the same shape but too small for the object. According to the publishers of the DAT, the differences in size are "large enough to be judged by [the precise] eye." You are cautioned, however, to take great care in looking for small differences in size.

Although you are presented with a drawing in which three sides are exposed, there are portions of the object that are not visible in the view that is displayed. The fourth rule states that *there are no irregular or surprising shapes in any portion of the object that are not in clear view as is presented in the three-dimensional rendering.* If, however, the object has symmetric indentations, the hidden portion will be symmetric with the part shown. As a rule, enough information will be presented to allow you to make an informed decision concerning the appropriate opening.

According to the last two rules, *the correct aperture is always the exact shape of the object's silhouette* and *in each group of apertures, there is only one aperture that can be used to pass the solid object.* These rules are clearly to your advantage. Unlike questions that challenge you to select the *best* answer, your task here is to select the *only* answer. Regarding the last rule, if you find that two openings appear to accommodate the object, you are probably overlooking a detail of form or have failed to recognize that one opening is too small. Consider, if you are stumped by multiple answer choices, that you are committing one of the above errors.

With all six of these rules in mind, the appropriate answer to the aperture passing question on page 194 is easily located. Careful consideration of the silhouette helps to eliminate choices B, D, and E. Choice A closely approximates "Entry 3: side/side," but the darkened oval shape is slightly misplaced. Choice C shows the correct aperture through which the object under consideration could pass (see "Entry 3: side/side," on page 195).

C. Lines as "Builders of the Form"

You need to practice the discipline of attending to lines as "builders of the form." There is a human tendency to approach an oddly shaped, irregular drawing with a mental stereotype of a familiar (household or geometric) form. A desire to deal with the familiar often overshadows the reality of what is presented. If you approach this section of the PAT by attending to lines as "followers of the form," you will unfortunately overlook quite a bit. Most likely you will never before have experienced the oddly shaped form in question. The bias to project ideas about familiar forms will undoubtedly cause you to overlook the actual lines in the drawing.

Keep in mind that all of the forms presented in the aperture-passing section are irregular. They are irregular in the sense that they are not easily describable and correspond only indirectly to familiar geometric shapes. For this reason, you need to take inventory of each line. Overlooking one subtle but important line is often the cause of error in this section. Practice attending to the details offered by each line in the following figure.

This is a highly complex figure. What makes it so difficult to deal with is the heavy reliance on the lines that is required in order to determine the many spatial planes.

Below is the same figure reproduced with visual cues and spatial guidelines.

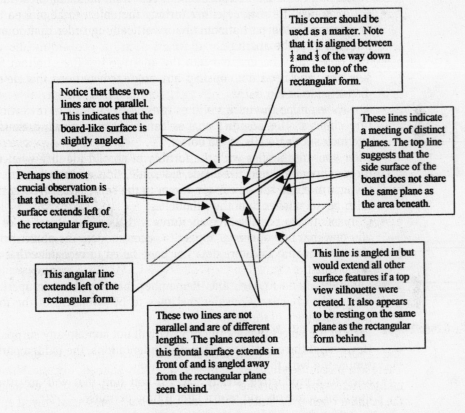

Notice that these two lines are not parallel. This indicates that the board-like surface is slightly angled.

This corner should be used as a marker. Note that it is aligned between $\frac{1}{2}$ and $\frac{1}{3}$ of the way down from the top of the rectangular form.

These lines indicate a meeting of distinct planes. The top line suggests that the side surface of the board does not share the same plane as the area beneath.

Perhaps the most crucial observation is that the board-like surface extends left of the rectangular figure.

This angular line extends left of the rectangular form.

This line is angled in but would extend all other surface features if a top view silhouette were created. It also appears to be resting on the same plane as the rectangular form behind.

These two lines are not parallel and are of different lengths. The plane created on this frontal surface extends in front of and is angled away from the rectangular plane seen behind.

Now consider the various silhouettes that would be produced from both side/side angles and from the top/bottom angle.

As you work through this section of the PAT, try to maintain a productive, steady pace. Do not let any one question drain you of too much time. If you find that you are stumped on a question, it is to your advantage to move on and return later if time permits. Often, a second consideration of a complex three-dimensional form will bring a fresh perspective if you allow yourself to concentrate on other forms in the meantime.

D. Review

- Although the object is presented in a particular position, it may be turned in any direction prior to insertion. The three-dimensional form will most often need to be turned or oriented in a position different from the initial presentation.
- You may need to imagine either turning the object to align a particular side, or rotating the object horizontally or vertically in order to accommodate the orientation of the aperture.
- The object may be inserted into the aperture top first, bottom first, or any side first. You need not consider any angular insertions that deviate from a distinct side or top entry.
- Always examine the intricate lines of the object prior to reviewing the aperture choices. The aperture shapes can bias your viewing, causing you to overlook subtle details of the object.
- After you are familiar with the form, you should identify what each of the three silhouettes looks like—side/side, side/side, and top/bottom. Recall that the aperture and the object are drawn to the same scale. Hence, the aperture must be no smaller than the silhouette.
- Only one of the possible five apertures will allow the object to be inserted. If you find that two openings appear to accommodate the object, you are probably overlooking a feature detail or have failed to recognize that an opening is too small.
- Carefully attend to each line. Remember that the forms in aperture passing are highly irregular. Consider the lines to be "builders of the form" rather than "followers of the form."
- Parts of the object that are out of view will not contain any surprising shapes. However, if the object has symmetric indentations, the hidden portion will be symmetric with the part shown.
- Keep to a productive, steady pace. If you find that you are stumped on a question, move on and return later if time permits.

Exercise 1
Examine the form presented in each framed box. After carefully studying the lines of the form, create a silhouette for every direction of viewing in the boxes below. Practice visualizing and representing each silhouette scaled to the size of the small image with arrows.

1.

2.

3.

4.

5.

6.

7.

8.

9.

10.

Exercise 2

This exercise follows the same format and directions that apply to the aperture-passing questions on the Perceptual Ability Test. Examine the figure shown to the far left. Then choose the aperture that would allow the object to completely pass through the opening if the proper side was inserted first.

9.

	A	B	C	D	E

10.

	A	B	C	D	E

ANSWERS TO EXERCISE 2

1. C, top/bottom entry

2. E, side/side entry

3. D, side/side entry

4. D, side/side entry

5. E, top/bottom entry

6. A, side/side entry

7. B, side/side entry

8. C, side/side entry

9. E, top/bottom entry

10. C, side/side entry

III. ORTHOGRAPHIC PROJECTIONS

A. Introduction

The second section of the PAT is orthographic projections. Here you will be shown two views of an object. Given the information presented by the two views, your task is to select the third view that correctly describes the object.

B. What Is an Orthographic Projection?

Engineers and architects heavily rely on orthographic projections when they draft plans for construction. Orthographic projections are sets of descriptive drawings that serve to portray and clarify the complexity and uniqueness of the objects being considered.

An orthographic projection is a series of two-dimensional views of an object. Below is an example of how an orthographic projection series is laid out.

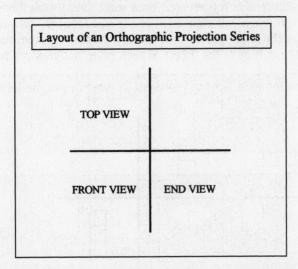

Layout of an Orthographic Projection Series

TOP VIEW

FRONT VIEW   END VIEW

The orthographic projections on the DAT are composed of three views: the top view, front view, and end view. Each of the views is rendered *without perspective*. In other words, each view is drawn as it would appear head on with its planes parallel to the viewer.

In the example of a brick below, examine both the labeled brick shown at the left and its corresponding orthographic projection at the right.

Notice the orientation of each projected image. It is as though the viewer examined each side in turn, walking around the object so that a perfect head-on view could be seen of each face (top, front, and end). Consider each display box (created by the crossed lines) to be a frame for the projection as seen from that particular viewing direction.

On the DAT, the projection layout is identical to that in the example above. The projection looking down at the object is displayed in the upper left hand corner of the projection layout and is labeled "TOP VIEW." The projection looking at the object from the front is displayed in the lower left corner and is labeled "FRONT VIEW." Lastly, the projection looking at the object from the end (or side) is displayed in the lower right corner and is labeled "END VIEW."

The use of both hidden and visible lines is a convention standard to the practice of creating and interpreting an orthographic projection. Visible lines are represented by the solid lines; hidden lines, by dashed lines. Most of the questions in this section of the PAT challenge your understanding and logical reasoning skills concerning the use of solid and dashed lines. Crucial to your success in this section is a strong understanding of when each of the two lines is used.

C. The Visible Line

As mentioned, a visible line is represented by a solid line. Visible lines are lines that are exposed to you when you view a particular side face on—simply put, visible lines are *visible* to you. Changes in form that are visible *only* from the view being considered and the outline of the object as seen from that view are represented by solid lines.

Examine the use of solid lines to represent visible lines in the following two examples.

TOP VIEW

FRONT VIEW   END VIEW

Study the figures carefully, and be sure that you are able to identify the correspondence between each projection line and the object. For clarification, refer to the following:

TOP VIEW

FRONT VIEW   END VIEW

TOP VIEW

FRONT VIEW   END VIEW

Now notice the slight modification of the second object that has occurred. Instead of a benchlike extension, this object now has a slide that extends from the central unit.

TOP VIEW

FRONT VIEW   END VIEW

Comparison between the projection series before and after modification reveals that only the front view changes. It is most important to understand why the end view does not change. Examine the line that is highlighted by the arrow in the figure below.

It may not be initially obvious why the end view does not change. To fully understand the use of the solid line (or the *visible line*), you must first understand how it is used in the end view of the modified object. In the figure, the slide extends from the flat surface that is just above it and is parallel to the plane on which the projection is rendered. Any deviation from this parallel plane results in a visible line at the point where the transition from parallel to angular takes place. Creases in the form that are visible from the projection view will always result in a solid line.

Lastly, the point should be made that, to fully describe some highly complex forms, additional projections may be necessary. For example, none of the views examined thus far addresses the wide hidden leg of the second example. In preparing for the PAT, you need be concerned only with mastering the three views discussed (top, front, and end). The end view will refer to the right side of the object in each projection series.

D. The Hidden Line

A hidden line is represented by a dashed line. Hidden lines refer to edges that cannot be seen because they are either inside or behind the object. These lines provide meaningful cues about an object's depth. In the following examples dashed lines indicate the presence of hidden lines.

In the first example, the drawing at left shows only a brick with an object on top and an oval on the side. The orthographic projection views reveal that these oval shapes are tubular and travel through the height and width of the brick.

In the second and third examples, notice that the width of the object can be identified by the vertical lines; solid and dashed, in the top view. The lengths of these lines match the width in the end view.

Now examine the following series:

Here, the front and end views are identical. Also notice that these views provide the information that the narrowest cylinder is the only form that extends through the entire height of the object. The widest cylinder rests on top of the square base with the middle cylinder passing through it. The middle cylinder also rests on the base.

Note: When a hidden line is exactly behind a visible line, the part of the dashed line that coincides with the solid (visible) line remains solid. When two hidden lines overlap, the resulting line remains dashed.

E. Completing the Orthographic Projection Series

On the Perceptual Ability Test, you will be provided with two of the three views discussed above. You will *not* be presented with a perspective drawing; but given the information contained in the views, you will be able to choose the appropriate view that completes the series.

On the PAT the orthographic projection series is laid out with two views and a question mark in place of the third, missing view. This section is much like trying to complete a puzzle. In the absence of a guiding image, you will need to examine each possibility in order to see what logically fits the given arrangement. It is highly unlikely that, by seeing the two views, you will be able to imagine the appropriate third view before examining the answer choices. There will be many third-view possibilities that could satisfy the conditions of the first two. Your job in this section is to examine the answer choices and identify the only correct view by eliminating the three incorrect choices.

Expect to see several types of each missing view question. The following is an example of an orthographic projection question as it would appear on the PAT:

Choose the correct END VIEW.

Your first strategy should be to identify the number of visible lines and hidden lines in one of the two views given. In this example, the top view has five horizontal lines. The top and bottom line are always exterior outlines, so the interest lies in the three interior lines. From top to bottom, the order of these lines is visible, visible, and hidden. With this information in mind, you should immediately begin eliminating incorrect answer choices. When examining the choices, take great care to count the sequence of visible and hidden lines in the proper order. As a rule, if you identify horizontal lines in the top view from top to bottom, their order of appearance in the end view will be from right to left. The first round of elimination leaves answers A and B as the only possible choices.

The next step is to use the information given by the other view in the same way. The front view has a total of four horizontal lines, two of which are interior visible lines. Choice A can now be eliminated because the front view that would correspond to its end view would have the following lines from bottom to top: visible, hidden, visible, and visible (not including the outlines). Choice B is the correct answer.

If after counting the number and pattern of visible and horizontal lines you have a match between two or more answer choices, verify for each choice that the lines are in the proper locations relative to each other and to the perimeter of the side being considered. For each group of projections, there will be only one answer that satisfies the conditions set forth by the two given views.

This strategy of identifying the number, order, and placement of appropriate lines can be highly effective and time saving. It will be necessary, however, to fully understand the logic of projected lines so that you can easily make transitions among different views.

If you find that you have difficulty with transitions among different types of absent views, it is suggested that you identify the projection series that you can most easily solve. Then, to remain clearly focused throughout this section, first solve the sets that you are most comfortable with; for example, solve all the problems that have a top and front view. Then return to all of one of the remaining types, for example, the front and end view problems. Lastly, address the questions of the third type (absent front view). This approach will help you to keep track of each perspective and will serve to "warm you up" for questions of greater challenge.

F. Review

- The orthographic projections on the PAT are composed of three views: the top view, front view, and end view. Each of the views is rendered without perspective.
- The end view refers to the right side of the object in each projection series.
- Visible lines are represented by solid lines, while hidden lines are represented by dashed lines.
- Changes in form that are visible only from the view being considered and from the outline of the object as seen from that view are represented by solid lines.
- Any deviation from the parallel viewing plane results in a visible line at the point where the transition from parallel to angular takes place. Creases in the form that are visible from the projection view always result in solid lines.
- Hidden lines, shown as dashed lines, refer to edges that cannot be seen because they are either inside or behind the object.
- When a hidden line is exactly behind a visible line, the part of the dashed line that coincides with the solid (visible) line remains solid. When two hidden lines overlap, the resulting line remains dashed.
- Your job in this section is to examine the answer choices and identify the only possible view by eliminating the three incorrect choices.
- When examining answer choices, take great care to count the sequence of visible and hidden lines in the proper order.
- The strategy of identifying the number, order, and placement of appropriate lines is highly effective and time saving.

Exercise 1

In each case, examine the three-dimensional image presented in the box. Then, to the right of each image, draw in the appropriate views. Use of a straightedge is suggested for this exercise.

1.

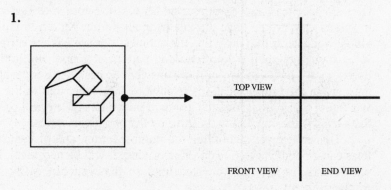

TOP VIEW

FRONT VIEW   END VIEW

2.

TOP VIEW

FRONT VIEW   END VIEW

3.

TOP VIEW

FRONT VIEW   END VIEW

ANSWERS TO EXERCISE 1

1.

TOP VIEW

FRONT VIEW   END VIEW

2.

TOP VIEW

FRONT VIEW   END VIEW

3.

TOP VIEW

FRONT VIEW   END VIEW

Exercise 2
Choose the correct view to complete each orthographic projection series.

1. Choose the correct END VIEW.

TOP VIEW

FRONT VIEW   END VIEW

A   B   C   D

2. Choose the correct TOP VIEW.

TOP VIEW

FRONT VIEW   END VIEW

A   B   C   D

3. Choose the correct FRONT VIEW.

TOP VIEW

FRONT VIEW   END VIEW

A   B   C   D

4.   Choose the correct FRONT VIEW.

ANSWERS TO EXERCISE 2
1. B   2. B   3. D   4. D

IV. ANGLE DISCRIMINATION

A. Introduction

The third part of the Perceptual Ability Test is angle discrimination. This is the only portion of the PAT that involves flat renderings representing two-dimensional space that you need not mentally rotate.

Angle discrimination questions ask you to rank angles by size, from smallest to largest. With practice, you will be able to sharpen your angle-estimation skills and thus to avoid pitfalls that are meant to complicate the task of discriminating between similar angles.

B. Angle Ranking

As a warmup to this section, spend some time reviewing the illustrations below. Begin by ranking the four angles in each of the following examples from smallest to largest.

Example 1:

The correct ranking is *B, C, A, D*. Most likely, you were able quickly to choose angle *B* as the smallest angle and angle *D* as the largest. Angles *A* and *C*, however, are relatively close in size. The first rule to follow in this section is to always begin by identifying the smallest and largest angles, which will generally be apparent upon initial inspection. Even if just the largest angle is obvious, your odds of answering correctly have been increased (more on this later).

Example 2:

The correct ranking is *B, A, D, C.*
The angles in the following example are closer in size.

Example 3:

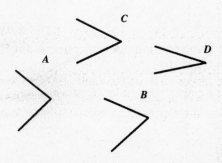

The correct ranking is *D, C, B, A.* In this example, the two angles closest in measurement are *B* and *A*. Angle *D* clearly appears smallest, but it is somewhat unclear which angle is largest.

In determining the rankings of two similar-appearing angles, refer to Exercise 1. One strategy that is often useful is called "parking the angle." When you have two angles of varying degrees, one angle (the larger angle) will always be able to "house" the other angle. In other words, the smaller angle can be inserted into the opening of the larger angle. Hence, the notion of *parking the angle* can help you identify the rankings of angles. To illustrate the application of this method, angle *C* from Example 1 above may be "parked" within angle *A* as follows:

Employment of the parking method depends largely on mental imagery. Asking the question, "Could angle *X* fit within angle *Y* or vice-versa?" often helps illuminate an intuitive hunch that one angle is smaller than the other. The concept of parking the angle applies also to angles with varying leg lengths. Basically stated, *a larger angle will always accommodate a smaller angle regardless of the*

length of the angles' legs. From Example 3, angle B is parked within angle A as shown below.

Exercise 1

In each of the following 10 sets of angles, determine which angle is larger.

ANSWERS TO EXERCISE 1

1. A   **2.** B   **3.** A   **4.** A   **5.** B   **6.** A   **7.** B   **8.** B   **9.** A   **10.** B

If you have identified several of the larger angles incorrectly, return to the angle sets repeatedly until you are able to perceive the subtle differences. It is often helpful to review these angle sets several times before moving on to further examples and explanations.

An angle is created by the joining of two distinct legs. Crucial to your success on the angle discrimination section is an understanding of the following rule: *The length of an angle's legs is independent of its angular measurement.* To fully grasp this rule, examine the angles below, which share the same angular measurement.

For most test-takers, confusion on this point arises from failure to recognize two main points. First, it must be understood that lines can be extended into space without disturbing the angle created by their junction. The three identical angles shown above can be imposed on each other as follows:

The three sets of legs (or rays) are extensions of the same angle.

Remember: The length of an angle's legs is independent of its angular measurement.

The second crucial point is concerned with how an angle is measured. On the DAT you will not be permitted to make use of any measuring device (including your fingers and test-taking materials). You must rely on visual acuity to "eyeball" relative sizes. One method of eyeing an angle is to examine the mouth at a set distance from the joining point of the legs. This technique can be helpful as long as you use great caution. To implement the procedure correctly, *you must compare all the angles at the same distance from the joining point.* The following figure illustrates this point.

½ inch   ½ inch

It can be inferred that the angle on the left is the larger angle. *When comparing angles, a greater measured distance between two legs will imply a larger angle if and only if the measurement is taken at the same distance from each angle's vertex.*

To practice your understanding of this rule, examine the two angles below.

When the horizontal dotted lines at the same distance from each angle's vertex are compared, it is readily apparent that the angle on the right is larger. Keep in mind that you will not be permitted to use any measurement devices on the DAT. The horizontal lines shown in the figures above are there to illustrate the viewing path that you may take when comparing angles.

C. Where to Look

Another useful method of angle comparison relies heavily on viewing only a discrete area of the angle, namely, the niche. The niche of the angle is the tightest part of the corner created by the two joining legs. This method also takes practice. Since your eye wants to traverse the extended lines away from the vertex, you must practice the restraint necessary to make angle comparisons at the niche. In the following examples, which highlight the viewing of an angle's niche, the angles are ordered from small to large:

Paramount to your success on the angle discrimination questions is a solid understanding of the basic laws and methods of angle comparison:

- Always begin by establishing a largest or smallest angle, or both if possible.
- Regardless of leg size, a smaller angle can always be inserted within the opening of a larger angle. Hence, the method of "parking an angle" can be useful in conceptualizing the task at hand.
- The length of an angle's legs is independent of its angular measurement.
- When comparing angles, a greater measured distance between two legs will imply a larger angle if and only if the measurement is taken at the same distance from each angle's vertex.

D. Complex Arrangements

The task of comparing angles is made slightly more complex by oblique positioning. Certainly it will not be possible to rotate the computer screen in order to view the angles at similar positions. For this reason, as you practice the comparison of angles, refrain from angling the book to accommodate your view of particular angles.

The following arrangement is made with identical angles. Notice how the oblique positioning of angles coupled with varying leg lengths affects your visual sensibility.

With repeated practice, you will overcome any tendency to allow distortions of angle orientation and leg length to interfere with your reasoning.

Exercise 2

The following exercise will help you overcome distortion interference. In each set of three angles, two angles are identical and one angle is different. Select the angle that is different from the other two angles; then determine whether it is smaller or larger.

A   *B*   *C*

1.

2.

3.

4.

5.

6.

7.

8.

9.

10.

ANSWERS TO EXERCISE 2

1. *B* (smaller) **2.** *C* (smaller) **3.** *B* (smaller) **4.** *A* (smaller) **5.** *C* (larger)
6. *B* (smaller) **7.** *A* (smaller) **8.** *A* (larger) **9.** *C* (smaller) **10.** *C* (larger)

You are not expected to score perfectly on this exercise. With continued exposure to these and other angle discrimination problems, however, you will develop the agility necessary to move from angle to angle with a keen eye.

E. Varied Leg Lengths in an Angle

You have now been exposed to a variety of angles positioned uniquely and having different leg lengths. Another form of perceptual interference is due to a mixed set of leg lengths in a given angle. If, however, you are careful to employ the techniques discussed thus far, you will find that angles with mixed leg lengths are actually helpful. Since your eye tends naturally to rush to the end of the line to make the angular comparison, the presence of a shorter leg helps you to avoid making an inaccurate comparison at the end of the line. Recall that, when comparing angles, a greater measured distance between two legs implies a larger angle *if and only if the measurement is taken at the same distance from each angle's vertex.*

A discrepancy between leg lengths in a given angle and between two angles that are compared should remind you of this crucial rule. To understand this concept fully, compare the two sets of angles presented below. In each case, angle *A* is the smaller angle. The measurements of both angles of set 1 match the corresponding angle measurements of set 2.

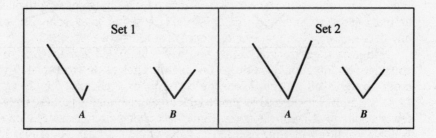

The shortened leg in angle *A* of set 1 dictates the reference position for comparison. The subtle difference in angle measurement between angles *A* and *B* is indicated in the following diagram.

Set 1

A   *B*

Again, the pitfall for most test-takers is that they make an inaccurate comparison at the end of the leg lengths, leading to an incorrect response. Below is an example of this *faulty* reasoning taken from set 2.

Set 2

A   *B*

F. General Strategy

Without becoming unduly suspicious, be aware that both the angles and answer choices on the PAT may tempt faulty reasoning. Rely heavily on the methods discussed, and rehearse the implementation of visual reasoning skills on angles you encounter.

Questions on the PAT show sets of four angles. You are asked to select, from four choices, the correct ranking of the angles from small to large. With a bit of test-taking logic and your heightened awareness of discriminating between like angles, you will be able to greatly improve your odds of scoring highly on these questions.

As already mentioned, you first should identify the smallest or largest angle, or both if possible. Then, before proceeding, examine the answer choices. Many times you will be able to eliminate one or two choices before examining the remaining angles. If the angle you selected as smallest is represented in two choices as the smallest angle, you can begin eliminating the other choices. Next examine whether the angle you think is largest is also listed as largest in one of the two choices you are considering. At this point, you may be able to select the correct answer.

Maintaining a fast pace throughout this section will allow you to concentrate longer on other items of the Perceptual Ability Test that require additional time. In order to stay organized while working quickly, it is recommended that you keep track of your angle discrimination decisions on the scratch paper provided. For example, upon your initial inspection for the largest and smallest angles, write down any decisions you can make before looking at the answer choices.

To keep track of choices that you have eliminated and answers you are still considering, you should jot down the answer choices on your scratch paper, and cross numbers off as you delete the corresponding choices. Simply writing "1," "2," "3," and "4" will enable you to stay organized, and it should take you only a few seconds to make these notes. Under test-taking circumstances, you can easily become confused in your decision making without these and similar brief notations. Most students who are skilled test-takers make use of minimal notes such as the ones suggested here.

Because of the computer format of the DAT, you will not be able to mark decision-making notations directly on the test. Hence, part of your preparation for the DAT should include practice in using scratch paper effectively. Below is an example of a typical PAT angle discrimination question and the use of scratch paper.

A. 1—3—4—2
B. 3—1—4—2
C. 3—1—2—4
D. 1—2—3—4

G. Review

- The length of an angle's legs is independent of its angular measurement.
- You must compare all the angles at the same distance from the joining point of the legs. When comparing angles, a greater measured distance between two legs will imply a larger angle if and only if the measurement is taken at the same distance from each angle's vertex.
- A useful method of angle comparison relies heavily on viewing only a discrete area of the angle, namely, the niche. The niche of the angle is the tightest part of the corner created by the two joining legs.
- When ranking angles, you first should identify the smallest or largest angle, or both if possible. Then begin eliminating answer choices.

Exercise 3
The following sets of angles are provided for your additional practice. They are structured in the same manner as angle discrimination problems from previous versions of the DAT. In each case, select the ranking that appropriately orders the angles from small to large.

1.

A. 1—3—2—4
B. 3—4—1—2
C. 2—1—4—3
D. 1—2—3—4

2.

A. 4—2—3—1
B. 2—4—3—1
C. 2—4—1—3
D. 4—3—2—1

3.

A. 4—1—2—3
B. 4—1—3—2
C. 1—4—2—3
D. 1—4—3—2

4.
1 2 3 4

A. 3—1—4—2
B. 1—3—4—2
C. 3—2—1—4
D. 1—3—2—4

5.
1 2 3 4

A. 3—1—4—2
B. 1—3—4—2
C. 3—2—1—4
D. 1—3—2—4

6.
1 2 3 4

A. 2—1—3—4
B. 2—3—1—4
C. 2—1—4—3
D. 2—3—4—1

7.
1 2 3 4

A. 4—3—2—1
B. 2—4—1—3
C. 4—2—3—1
D. 2—4—3—1

8.
1 2 3 4

A. 2—4—1—3
B. 1—2—3—4
C. 4—3—2—1
D. 3—2—1—4

9.
1 2 3 4

A. 2—1—3—4
B. 2—4—3—1
C. 1—2—3—4
D. 2—1—3—4

10.
1 2 3 4

A. 4—1—2—3
B. 1—4—2—3
C. 1—4—3—2
D. 4—1—3—2

ANSWERS TO EXERCISE 3

1. C, 2 – 1 – 4 – 3
2. B, 2 – 4 – 3 – 1
3. D, 1 – 4 – 3 – 2
4. D, 1 – 3 – 2 – 4
5. A, 3 – 1 – 4 – 2

6. D, 2 – 3 – 4 – 1
7. D, 2 – 4 – 3 – 1
8. B, 1 – 2 – 3 – 4
9. B, 2 – 4 – 3 – 1
10. C, 1 – 4 – 3 – 2

V. PAPER FOLDING

A. Introduction

The fourth section of the perceptual ability test is paper folding. Beginning with a square, you are presented with a series of progressive folds that the initial square undergoes. After the folds have been completed, a hole is punched somewhere in the final form. The task of this section is to mentally unfold the paper and determine the precise positioning of the one or more holes resulting from the punch.

B. Rules

The parameters of paper folding are straightforward:

- The initial paper will always be square.
- The paper will never be twisted.
- The orientation of the paper will remain the same.
- All folds will result in forms that are contained within the imaginary perimeter of the initial square.
- Dashed lines indicate the absence of paper due to a fold.
- Solid lines indicate either a crease or the paper's edge.
- Only after all folds have been completed will a hole be punched.
- One or more holes may be punched.
- The hole may penetrate one layer or multiple layers of the paper.

Success on the paper-folding section relies heavily on the understanding of a few basic principles. With practice, you should be able to answer the paper-folding questions in a short time and with little error.

C. Format of the Folding Sequence

The paper-folding sequence is presented as a series of two to four images arranged side by side. The series is laid out progressively, beginning with the first fold, then the second, and so on. Although not shown, the starting form is always assumed to be a square. The final image of the sequence is identical to the next to last image but shows the placement of the hole punch.

Below is an example of a typical paper fold sequence.

The dashed lines indicate absence of the paper (due to folding) from the original square. A solid line marks either a crease in the paper (seen only from frontal viewing) or the paper's edge. In the last image, the circle marks the location of the hole punch.

The following illustration includes guide arrows for clarification.

In this sequence, there are three folds. Prior DATs indicate that you can expect to see mostly two- and three-fold sequences.

D. The Punch Grid

Presented with the folding sequence are five possible answers as to where the punched holes are located on the paper. These choices are presented in the form of punch grids. The blackened circles on the grid indicate the locations of punched holes. Below are five possible answer choices for the sequence presented above.

A   B   C   D   E

The punch grid is a standard configuration that is used in all types of folding sequences. Examination of the general punch grid offers important information concerning the nature of the types of folds that can be used in folding series.

The punch grid is composed of 16 possible holes, evenly arranged in rows and columns. A folding pattern will never result in hole punches that stray from the possibilities offered in the punch grid. With this fact in mind, it is evident that the folds must maintain the integrity of the four ordered rows and columns.

Exercise 1

The following exercise will help you better understand the relationship between folding patterns and punched hole outcomes. Remove the exercise punch grids found on pages 233–238. Using these punch grids and a handheld hole puncher, complete each of the following folding patterns and punch a hole in the place as indicated. Blacken the appropriate holes of the answer punch grid for each sequence *after* unfolding the hole-punched exercise punch grid.

1.

7.

8.

9.

10.

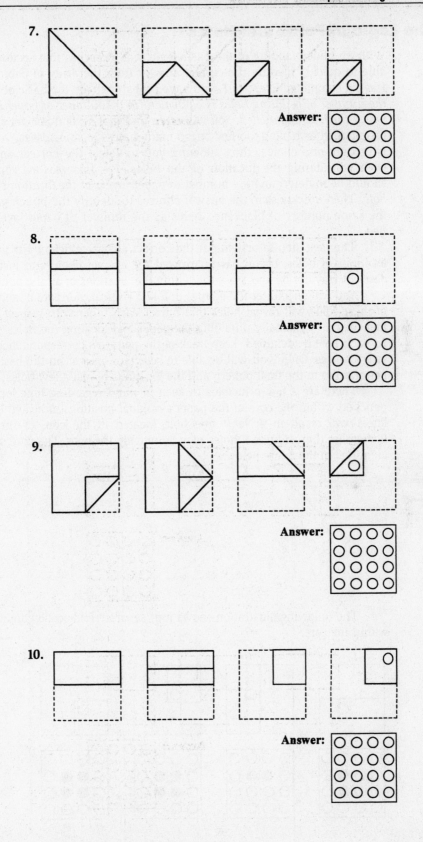

E. The Logic of Folds and Holes

With an understanding of the basic logic that underlies this section, you will be able to quickly identify the correct answer from the array of choices presented. Having completed Exercise 1, you have probably made the basic observation that *the number of resulting holes is equivalent to the number of paper layers through which the hole is punched.* You will often find that several answer choices can be disregarded as having too few or too many holes. In some cases, you may be left with only one choice, thus allowing you to select the correct answer without even considering the location of the holes. For this reason, your initial step should be to determine the number of paper layers *at the location of the punched hole.* Then quickly scan the answer choices to identify the punch grids that have the same number of blackened holes as the number of paper layers you identified.

The next step in arriving at the correct answer efficiently is to pinpoint the locations of holes. If you have narrowed the answer choices to just a few candidates, it may not be necessary to identify the locations of all the points.

You will encounter three types of folds: vertical, horizontal, and diagonal. All of these folds will reveal holes that mirror each other with respect to the line of fold. Begin by mentally unfolding the paper and locating the holes one at a time. As each hole is identified, keep track of the pattern's correspondence with the answer choices. Often you will be able to select an answer on the basis of the number of holes in the final pattern and the locations of just a few holes.

There are a few principles to keep in mind regarding hole location. A hole punched within the core of the paper's original position (indicated by the dashed lines) will result in at least one hole located in the core of the punch grid. Remember that additional holes may lie outside the core. The core of the paper is identified in the figure below.

The following illustration shows four separate folds each containing a punch within the core.

As previously mentioned, although a hole may be punched within the core, holes may also occur around the perimeter of the paper. For example, examine the following sequence:

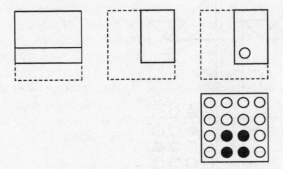

As a general rule, if the final form has a hole punched within the core of the form created by the original square (indicated by the dashed lines), the resulting punch grid will have at least one core hole. This general rule may be used to eliminate improbable answer choices.

Holes punched around the perimeter of the original square will result in forms that have at least one perimeter hole. Perimeter hole punches may be located in any of the positions indicated below.

The restraint that the paper must stay within the confines of the original square makes it difficult to obtain an interior core hole from a perimeter punch. With this restriction, the only way to obtain interior core holes from a perimeter punch is to have a folding segment that quarters the length or width of the paper to the edge of the original square. Examples of the resulting forms are seen in the figure below.

Most of the folds necessary to create an interior core hole from a punch around the perimeter would resemble those in the following sequence:

Note: This folding pattern violates the folding restrictions.

F. Review

- First establish how many paper layers were penetrated by the hole punch. Eliminate answer choices that have too few or too many holes.
- Identify the locations of the punched holes. Remember that each fold will produce mirrored holes with respect to the line of fold.
- If the final form has a hole punched within the core of the form created by the original square (indicated by the dashed lines), the resulting punch card will have at least one core hole.
- Holes punched around the perimeter of the original square will result in forms that have at least one perimeter hole and generally no core hole (see the illustration above for exceptional folds).

Exercise 1

The following folding sequence questions are provided for your additional practice.

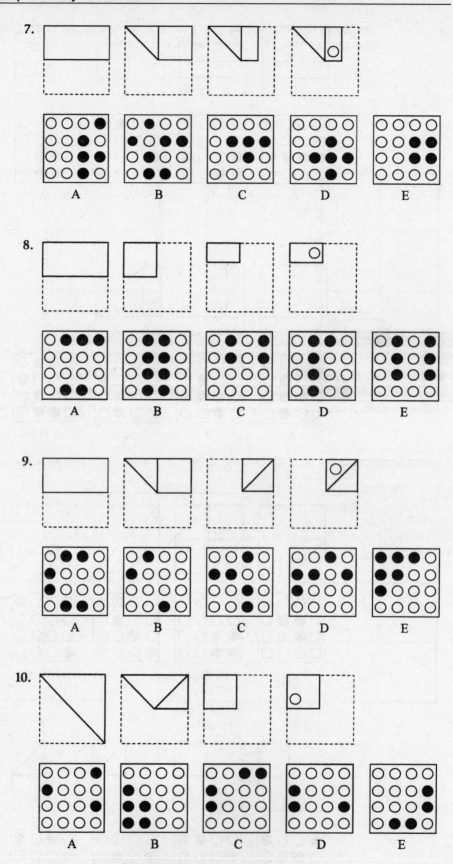

7.

A B C D E

8.

A B C D E

9.

A B C D E

10.

A B C D E

ANSWERS TO EXERCISE 1
1. D **2.** B **3.** D **4.** C **5.** C **6.** A **7.** E **8.** B **9.** A **10.** E

The following punch grids are provided for use in the folding exercises. Using scissors, cut along the perimeter of each grid.

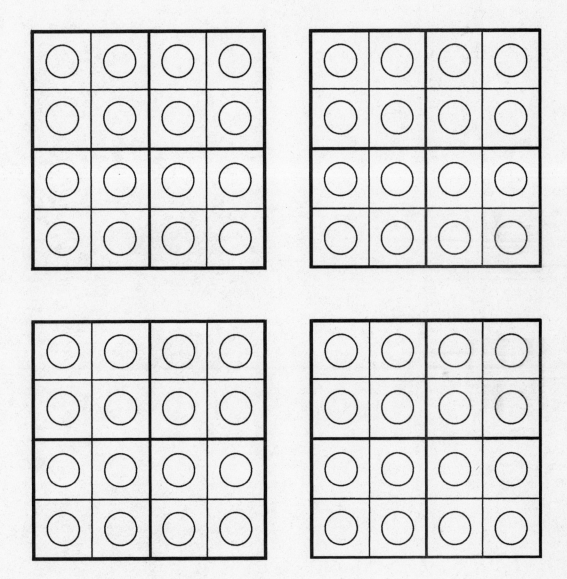

VI. CUBES

A. Introduction

The fifth section of the Perceptual Ability Test involves counting the painted surfaces of cubes. In this section, you will be presented with formations of stacked cubes. Groups of questions will correspond to the cube formations. The questions will ask you to determine how many cubes have a particular number of painted surfaces.

What distinguishes this section is the ease with which an answer can be quickly generated. For most test-takers, this section presents the fewest difficulties. In fact, with careful preparation and strategy, you can expect to answer these questions both efficiently and accurately. Because of the relative ease of this section in comparison to the other perceptual ability sections, you are cautioned to *not overlook* the use of strategy and preparative measures necessary for exceptional scoring. A high score on this group of questions will play an important role in achieving an overall high score on the PAT. Remember as you review for the cube questions that you are aiming for a nearly perfect score on these questions, which count no less than other, seemingly more difficult questions in the perceptual ability section of the DAT.

B. Cube Counting

Below is an example of a basic cube formation. This example is used to illustrate the basic assumptions that should underlie your reasoning throughout the cube section. The cube formations on the actual test will not be labeled and will be more complex than the simple example that follows. Further testlike examples will be offered after the introductory explanations.

Notice that there appear to be three cubes in the above formation. In this section, you must pay careful attention to any hidden or obscured cubes. Realizing that cube *A* is above cubes *B* and *C*, you should infer that there exists cube *D*, which is out of view. Hence, there are four cubes in this simple formation. The assumption of *necessary support,* that is, that any cube above the first level must be supported by underlying cubes, is the first crucial assumption that you should make throughout this section.

To review your understanding of this basic assumption, practice counting the number of cubes in the following formation.

If you counted 18 cubes, you have answered correctly. If you failed to identify all 18 cubes, chances are that you either lacked organization as you counted or you did not attend to the assumption of necessary support. An organized count might begin at the top and work downward. (Additionally, for more complex arrangements, the direction of count would move from left to right for each level.) In this fashion, you would first identify the top 3 cubes. Then, following the assumption of necessary support, you would identify the 3 hidden cubes plus the additional 3 visible cubes on the second level. Thus, the second level has a total of 6 cubes. The bottom level has 6 hidden and 3 visible cubes, totaling 9 cubes. The grand total is 3 + 6 + 9 = 18.

Again, practice arriving at a total cube count by using the following formation.

The correct answer is 10 cubes (1 + 3 + 6 = 10).

The second assumption that you should make in dealing with the cube section is that an *empty "ceiling" implies that there are no hidden cubes beneath.* For example, in the following formation examine the columns beneath the arrows. Of course, in real life a cube *could* exist on the first level that is out of view. On the PAT, however, an empty ceiling (top level) implies an empty column if the column is entirely out of view.

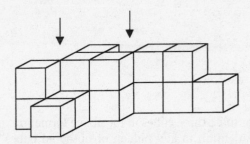

In the figure shown above, there are 6 cubes on the top level and 9 cubes on the bottom level. Here, the arrows draw your attention to empty columns. On the PAT, however, there will not be arrows to indicate empty columns. You will need to rely on your knowledge of the two assumptions discussed above in order to make appropriate judgments concerning the absence or presence of cubes out of view.

Now, try a more complex arrangement.

The correct answer is 21 cubes.

The initial counting of cubes is an important step that should precede any reasoning concerning the painted surface questions. Although no questions will ask you to simply identify the total number of cubes, an initial cube count takes little time and helps you avoid the trap of failing to identify hidden cubes. Additionally, the cube count will serve as a self-check in figuring your answers.

Exercise 1

The following cube formations are provided to help you achieve greater speed and accuracy in counting cubes. Exercise 1 in Section F will also refer to these 10 formations.

How many cubes are there in each formation?

1.

2.

3.

4.

5.

6.

7.

8.

9.

10.

Compare your cube count totals with the answers provided below:

ANSWERS TO EXERCISE 1

1. 8   **2.** 7   **3.** 9   **4.** 11   **5.** 10   **6.** 20   **7.** 15   **8.** 12   **9.** 14   **10.** 11

C. Counting Painted Surfaces

The task in the cube section of the PAT is to count painted surfaces. Imagine that the formation below has been painted with white paint on all exposed sides. The exposed sides are the sides that would reflect light if light were projected from the front, the back, and the left and right sides of the formation.

What is the total number of painted surfaces (or cube sides) in the formation shown below?

The total number of painted surfaces (or cube sides) of this formation is 15. In counting, it is a common mistake to overlook the exposed sides of blocks that are not visible to the respondent.

Below is a block separation of the basic figure considered above. Notice that the blackened areas are the surfaces that either sit on the imaginary floor or are shared between two blocks. These blackened areas are never to be counted as painted surfaces.

Actual painted surface questions that have appeared on previous DAT exams had this form:

In figure X, how many cubes have
A. one of their exposed sides painted?
B. two of their exposed sides painted?
C. four of their exposed sides painted?

On the test approximately three painted surface questions refer to each formation. For this reason, it is crucial to follow a consistent methodology when counting painted surfaces. Failure to accurately identify all the cubes in a particular formation could result in incorrect responses to several questions.

Note that no cube should ever have six painted surfaces. Although there are six surfaces to a cube, the cube will always be resting against the imaginary floor or another cube. Also note that there will be instances in which a given cube will have no painted surface. This will occur when there are neighboring cubes on all sides and another cube rests above the cube in question. In general, your success in counting painted surfaces will depend on your ability to mentally meander around the far corners of the arrangement that are out of view. As is true for all sections of the DAT, with practice you will notice improvement.

Since the DAT will be administered on the computer, you will need to make good use of available scratch paper. The painted cube questions, perhaps more than any other type, will reflect your ability to remain organized under test-taking circumstances.

D. Strategy

As stated previously, you should count the total number of cubes before addressing the issue of painted surfaces. (Remember to use an organized count—top down, left to right, and back in space.) This preliminary count will serve two purposes. First, it will help you identify all the obscured or hidden cubes. Second, the total cube count will serve as a self-check when you tally the numbers of painted surfaces. After establishing a total count, begin identifying (by cube) the number of painted surfaces on each cube. Follow the same pathway that you used to count the number of cubes (top down, left to right, and back in space). On your scratch paper create a vertical list that assigns a number of painted surfaces to each cube.

After counting the cube surfaces in the top level, draw a horizontal line to indicate the counting of cubes in a new level. Insert a horizontal line after each level. Finally, before answering the questions, check that the number of cubes you have tallied matches the total cube count that you identified initially.

To review the suggested counting methodology, consider the following example:

Although it is tempting to "break up" the cube formation into different sections for counting purposes (for example, to group the far left, middle, and right sections), this is *not* recommended. It takes only a few seconds to carry out the top down, left to right, and back in space procedure, and a consistent direction of count helps you to remain accurate from formation to formation despite the differences between formations. The use of an organized procedure such as the one recommended above and illustrated below helps ensure that you will properly identify all hidden cubes.

On your scratch paper, note the total cube count before proceeding. Next, begin your vertical list of numbers that correspond to painted surfaces. For the above example, the list would be written as follows:

```
5        (top level)
___

4
3        (middle level)
5
___

2
2
4        (bottom level)
2
2
3

         total cubes= 10
```

As mentioned previously, the cube count serves as a means of self-checking. Before responding to questions, verify that the number of cube surfaces you have identified matches the total number of cubes. If you find that you have made a mistake at some point, recheck your scratch work level by level (as separated by the horizontal lines in your list) to find where the skipped item was omitted.

At this point, you are ready to efficiently answer questions regarding the numbers of painted surfaces. Consider the following questions:

> In the figure above, how many cubes have two of their exposed sides painted?
> How many cubes have three of their exposed sides painted?
> How many cubes have four of their exposed sides painted?
> How many cubes have five of their exposed sides painted?

A helpful method for combing your list is to employ a circle, the letter X, and a squiggle to identify like numbers. A basic method of this sort helps avoid the fatal flaw of overlooking a crucial number. Failure to identify how many cubes share a certain number of painted sides can lead to incorrect responses on the test. Using an active rather than a passive method at each stage of developing your final answer will enable you to avoid mistakes.

Below is an example of the circle, X, and squiggle method for establishing the final answers to the questions given above. You can develop additional forms of notation that catch your eye at a glance.

How many have two sides painted? 4
How many have three sides painted? 2
How many have four sides painted? 2
How many have five sides painted? 2

E. Review

- According to the assumption of necessary support, any cube above the first level must be supported by underlying cubes.
- An empty ceiling (top level) implies an empty column if the column is entirely out of view.
- The initial counting of cubes is an important step that should precede any reasoning concerning painted surface questions.

Exercise 1

Practice is necessary to develop speed and accuracy in the employment of the various methods discussed above. Turn to pages 241–242, and answer the following questions for each of the 10 formations:

a. How many cubes have one exposed side painted?
b. How many cubes have two exposed sides painted?
c. How many cubes have three exposed sides painted?
d. How many cubes have four exposed sides painted?
e. How many cubes have five exposed sides painted?

ANSWERS TO EXERCISE 1

1. 0, 1, 2, 4, 1   (Note: One cube has no painted surface.)
2. 0, 1, 2, 3, 1
3. 0, 1, 3, 4, 1
4. 0, 2, 3, 4, 2
5. 1, 2, 5, 1, 1
6. 3, 7, 6, 1, 2
7. 1, 6, 3, 3, 1
8. 2, 3, 4, 2, 1
9. 1, 3, 4, 5, 0
10. 0, 0, 4, 4, 1   (Note: Two cubes have no painted surface.)

VII. FORM DEVELOPMENT

A. Introduction

The last section of the Perceptual Ability Test is form development. In this section, you are presented with a flat pattern that is to be folded into a three-dimensional form. Your task is to select the appropriate three-dimensional rendering of the flattened image from four possible choices.

This section has the power to consume a tremendous amount of valuable test time. One of your many goals for this section is to be able to recognize when it is prudent to skip questions too difficult to be solved at first try. Although form development is a challenge for most test-takers, it offers the opportunity to integrate the skills mastered for other sections of the PAT. This section need not be construed as formidable; careful use of strategy will enhance your ability to recognize the appropriate answer without delay.

B. The Flattened Image

The flattened image is a rendering of what you would have if a three-dimensional object was opened at its edges with each surface "unwrapped" and the whole form flattened on one plane. The following is an example of a flattened image.

Notice that the flattened image is one complete unit. Although sides have been cut at the edges, each panel has at least one edge joined with another surface. On some flattened images, shaded regions or designs mark the surfaces. Keep in mind that each line that is part of the flattened image indicates one of the following: (1) a bend, (2) an edge, or (3) the outline of a shaded region.

C. Construction of the Three-Dimensional Image

Your task in the form development section is to select the correct or appropriate three-dimensional image constructed from the flattened figure. The three-dimensional figures will be rendered as isometric drawings. An isometric drawing is a representational drawing in which all faces of the image are shown with equal inclination and all the lines are drawn to their true lengths. Below is an example of a three-dimensional construction of the flattened image shown above.

The orientation of the three-dimensional image will vary from question to question. After the form is constructed, it may be turned on its side or upside down. The following two examples illustrate how the same flattened image may be represented three dimensionally in two different ways.

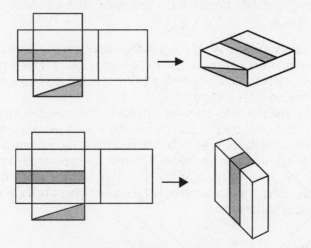

Likewise, there is no standard orientation of the flattened image that relates to the direction of fold used to construct the three-dimensional image. In the following example, the flattened pattern is oriented in four different positions. What is later perceived as the figure's top may seem to be a likely bottom when viewing the flattened image.

Any of the flattened images above could be used to describe *all* of the following three-dimensional forms:

Often, the orientation of the flattened image biases your thinking in regard to where the folding begins and how you conceive of the folding direction. Such a bias may interfere with the ability to regard certain answer choices as possible accurate renderings. For this reason, it is important to develop a strategy that leads you to the correct answer regardless of the orientation or positioning of the flattened form or of the three-dimensional answer choices.

D. Attention to Detail

Perhaps the quickest way to identify an appropriate three-dimensional rendering of the flattened form is to utilize details of each drawing (flattened figures and three-dimensional answer choices). Consider the following flattened form and corresponding answer choices:

In this example, the details that stand out are the shaded half-circles and the shaded rectangle. *Whenever shading is used, first examine the answer choices to eliminate any that have an inappropriate positioning of the shaded region or design.* Take note of the precise positioning of a shaded region. It is not necessary to initially check each design for the positioning of each shaded region. Often you can eliminate several choices by checking the positioning of just one shaded region. As you narrow the choices, you can expand the degree of detail on which you will base your final judgment. In the example above, the first detail check might be to scan for the distance between the half-circle and the rectangular figure. Noticing that both half-circles are positioned closer to the blank hexagon than to the hexagon with the rectangle, you can eliminate choices A, B, and D. With little effort, you realize that the correct answer is C. This answer was arrived at without considering the angle of view or the spacing between marked sides. By keeping to a simplistic plan such as detail scanning, you save a tremendous amount of time and energy.

Although detail scanning is extremely helpful in questions that contain shaded regions or designs, in other questions you will be confronted with complex flattened images that contain no distinct feature markings.

E. Complex Forms

Some flattened forms will be difficult to visualize in three dimensions. The shape may be unusual, or the number of folds necessary to arrive at the final form may be unusually high. The form below would be considered complex in both regards.

In such cases, rather than spending time trying to visualize the totality of the final three-dimensional form, concentrate on the elimination of unlikely answer choices. To begin the process of elimination, it is necessary to identify a reference shape in the flattened form. This reference shape should be easy to locate and unique in some regard.

One of many reference shapes that may be used is shown below.

This particular form happens to be the largest unfolded portion of the flattened figure. It is also appears twice in the flattened image. Often, a pair of identical large regions serves the three-dimensional image as the sides or the top and bottom.

Once you have identified the reference shape you wish to use, examine the answer choices. Check each choice to see whether the shape is reproduced correctly, the neighboring sides make logical sense given the joining shapes in the flattened form, and the shape is repeated the correct number of times.

Now, considering the form given above, try these strategies on the answer choices below.

A.   B.

C.   D.

The correct answer is D.

F. Review

- The orientation of the three-dimensional image will vary from question to question. After the form is constructed, it may be turned on its side or upside down. Likewise, there is no standard orientation of the flattened image in relation to the direction of fold used to construct the three-dimensional image.
- Each line that is part of the flattened image indicates one of the following: (1) a bend, (2) an edge, or (3) the outline of a shaded region.
- Whenever shading is used, first search your answer choices to eliminate any that have an inappropriate positioning of a shaded region or design. Remember that it is not necessary to initially check each design for the positioning of every shaded region. You are often able to eliminate several choices by checking the positioning of just one shaded region.
- When confronted with a complex form, concentrate on the elimination of unlikely answer choices. To begin the process of elimination, identify a reference shape in the flattened form. Check each answer choice to see whether the shape is reproduced correctly, the neighboring sides make logical sense given the joining shapes in the flattened form, and the shape is repeated the correct number of times.
- Use your time carefully. Do not allow yourself to dwell on any one question. Skip a question if you cannot effectively eliminate answer choices at the first try.

Exercise 1

The following exercise makes use of both folding and design location skills. Paying particular attention to the locations of design markings, examine each flattened image. Below each flattened image, you will see an incomplete three-dimensional rendering. Add the appropriate marking to each cube so that it accurately represents the flattened image.

Items 1 – 4

Items 5 – 8

Items 9 – 12

ANSWERS TO EXERCISE 1

1. Shaded circle	2. Shaded ring	3. White circle
4. Shaded square	5. White square	6. Shaded square
7. White ring	8. Shaded ring	9. White circle or white ring
10. (Blank)	11. Shaded circle	12. Shaded ring

Exercise 2

This exercise is formatted identically to the way in which form development questions appear on the DAT. In each case, choose the correct three-dimensional representation of the flattened image shown at left.

1.

2.

3.

4.

5.

ANSWERS TO EXERCISE 2

(It is suggested that you complete Exercise 3 before checking your answers to Exercise 2.)

1. C **2.** D **3.** A **4.** B **5.** D

Exercise 3

On the following pages you will find reproductions of all the flattened forms discussed in the form development section. Carefully cut out each form and create three-dimensional forms by folding the cutouts. Then use the three-dimensional figures to review the strategic discussions and Exercises 1 and 2.

Carefully remove each flattened figure by cutting around its perimeter. Then construct a three-dimensional form by folding. Clear tape may be used to fasten the sides.

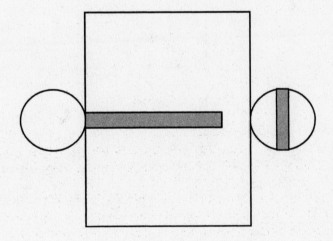

READING COMPREHENSION TEST REVIEW

OUTLINE

I. INTRODUCTION

This review will provide information on how to prepare for and take the Reading Comprehension Test (RCT) of the DAT. *Unlike reading comprehension sections on any other standardized exams, all of the reading comprehension passages on the DAT will be heavily technical and scientific.*

The RCT consists of three passages of about 1,300–1,500 words each. Dental school professors are hired by the ADA to write the passages on the actual DAT. These passages are representative of the type of material you will encounter in your first year of dental school. Following each passage are 16 or 17 multiple-choice questions for a total of 50 questions. You will have 60 minutes to complete this section.

II. THE IMPORTANCE OF READING COMPREHENSION

The Reading Comprehension Test is often regarded as the least important section of the DAT. There is some truth behind this view since most Admissions Committees tend to look for high marks on the sciences and the Perceptual Ability Test. However, reading comprehension also may be considered the most important section because your ability to read quickly and to comprehend what you have read will be a determining factor in how well you do in dental school.

During the first year of dental school you will be assigned more reading than you can possibly finish. You must be able to determine what readings are important, to read them at a good pace, and to retain a fair amount of what you have read. This is not to say that dental school is impossibly difficult, but rather that your ability to read well will be tested on a daily basis.

III. AN EASY TEST AND A HARD TEST

In one respect, you can think of the Reading Comprehension Test as the easiest part of the DAT. Just think: you do not need any outside knowledge, and all of the answers are provided in the passages. All that is required of you is to read the question, find the answer in the passage, and then mark the correct choice on the answer sheet. What could be easier?

As easy as the RCT is, it is also the test on which many people run into problems. The main problem is lack of time. It is not uncommon for test takers to find themselves with 1 minute left and five questions unanswered. This situation occurs, not because the questions are too difficult, but because the students did not have an efficient method for finding information in the passage.

IV. WHY SOME STUDENTS DO POORLY

Many students believe that they do poorly on this test because they are slow readers, but this is not always the case. What is more important is how carefully you read and then how skillfully you go about finding the answers to the questions. Speed reading is not necessary for this section and may actually be counterproductive since many small facts may be missed.

There are only three passages on the exam, and each one is not excessively long. Therefore, even if you do not consider yourself a fast reader, you should still have no problem finishing the test. Where the majority of test takers lose the most time is in locating the answers in the text. It is imperative that you develop a method that allows you to read the passage, locate in the passage the answers to the questions, and then have 2–5 minutes left at the end to return to any questions you have skipped.

V. YOU CAN IMPROVE

It is completely reasonable to believe that with a little practice anyone can improve on the Reading Comprehension Test. You just have to be willing to put in some time. It is understandable that, with all the subjects you have to study, reading comprehension is probably not at the top of your list. You must learn, however, to budget your time and to set aside a certain amount of time each week to practice for this test.

You must remember that, just as with the other tests, practice will improve your RCT score. Just reading a lot will not guarantee a good score—although it will help. You must learn to quickly recall where you saw items in a passage so as to not waste time hunting for them.

VI. METHODS FOR READING COMPREHENSION

Many methods have been proposed to help students achieve higher scores on the Reading Comprehension Test. All of these methods have positive and negative aspects, just as the one proposed in the next section surely does. It will be helpful now to mention a few alternative methods and to explain why each is good and not so good.

One method suggests that you read the questions before reading the passage. This approach will help you in that it will provide you with some idea of what questions are being asked. Then, while reading the passage, you can be on the lookout for the answers to those questions. Thus, you may even be able to answer some of the questions while you are reading. There are, however, two drawbacks to this method. First, it is time consuming. If you have to read the questions twice, once before you read the passage and once after, you are wasting time. A second problem with this method is that there are 16 or 17 questions per passage. It is unlikely that you will be able to remember more than five or six of the questions while reading the passage.

A second method asks that you skim the passage once before reading. Skimming generally means that you read the first and last lines of each paragraph to try to get the main idea of the passage. This approach can be very useful, especially since there are usually a couple of questions that ask about the main idea. However, just as with the first method, this is time consuming. If you are having trouble making it through the RCT just reading each passage once, skimming is not likely to help you. A word of warning: If you decide to use this method, you must read the passage in its entirety after you have skimmed it. Do not just skim! Most questions pertain to specific facts that will be missed without careful reading.

A third method involves the order in which you answer the questions. However, all of the questions must be answered, and all of them carry the same point value. If there were a quick way to find the easiest questions, so that these could be answered first, then this method would be worthwhile. Your best bet is to answer the questions in the order they are given, reading the question first and then the answer choices. This approach is less confusing, and you will be less likely to make a mistake when keying in your responses.

A final method suggests a system for marking the passage. The test taker is advised to mark the passage as he or she reads. Since this method is impossible on the computer, it is not discussed here.

VII. THE "KEY" METHOD

This section will provide you with a detailed explanation of one possible method for taking the Reading Comprehension Test. As mentioned previously, this approach may not work for everyone. There are, however, two main reasons why this method is preferable to the ones just discussed. The first reason is that it is easy to learn. With just a little practice you should be able to decrease the time required to complete the RCT while increasing the number of correct answers that you get. The second reason is that the method is easy and fast to use. It is not time consuming, and there is nothing extra that you will have to remember for test day.

This method is based on key elements, words, or numbers, which will be referred to as keys. Keys are any words that are important. The challenge is to determine which ones are important. Some obvious examples are scientific words or other words with which you are unfamiliar, such as *odontoblast* or *chondrocyte*. You don't have to worry what these words mean. If a word is important, it will be defined in the passage. Other keys to look for are numbers or statistics because they often sum up the results of a study or give important data. Aside from these, it is up to you to determine what is important and therefore is a key. Don't worry—there are examples later on that will help to clarify what you should be looking for.

When you begin the RCT, the first thing you should do is read the first passage.

Do not skim it, make sure you read every word. Use the following guides to create your *List of Keys*:

- As you read, look for keys and jot them down.
- Use a clean piece of scratch paper for each of the three passages.
- Jot keys down in sequential order.
- Draw a short horizontal line in the left-hand margin to indicate paragraph breaks.
- For keys that are excessively long (10 letters or more) create your own form of shorthand to save time.

You will receive plenty of scratch paper at the Sylvan Learning Center. If for any reason you do not have ample paper, *ask for more!* When writing keys, you must be careful to include only what is important; writing too many keys, wastes time and can lead to confusion later on. When creating your list of keys, choose for each key the one or two words that are most important.

Consider this sentence: "The olfactory nerve is the shortest of the twelve cranial nerves, spanning as several small bundles the short distance through the cribiform plate between the olfactory epithelium and the expanded olfactory bulb." It is easy to see that this sentence is important because it presents a term, *olfactory nerve*, and then a description of the nerve. If this were a text to be used for study purposes, you would highlight the entire sentence. On the DAT, however, you would just jot down the key, in this case *olfactory nerve* (or a shorthand version, *olfact n.*). This will allow you to find the description of the nerve quickly if it appears in a question later on. For this sentence you could also jot down *olfactory bulb* and *olfactory epithelium* (in shorthand, *olfact bulb/epith*); however, no information is given for these terms, so it may be better to skip them and go on. Continue this process until you have completed the passage then move on to the questions.

Exercise 1

Read the following passage carefully and create a practice list of keys. Then compare your keys to those in the answer.

Achieving effective and predictable anesthesia of the mandibular arch has long been a formidable challenge for the dental professional. It is reported that the success rate for the inferior alveolar nerve block is 80% to 85%. Variations in the height of the mandibular foramen location coupled with the depth requirement of the needle penetration serve to reduce the success rate of the inferior alveolar nerve block. The density of the mandibular bone makes it imperative that the anesthetic solution be deposited to within 1 mm of the target nerve.

Alternatives to the traditional inferior alveolar block have been proposed. The Gow-Gates and Vazirani-Akinosi blocks provide regional anesthesia to the pulps of the mandibular teeth in a quadrant. The mandibular anterior teeth can be easily anesthetized with the incisive nerve block. It is a valuable alternative to the inferior alveolar nerve block when treatment is limited to these teeth; however, anesthesia of the mandibular molars is usually approached with a block injection.

Supplemental mandibular anesthesia techniques include the PDL injection. Although this supplemental injection can be used in either arch, it is most often used to anesthetize mandibular teeth.

ANSWER TO EXERCISE 1

List of Keys

anesthesia of mand.

success rate	inf. <u>alveolar</u> n. block	80% to 85%.
height	mandibular foramen	
depth requirement	needle penetration	reduce the success rate
density mand. bone	anesth. sol. be deposited	

Gow-Gates and Vazirani-Akinosi
mandibular anterior teeth
incisive nerve block

Supplemental mandibular anesthesia
PDL injection

Start with the first question. Read the question and, as you did with the passage, look for a key. If you find one, try to match it with one of the keys you have listed from the passage. If you find a match, look for the corresponding answer choice. If you don't find a match, or an appropriate answer to the question, read the answer choices given and look for more keys. Then, once again, match those keys with ones you listed for the passage.

There is one more thing that you must do when reading each question: You must determine exactly what the question is asking. First try to figure out whether the question is asking for a specific fact or for a general understanding of the passage. If the question is asking for specific information, use your keys to find the answer. An example of this type of question could be: Which is the shortest cranial nerve? If, on the other hand, the question is asking for more general knowledge of the passage, keys may not be as helpful. *For these types of questions you will have to rely on your ability to comprehend what you have read.* Questions that require general understanding can pose more of a challenge for some test takers, and therefore it may be wise to skip them the first time around and return to them later. Be aware, though, that if you leave the general questions until the end of the test, you may not remember what the passage was about when you try to answer them. Your best bet is to answer as many of the questions as you can the first time through. If, however, you can not pick the correct answer, select the mark key on the screen and return to it later. If you have a best guess, mark it.

Exercise 2
Answer the following questions, using the passage from Exercise 1 to find the answers.

1. Which of the following could be used in place of a traditional inferior alveolar nerve block to anesthetize mandibular molars?
   A. PDL injection
   B. incisive nerve block
   C. mental nerve block
   D. Vazirani-Akinosi block
   E. greater palatine nerve block

2. For an inferior alveolar nerve block the anesthetic solution should be placed?
   A. in the PDL
   B. directly on the target nerve
   C. in the mandibular bone
   D. no more than 1 mm from the target nerve
   E. no less than 1 mm from the target nerve

3. A PDL injection is most often used for
   A. anesthetizing mandibular bone
   B. anesthetizing mandibular teeth
   C. a Gow-Gates block
   D. primary mandibular anesthesia
   E. anesthetizing maxillary teeth

4. The success rate of the incisive nerve block is
   A. 80% to 85%
   B. dependent on the anesthetic used
   C. higher than that of an alveolar nerve block
   D. not given in the passage
   E. 60% to 70%

ANSWERS TO EXERCISE 2

1. Correct answer: **D.** For this question the key is "in place of." Refer to the passage for this phrase or one that is close to it. The closest match is "Alternatives." Now read the sentence in the passage that contains the key. Since no answer is given there, read the next sentence. Now check the answer choices. You could also read over the answer choices before reading the sentence in the passage. Either way is fine, so choose whichever works better for you.

2. Correct answer: **D.** Use the same method as above. Make sure to read the answer choices carefully. Answers D and E differ by only one word and can easily be confused.

3. Correct answer: **B.** The key is "PDL injection."

4. Correct answer: **D.** For this question there are two keys, "success rate" and "incisive nerve block." It is important that you locate all keys in the question; otherwise, you will end up with an incorrect answer. If you took only "success rate" as the key, you might choose A as the correct answer. That would be correct if you had been asked about the success rate of inferior alveolar nerve blocks. Since no success rate was given for incisive blocks, answer D is the correct choice.

VIII. PRACTICE PASSAGE

Now try this practice passage. As you read the passage, create a list of keys on the scratch paper provided (see page 273). Then use the keys to help you answer the questions that follow.

(Time limit 20 minutes)

Changes in Tissues Overlying Teeth

The initial change seen in the tissues overlying the teeth before eruption of the crown is the alteration of the connective tissue of the dental follicle to form a pathway for the erupting tooth. Usually, this is more prominent in erupting permanent teeth. Histologically, the coronal part of the dental follicle becomes heavily populated by numerous monocytes in parallel with osteoclasts to participate in bone resorption and formation of the eruption pathway. The future eruption pathway appears as a zone in which connective tissue fibers have disappeared, cells have degenerated and decreased in number, blood vessels have become fewer, and terminal nerves have broken up and degenerated. These changes are probably the partial result of the loss of blood supply to this area, as well as the release of enzymes that aid in degradation of these tissues. Clinically, tooth eruption may be accompanied by discomfort or pain, irritability, and/or a slight temperature increase. An altered tissue space or compartment overlying the tooth becomes visible as an innervated, funnel-shaped area. In the periphery of this zone, the follicle fibers direct themselves toward the mucosa and are defined as the gubernaculum dentis or gupernacular cord. Some authors believe that this structure guides the tooth in its eruptive movements.

For successful tooth eruption, there must be some resorption of the overlying bony crypt, which is in a constant state of remodeling as the tooth germ enlarges and the face grows anteriorly and laterally. The eruptive process can be considered part of this remodeling growth. Osteoclasts differentiate and resorb a portion of the bony crypt overlying the erupting tooth. The eruption pathway, which at first is small, increases in dimension, allowing movement of the tooth to the oral mucosa. Although the eruption of most permanent teeth is similar to that of primary teeth, the overlying primary teeth are an additional complication. The eruptive pathway of permanent incisors and cuspids is lingual to the corresponding primary teeth. This area shows a pronounced enlargement to accommodate the advancing crown.

Small foramina in the mandible and maxilla are evidence of eruption pathways of the anterior permanent teeth. These openings, the gubernacular foramina, are found lingual to the anterior primary teeth and are the sites of the gubernacular cords. The premolars are between the roots of the primary molars. Root resorption in primary teeth proceeds in much the same manner as bone resorptions. When the roots are fully resorbed, the attachment of the primary crown is lessened and the crown is shed. This produces an eruption pathway for the premolars. Most roots resorb completely; the primary pulps degenerate as well. During the period of mixed dentition (around 6 to 12 years of age), when both primary and permanent teeth are in the mouth, the phenomena of root resorption and tooth formation proceed side by side. These changes occur while the teeth still maintain chewing efficiency.

When the tooth nears the oral mucosa, the reduced enamel epithelium comes into contact with the overlying mucosa. Simultaneously, the oral epithelial cells and reduced enamel epithelial cells proliferate and fuse into one membrane. Further movement of the tooth stretches and thins the membrane over the crown tip. At this stage the mucosa become blanched because of a lack of blood supply to the area. Very soon, the tips of the teeth penetrate the area and appear in the oral cavity. Eruption is a gradual, as well as an intermittent, process. The tooth will erupt slightly, remain stationary for some time, and then erupt again. In this manner, the supporting tissues are able to make adjustments to the eruptive movements. Each eruptive movement results in more of the crown appearing in the oral cavity and further separation of the attachment epithelium from the enamel surface. Recent observations of human premolar eruption revealed that eruptive activity occurred mostly at night with a marked slowing or cessation during the day.

Changes in Tissues Around Teeth

The tissues around the teeth also undergo change during tooth eruption. Initially, the dental follicle is composed of delicate connective tissue. Gradually, as eruptive movements commence, collagen fibers become prominent, extending between the forming root and the alveolar bone surface. The first noticeable periodontal fiber bundles appear at the cervical area of the root and extend at an angle coronal to the alveolar process. At the same time, the alveolar bone of the crypt is remodeled to accommodate the forming root. As the large crown moves occlusally, the bone fills in to conform to the smaller root diameter. As eruption proceeds, other collagen fiber bundles become visible along the forming root. The area becomes more densely populated with fibroblasts. A special type of fibroblast, the myofibroblast, is said to have contractile capabilities. It has been reported to be present in the periodontal ligament. If present, the myofibroblast, could aid in the force needed in tooth eruption. All ligament cells and fibers are currently believed to be important in the eruptive process. During eruptive movements, collagen formation and fiber turnover are very rapid (possibly 24 hours). Very early in the eruptive process, perforating givers attach to the cementum on the root surface and to the alveolar bone. Some fibers release as the tooth moves, then reattach to stabilize the tooth. In this manner, the tooth-stabilizing process is performed by the same group of fibers throughout tooth eruption. The fibroblasts are the cells active in formation and degeneration of collagen fibers. Alveolar bone remodeling is continuous during eruption. As the tooth moves occlusally, the alveolar bone increases in height and changes shape to accommodate passage of the crown. Because tooth crown has migrated occlusally, new bone is deposited around the root to reduce the size of the crypt. Above and around the crown, osteoclastic and osteoblastic actions occur. These actions are coordinated during the entire eruption process, as well as throughout life.

Changes in Tissues Underlying Teeth

Changes also occur in the follicular tissue underlying the developing tooth. These changes take place in the soft tissue and the fundic bone (bone surrounding the apex of the root). As the tooth erupts, space is provided for the root to lengthen, primarily because of the crown moving occlusally and the increase in height of the alveolar bone. Changes in the fundic region are thus believed to be largely compensatory to the lengthening of the root. During the preeruptive and early eruptive phases, the follicular fibroblasts and fibers lie in a plane parallel to the base of the root. The root moves more rapidly in the socket during prefunctional eruption than at any other period. Fine bony trabeculae appear in the fundic area. They compensate for tooth eruption and provide some support to the apical tissues. Some authors describe this as a bony ladder. The ladder becomes more dense as alternate layers of bone plates and connective tissue are laid down. At the end of the prefunctional eruptive phase, when the tooth comes into occlusion, about one third of the enamel remains covered by the gingiva, and the root is incomplete. At this time, the bony ladder is gradually resorbed, one plate at a time, to make space for the developing root tip. Root completion continues for a considerable time after the teeth have been in function; this process takes from 1 to 1.5 years in primary teeth and from 2 to 3 years in permanent teeth.

LIST OF KEYS

Questions

1. At what time is the crown of a primary tooth lost?
   A. when the underlying permanent tooth is fully formed
   B. when the crown is fully resorbed
   C. when the root is fully resorbed
   D. when the periodontal ligament is fully resorbed
   E. when the underlying permanent tooth erupts

2. What becomes prominent in the dental follicle during eruption?
   A. osteoclasts
   B. delicate connective tissue
   C. fundic bone
   D. erythrocytes
   E. collagen fibers

3. What is responsible for resorption of the bony crypt overlying the erupting tooth?
   A. reduced enamel epithelial cells
   B. osteoblasts
   C. dental follicle cells
   D. eruptive forces
   E. osteoclasts

4. As a tooth erupts, what happens to the alveolar bone?
   A. It remains constant.
   B. It increases in height.
   C. It decreases in height.
   D. It becomes more dense.
   E. It becomes less dense.

5. What makes up the bony ladder?
   A. bony trabeculae
   B. fundic bone
   C. compact bone
   D. osteoclasts
   E. cementum

6. What forms the gubernacular cord?
   A. osteoblasts
   B. follicle fibers
   C. the periodontal ligament
   D. oral epithelial cells
   E. monocytes

7. When do premolars show the most marked eruption?
   A. during periods of increased stress
   B. at no particular time; eruption is constant
   C. at night
   D. during mastication
   E. during the day

8. What is the bone surrounding the apex of the root called?
   A. alveolar bone
   B. periodontal bone
   C. fundic bone
   D. bony crypt
   E. follicular bone

9. What makes the myofibroblast unique?
   A. It can resorb bone.
   B. It aids in bone formation.
   C. It has immunological capabilities.
   D. It has contractile capabilities.
   E. It aids in pulp formation.

10. Once a permanent tooth has come into occlusion, what portion
    of the enamel is exposed?
    A. 1/2
    B. 1/3
    C. 2/5
    D. 2/3
    E. 1/5

11. What is necessary for successful tooth eruption?
    A. root formation
    B. enamel
    C. formation of the gubernacular dentis
    D. formation of the fundic bone
    E. resorption of overlying bone

12. What happens to oral epithelial cells and reduced enamel
    epithelial cells as the erupting tooth nears the oral mucosa?
    A. They fuse.
    B. They resorb.
    C. They remain the same.
    D. They form the enamel.
    E. They form the periodontal ligament.

13. Where is the eruption pathway of permanent incisors and cuspids
    in relation to corresponding primary teeth?
    A. facial
    B. distal
    C. lingual
    D. mesial
    E. The pathways are the same.

14. Where are the first periodontal fiber bundles seen?
    A. at the cervical area of the root
    B. at the apex of the root
    C. on the crown
    D. in the dentin
    E. within the bony crypt

15. What are changes in the fundic region attributed to?
    A. lengthening of the crown
    B. dentin formation
    C. tooth eruption
    D. loss of primary teeth
    E. lengthening of the root

16. During what ages does mixed dentition occur?
    A. 10–15 years
    B. 6–12 years
    C. 4–8 years
    D. 6–12 months
    E. There is no set age range.

PRACTICE PASSAGE ANSWER KEY
1. C   2. E   3. E   4. B   5. A   6. B   7. C   8. C   9. D   10. D   11. E   12. A
13. C   14. A   15. E   16. B

Quantitative Reasoning Test Review

OUTLINE

XI. Trigonometry

   A. The Cartesian Coordinate System
   B. Trigonometry of the Right Triangle
   C. The Trigonometric Functions
   D. The Trigonometric Identities

XII. Applied Mathematical Problems

   A. Percent Word Problems
   B. Ratio and Proportion Word Problems
   C. Word Problems Involving Distance, Rate, and Time
   D. Word Problems Involving the Work Rates of Two Individuals
   E. Word Problems Using Odd and Even Integers
   F. Word Problems Involving Ages

I. INTRODUCTION TO QUANTITATIVE REASONING

The Quantitative Reasoning Test (QRT) contains 40 items. You will have 45 minutes to complete this last section of the DAT. To prepare successfully for the QRT, you need to develop your ability to reason with numbers, to manipulate numerical relationships, and to deal intelligently with quantitative materials.

Each test item is a question or an incomplete statement followed by suggested answers or completions. Read the test item and decide which choice is the best. In preparing for the test, the use of calculators, rulers, measuring devices, mathematical tables, and other study aids is not recommended because these aids are not permitted in the testing center.

II. SCOPE OF EXAMINATION

It is important to keep in mind that the goal of your review of quantitative reasoning is to score well on this section of the DAT. Mastering the fundamental concepts outlined in the scope of examination is the best method of preparation for the QRT. The following is the scope of examination, as defined by the ADA Department of Admission Testing:

- Algebraic equations
- Fractions
- Conversions (ounces, pounds, inches, feet)
- Percentages
- Exponential notation
- Probability and Statistics
- Geometry
- Trigonometry
- Applied Mathematics Problems

Check off each topic on the outline as you review the material. Doing so will ensure that you have covered all the topics outlined in the ADA's scope of examination at the end of your review.

III. FRACTION SIMPLIFICATION AND OPERATIONAL MATH WITH FRACTIONS

A fractional number is a ratio of two numbers expressed as $\frac{x}{y}$, in which x can be any positive or negative number and y can be any positive or negative number except zero. A fraction is made up of two parts, the numerator and the denominator. In $\frac{4}{9}$ the numerator is 4, which indicates how many of the 9 equal parts are considered. In $\frac{3}{8}$, 8 is the denominator which indicates the number of equal parts.

When the numerator is less than the denominator, the fraction is called a proper function, otherwise the fraction is an improper fraction.

Proper fractions: $\frac{1}{4}, \frac{3}{5}, \frac{5}{8}, \frac{6}{9}$

Improper fractions: $\frac{4}{3}, \frac{6}{4}, \frac{8}{5}, \frac{9}{7}$

Equivalent Fractions

The value of a number is unchanged if you multiply or divide the number by 1. In a fraction, multiplying the numerator and denominator by the same nonzero number is the same as multiplying the fraction by 1; therefore, the fraction is unchanged. Similarly, dividing the numerator and denominator by the same nonzero number leaves the fraction unchanged.

Example:

Multiply $\frac{1}{3}$ by $\frac{2}{2}$.

$$\frac{1 \times 2}{3 \times 2} = \frac{2}{6}$$

Reducing Fractions

Generally speaking, when you work with fractions on the DAT, you'll need to put them in *lowest terms.* That means that the numerator and the denominator are not divisible by any common integer greater than 1. For example, the fraction $\frac{1}{2}$ is in lowest terms; but the fraction $\frac{2}{8}$ is not, since 2 and 8 are both divisible by 2. The method used to put such a fraction in lowest terms is called reducing.

Example:

Reduce $\frac{18}{27}$.

$$\frac{18}{27} = \frac{2 \times 9 \div 9}{3 \times 9 \div 9} = \frac{2}{3}$$

Addition and Subtraction of Fractions

Two fractions can't be added or subtracted directly unless they have the same denominator. Therefore, before adding or subtracting, you must find a common denominator. A common denominator is a common multiple of the denominators of the fractions. The *least common denominator* (LCD) is the least common multiple—in other words, the smallest positive number that is a multiple of all the terms.

Example:

Find the LCD of $\dfrac{1}{4}$ and $\dfrac{1}{5}$.

$\dfrac{1}{4}$ = 4, 8, 12, 20, 24

$\dfrac{1}{5}$ = 5, 10, 15, 20, 25

LCD = 20

Example:

Solve: $\dfrac{5}{6} + \dfrac{3}{4} - \dfrac{7}{8}$.

$\dfrac{5}{6} + \dfrac{3}{4} - \dfrac{7}{8} = \dfrac{20}{24} + \dfrac{18}{24} - \dfrac{21}{24} = \dfrac{20 + 18 - 21}{24} = \dfrac{17}{24}$.

Multiplication of Fractions

To multiply two or more fractions, multiply their numerators to obtain the numerator of the product, then multiply the denominators to obtain the denominators of the product.

Example:

Multiply: $\dfrac{9}{10} \times \dfrac{5}{4} \times \dfrac{2}{3}$.

Calculations are greatly simplified if the fractions are put in simplest terms by cancellation of common factors. Express all the numerators and denominators in the factored form, cancel the common factors, and carry out the multiplication of the remaining factors. Cancellation lets you work with smaller rather than larger numbers in the numerator and denominator, thus decreasing the chances of error.

$$\dfrac{9}{10} \times \dfrac{5}{4} \times \dfrac{2}{3} = \dfrac{3 \times 3}{2 \times 5} \times \dfrac{5}{2 \times 2} \times \dfrac{2}{3} = \dfrac{3}{2} \times \dfrac{1}{2} \times \dfrac{1}{1} = \dfrac{3}{4}$$

Division of Fractions

Dividing is the same as multiplying by the *reciprocal* of the divisor. To get the reciprocal of a fraction, just invert the fraction by interchanging the numerator and the denominator. The reciprocal of fraction $\dfrac{x}{y}$ is $\dfrac{y}{x}$. It is important to emphasize that division by zero is impossible, therefore a fraction cannot have zero as a denominator.

Example:

Divide: $\dfrac{3}{5} \div \dfrac{2}{5}$.

$\dfrac{3}{5} \div \dfrac{2}{5} = \dfrac{3}{5} \times \dfrac{5}{2} = \dfrac{3}{2}$

Complex Fractions

A complex fraction is a fraction that contains one or more other fractions in its numerator or denominator. Treat the numerator and denominator separately. Combine the terms in each to get a single fraction on the top and a single fraction on the bottom. You are left with the division of the two fractions, which you perform by multiplying the top fraction by the reciprocal of the bottom one.

Example:

Divide: $\dfrac{\dfrac{7}{9} - \dfrac{1}{6}}{\dfrac{1}{3} + \dfrac{1}{2}}$

$$\frac{\dfrac{7}{9} - \dfrac{1}{6}}{\dfrac{1}{3} + \dfrac{1}{2}} = \frac{\dfrac{14}{18} - \dfrac{3}{18}}{\dfrac{2}{6} + \dfrac{3}{6}} = \frac{\dfrac{11}{18}}{\dfrac{5}{6}} = \frac{11}{18} \times \frac{6}{5} = \frac{11}{15}$$

Mixed Numbers

A mixed number is a number consisting of an integer and a fraction. For example, $5\frac{1}{4}$, $3\frac{2}{3}$, $8\frac{5}{6}$ are all mixed numbers. Fractions whose numerators are greater than their denominators may be converted into mixed numbers, and vice versa.

Example:

Convert $\dfrac{19}{3}$ to a mixed number.

$$\frac{19}{3} = \frac{18}{3} + \frac{1}{3} = 6\frac{1}{3}$$

Example:

Convert $5\frac{3}{4}$ to a fraction.

$$5\frac{3}{4} = 5 + \frac{3}{4} = \frac{20}{4} + \frac{3}{4} = \frac{23}{4}$$

Comparing Positive Fractions

If the numerators of two fractions are the same, the fraction with the smaller denominator will have the larger value because the numerator is divided into a smaller number of parts. If the denominators are the same, the fraction with the larger numerator will have the larger value. If neither the numerators nor the denominators are the same, express all of the fractions in terms of some common denominator. The fraction with the largest numerator will be the largest.

IV. PERCENT, DECIMAL, AND FRACTION CONVERSIONS

Percents are among the math relationships appearing most often on the DAT. Percent means "part of 100," one one-hundredth. Therefore, 21 percent (21%) means 21 hundredths, or 0.21, or $\dfrac{21}{100}$.

Percent is a special type of fraction with 100 as the denominator. A percent may always be reduced to a fraction, and then this fraction may in turn be expressed in decimal form. Thus, 25% represents the same fractional measure as $\dfrac{25}{100}$ or $\dfrac{1}{4}$, or the same decimal measure as 0.25.

Decimal to Percent Conversion

To convert a decimal fraction to an equivalent percent, multiply the decimal fraction by 100. To do this, move the decimal point two places to the right.

Example:

Express 0.45 as a percent.

$0.45 \times 100 = 45\%$

Fraction to Decimal Conversion

To convert a percent to a decimal fraction, divide the numerator by the denominator.

$$\frac{1}{4} = 0.25 \qquad \frac{1}{8} = 0.125 \qquad \frac{1}{5} = 0.20 \qquad \frac{4}{5} = 0.80$$

$$\frac{1}{2} = 0.50 \qquad \frac{3}{8} = 0.375 \qquad \frac{2}{5} = 0.40 \qquad \frac{3}{16} = 0.1875$$

$$\frac{3}{4} = 0.75 \qquad \frac{5}{8} = 0.625 \qquad \frac{3}{5} = 0.60 \qquad \frac{7}{8} = 0.875$$

Fraction to Percent Conversion

To convert a fraction to a percent, convert the fraction so that its denominator is 100. The numerator of the new fraction is the percent.

Example:

Express $\frac{8}{25}$ as a percent.

Multiply by $\frac{4}{4}$: $\frac{8}{25} \times \frac{4}{4} = \frac{32}{100} = 32\%$

$$\frac{1}{5} = 20\%$$

$$\frac{2}{5} = 40\% \qquad \frac{1}{6} = 16\frac{2}{3}\% \qquad \frac{1}{8} = 12\frac{1}{2}\%$$

$$\frac{1}{2} = 50\% \qquad \frac{1}{3} = 33\frac{1}{3}\% \qquad \frac{3}{8} = 37\frac{1}{2}\%$$

$$\frac{3}{5} = 60\% \qquad \frac{2}{3} = 66\frac{2}{3}\% \qquad \frac{5}{8} = 62\frac{1}{2}\%$$

$$\frac{4}{5} = 80\% \qquad \frac{5}{6} = 83\frac{1}{3}\% \qquad \frac{7}{8} = 87\frac{1}{2}\%$$

Word Problems Using Percent

Most percent problems can be solved by using one formula:

Percent × Whole = Part

This formula has three variables: percent, whole, and part. In percent problems, the *whole* usually follows the word *of* or a preposition; the *part* usually follows the word *is* or another verb. The percent can be represented as the ratio of the part to the whole, or the *is* to the *of*.

A percent problem usually gives you two of the variables and asks for the third. On the DAT, it is usually easiest to change the percent to a common fraction and solve from there.

Example:

What is 25% of 56?

Here you are given the percent and the whole. To find the part, change the percent to a fraction, then multiply. Use the formula above.

Since $25\% = \frac{1}{4}$ you are really asking what one-fourth of 56 is.

$$\frac{1}{4} \times 56 = 14$$

Example:

21 is $33\frac{1}{3}$ of what number?

Here you are given the percent and the part and are asked for the whole. If *Percent* × *Whole* = *Part*, then

$$Whole = \frac{Part}{Percent}$$

Since $33\frac{1}{3}\% = \frac{1}{3}$:

$$= \frac{21}{\frac{1}{3}} = 21 \times \frac{3}{1} = 63$$

Example:

24 is what percent of 8?

Here you are given the whole and the part and asked for the percent.

$$Percent = \frac{Whole}{Part}$$

Since the part and the whole are both integers, and you are looking for a percent, you will have to make the answer into a percent by multiplying by 100.

$$Percent = \frac{24}{8} \times 100 = 3 \times 100 = 300\%$$

Word Problems Using Percent Change

Percent change, percent increase, and percent decrease are special types of percent problems in which the difficulty lies in making sure to use the right numbers to calculate the percent.

$$Percent\ increase = \frac{Amount\ of\ increase}{Original\ amount} \times 100\%$$

$$Percent\ decrease = \frac{Amount\ of\ decrease}{Original\ amount} \times 100\%$$

Example:

An item is priced 20 percent more than its wholesale cost. If the wholesale cost was $800, what is the price of the item?

The original amount is $800, and the percent increase is 20%. Change 20% to a fraction, $\frac{1}{5}$, and use the formula.

$$Amount\ of\ increase = Percent\ increase \times Original\ amount$$

$$= 20\% \times \$800$$

$$= \frac{1}{5} \times \$800 = \$160$$

To find the new amount (the new selling price):

$$New\ amount = Original\ amount + Amount\ of\ Increase$$

$$= \$800 + \$160 = \$960$$

On some problems, you'll need to find more than one percent or to find a percent of a percent. You can't add percents unless they are percents of the same amount.

Example:
A $100 chair is increased in price by 50 percent. If the chair is then discounted by 50 percent of the new price, at what price will it be offered for sale?

First, you know that the price of the chair is increased by 50%. That is the same as saying that the price becomes (100% + 50%), or 150%, of what it originally was. 150% of $100 is equal to $\frac{3}{2} \times$ $100, or $150. Then, this price is reduced by 50%. Since 50% $\times$ $150 = $75, the final price of the chair is $150 – $75 = $75.

V. EXPONENTIAL NOTATION; CONVERSION TO AND FROM EXPONENTIAL NOTATION

A number is said to be in scientific notation if it is expressed as the product of a number between 1 and 10 and some integral power of 10. For example, 10,000 is written in scientific notation as 1.0×10^4 or, more simply, as 10^4; 0.001 is written as 10^{-3}; $2,378 = 2.378 \times 10^3$; $0.000398 = 3.98 \times 10^{-4}$.

Since the decimal point of any number can be shifted at will to the left or to the right by multiplying by an appropriate power of 10, any number can be expressed in exponential notation. In general, x is any number; we write $x = a \times 10^z$, where a is a number between 1 and 10 and z is an integer, positive or negative.

Example:
Write 10,000 in exponential notation.

The decimal point in 10,000 is after the last zero. The first significant number is 1. Move the decimal point to the left four places (1.0000). Multiply by 10^4 to obtain the number in exponential notation: $10,000 = 1.0 \times 10^4$, or, more simply, 10^4.

Example:
Write 0.0002367 in exponential notation.

Move the decimal point to the right four places. The resulting number is $0.0002367 = 2.367 \times 10^{-4}$.

VI. POWERS AND ROOTS

In the term $4x^2$, 4 is the *coefficient*, x is the *base*, and 2 is the *exponent*. The exponent refers to the number of times the base is multiplied by itself, or how many times the base is a factor. For instance, in 2^3, there are three factors of 2: $2 \times 2 \times 2 = 8$.

When a number is multiplied by itself twice, the result is called the *square* of that number; for example x^2 is x squared. When a number is multiplied by itself three times, the result is called the *cube* of that number, for example x^3 is x cubed.

To multiply two terms with the same base, keep the base and add the exponents.

For example: $4^3 \times 4^5 = 4^{3+5} = 4^8$

To divide two terms with the same base, keep the base and subtract the exponent of the denominator from the exponent of the numerator.

For example: $x^5 \div x^3 = \dfrac{x^5}{x^3} = x^{5-3} = x^2$

To raise a power to another power, multiply the exponents.

For example: $(5^3)^2 = 5^{2\times3} = 5^6$

Any nonzero number raised to the zero power is equal to 1: $x^0 = 1$ if $x \neq 0$. The quantity 0^0 is undefined.

A negative exponent indicates a reciprocal. To arrive at an equivalent expression, take the reciprocal of the base and change the sign of the exponent. $x^{-n} = \dfrac{1}{x^n}$.

For example: $3^{-4} = \dfrac{1}{3^4} = \dfrac{1}{81}$

A fractional exponent indicates a *root*: $(x)^{\frac{1}{n}} = \sqrt[n]{x}$ (Read as "the nth root of x." If no n is present, the radical sign signifies a square root.)

For example: $9^{\frac{1}{2}} = \sqrt{9} = 3$

Every positive number has two square roots, one positive and one negative. The positive square root of 16 is 4, since $4^2 = 16$; and the negative square root of 16 is –4, since $(-4)^2 = 16$ also.

By convention, the symbol $\sqrt{\ }$ (radical) means the *positive* square root only.

For example: $\sqrt{25} = +5$; $-\sqrt{25} = -5$

In performing the four basic arithmetic operations, radicals are treated in much the same way as variables.

Addition and Subtraction of Radicals
Only like radicals can be added to or subtracted from one another.

For example: $3\sqrt{2} - 4\sqrt{3} + 5\sqrt{2} + 2\sqrt{3} = (3\sqrt{2} + 5\sqrt{2}) + (2\sqrt{3} - 4\sqrt{3})$
$$= 8\sqrt{2} + (-2\sqrt{3})$$
$$= 8\sqrt{2} - 2\sqrt{3}$$
$$4\sqrt{2} - \sqrt{2} + 2\sqrt{3} = (4\sqrt{2} - \sqrt{2}) + 2\sqrt{3}$$
$$= 3\sqrt{2} + 2\sqrt{3}$$

Multiplication and Division of Radicals
To multiply or divide one radical by another, multiply or divide the number outside the radical signs, then the numbers inside the radical signs.

For example: $3\sqrt{5} \times 4\sqrt{3} = (3 \times 4) \circ (\sqrt{5} \times \sqrt{3}) = 12\sqrt{3 \times 5} = 12\sqrt{15}$
$$9\sqrt{15} \div 3\sqrt{5} = (9 \div 3) \circ (\sqrt{15} \div \sqrt{5}) = 3\sqrt{\dfrac{15}{5}} = 3\sqrt{3}$$
$$\dfrac{6\sqrt{18}}{3\sqrt{6}} = \left(\dfrac{6}{3}\right)\left(\dfrac{\sqrt{18}}{\sqrt{6}}\right) = 2\sqrt{\dfrac{18}{6}} = 2\sqrt{3}$$

If the number inside the radical is a multiple of a perfect square, the expression can be simplified by factoring out the perfect square.

For example: $\sqrt{48} = \sqrt{16 \times 3} = \sqrt{16} \times \sqrt{3} = 4\sqrt{3}$

VII. THE TWO COMMON SYSTEMS OF MEASUREMENT

The DAT candidate is expected to understand and operate in either the metric system of measurement or the system of common British units. You may be required to perform conversions from one system to the other.

A. The Common British System

You should know the following equivalences and abbreviations:

1 yard (yd.) = 3 feet (ft.) = 36 inches (in.)
1 foot = 12 inches
1 mile (mi.) = 5,280 feet = 1,760 yards
1 pound (lb.) = 16 ounces (oz.)
1 ton (T.) = 2,000 pounds
1 gallon (gal.) = 4 quarts (qt.) = 8 pints (pt.)
1 quart = 2 pints
1 pint = 16 fluid ounces

This table of equivalencies permits conversions within the British system.

Example:
How many ounces are there in 2 tons?

$$2 \text{ tons} \times \frac{2,000 \text{ lb.}}{\text{ton}} \times \frac{16 \text{ oz.}}{\text{lb.}}$$

$2 \times 2,000 \times 16$ oz. $= 64,000$ oz.

Note that the names of units that appear once in the numerator and once in the denominator are canceled. This cancellation leaves only the name of the unit, *oz.*, in which the answer is expressed.

B. The Metric System

The basic units for the metric system are as follows:

length: meters (m)
volume: liters (L)
mass: grams (g)

The following prefixes are attached to the names of the basic units to denote other units whose size equals the basic unit multiplied or divided by a power of 10:

pico- (p) $= 10^{-12}$
nano- (n) $= 10^{-9}$
micro- (μ) $= 10^{-6}$
milli- (m) $= 10^{-3}$
centi- (c) $= 10^{-2}$
deci- (d) $= 10^{-1}$
kilo- (k) $= 10^{3}$
mega- (M) $= 10^{6}$

Thus, a kilometer (km) is 10^3 or 1,000 times as large as a meter. A centimeter (cm) is 10^{-2} times a meter or $\frac{1}{100}$ the size of a meter. A milligram (mg) is 10^{-3} times the size of a gram or $\frac{1}{1000}$ the size of a gram.

VIII. ALGEBRAIC EQUATIONS

A *term* is a numerical constant or the product (or quotient) of a numerical constant and one or more variables.

For example: $5x$, $3abc$, $\dfrac{2x}{y}$

An *algebraic* expression is a combination of one or more terms. The terms in an expression are separated by either $+$ or $-$ signs.

For example: $5xy$, $3ab + 2cd$.

In the term $5xy$, the numerical constant 5 is called a coefficient. In a simple term such as z, 1 is the coefficient.

A number without any variables is called a *constant term*. An expression with one term, such as $5xy$, is called a *monomial;* one with two terms, such as $6a - 2b$, is a *binomial*. The general name for expressions with more than one term is *polynomial*.

Substitution is a method used to evaluate an algebraic expression or to express an algebraic expression in terms of other variables.

Example:
Evaluate $x^2 + 3x + 3$ when $x = -3$.

Replace every x in the expression with -3, and then carry out the designated operations.

$$x^2 + 3x + 3 = (-3)^2 + 3(-3) + 3 = 9 + (-9) + 3 = 3$$

Example:
Express $\dfrac{a + b}{2a}$ in terms of x and y if $a = 2x$ and $b = 3y$.

Replace every a with $2x$ and every b with $3y$:
$$\frac{a + b}{2a} = \frac{2x + 3y}{2(2x)} = \frac{2x + 3y}{4x}$$

A. Linear Equations

An *equation* is an algebraic sentence that says two expressions are equal to each other. The two expressions may consist of numbers, variables, and arithmetic operations to be performed on these numbers and variables. To solve for some variable, manipulate the equation until that variable is isolated on one side of the equal sign, leaving any numbers or other variables on the other side. Of course, you must be careful to manipulate the equation only in accordance with the *equality postulate:* Whenever an operation is performed on one side of the equation, the same operation must be performed on the other side. Otherwise, the two sides of the equation will no longer be equal.

A *linear* or *first-degree equation* is an equation in which all the variables are raised to the first power. To solve such an equation, perform operations on both sides of the equation in order to get the variable for which you are solving alone on one side. The operations you can perform without upsetting the balance of the equation are addition and subtraction, and multiplication or division by a number other than zero. Typically, at each step in the process, you will need to use the reverse of the operation that is being applied to the variable in order to isolate the variable.

Example:

If $3x - 8 = x + 6$, what is x?

1. To get all the terms with the variable on one side of the equation, first add $-x$ to each side. Then combine the terms.

$$3x - 8 = x + 6$$
$$3x - x - 8 = x - x + 6$$
$$2x - 8 = 6$$

2. To get the constant terms on the other side of the equation, add $+8$ to each side.

$$2x - 8 + 8 = 6 + 8$$
$$2x = 14$$

3. Isolate the variable by dividing both sides by its coefficient.

$$\frac{2x}{2} = \frac{14}{2}$$
$$x = 7$$

You can easily check your work when solving this kind of equation. The answer you arrive at represents the value of the variable that makes the equation hold true. Therefore, to check that your answer is correct, just substitute this value for the variable in the original equation. If the equation holds true, you've found the correct answer.

Equations with fractional coefficients can be a little more tricky. They can be solved using the same approach, although this often leads to rather involved calculations. Instead, an equation of this type can be transformed into an equivalent equation that does not involve fractional coefficients.

Example:

Solve for x: $\dfrac{5x + 7}{2} = 8 + x$.

1. Multiply both sides of the equation by the lowest common denominator (LCD). Here the LCD is 2.

$$2\left(\frac{5x + 7}{2}\right) = 2\left(\frac{8 + x}{1}\right)$$

2. Clear the parentheses using the distributive property.

$$5x + 7 = 2(8 + x)$$
$$5x + 7 = 16 + 2x$$

3. Get all the terms with the variable on one side. Combine like terms.

$$5x - 2x = 16 - 7$$
$$3x = 9$$

4. Isolate the variable by dividing both sides by its coefficient.

$$x = \frac{9}{3} = 3$$

B. Inequalities

An *inequality* is a statement that two quantities are not equal.

Inequality symbols

The following symbols are used to denote inequality:

>   greater than
<   less than
≥   greater than or equal to
≤   less than or equal to

Solving Inequalities

The same methods are used to solve inequalities as are used in solving equations, with one exception: If the inequality is multiplied or divided by a negative number, the direction of the inequality is reversed. Thus, if the inequality $-5x < 10$ is multiplied by -1, the resulting inequality is $5x > -10$.

Example:
Solve for x: $3x - 16 > 4x + 12$.

$$3x - 4x - 16 > 4x - 4x + 12$$
$$-x - 16 + 16 > 12 + 16$$
$$-x > 28$$
$$x < 28$$

C. Simultaneous Equations

Two different equations with two variables (that is, *simultaneous equations*) can be combined to obtain a unique solution set. Isolate the variable in one equation, then plug that expression into the other equation.

Example:
Find the values for x and y if $x = 9 - 2y$ and $2x - 3y = 4$.

1. You know that $x = 9 - 2y$.
   Substitute $9 - 2y$ for x
   in the second equation.

   $$2x - 3y = 4$$
   $$2(9 - 2y) - 3y = 4$$
   $$18 - 4y - 3y = 4$$

2. Solve for y.

   $$-7y = -14$$
   $$y = 2$$

3. To find the value of x,
   substitute 2 for y in the
   first equation and solve.

   $$x = 9 - 2y$$
   $$= 9 - 2(2)$$
   $$= 5$$

IX. PROBABILITY AND STATISTICS CONCEPTS

Here is the classic definition of probability: The probability of event A equals the number of favorable outcomes of A divided by the total number of outcomes.

$$P(A) = \frac{Favorable\ outcomes}{Total\ outcomes}$$

To use this definition, we must be dealing with equally likely, mutually exclusive events. When two or more outcomes of an experiment cannot occur at the same time, the outcomes are said to be *mutually exclusive*. If no outcome is any more likely to occur than any other, the outcomes are said to be *equally likely*.

For instance, consider an ordinary deck of playing cards. If an experiment consists of drawing one card at random from the well-shuffled deck, then there are 52 equally likely outcomes because any one of the 52 cards may be drawn. It is logical to decide that the outcomes are equally likely because, if the deck is well shuffled and a card is drawn at random, there is no reason to expect any card to be more likely to be drawn than any other. Moreover, on any draw of a single card, just one card and no other will be picked, so the outcomes are mutually exclusive.

Example:
Find the probability of drawing a black card in a single random draw from a well-shuffled deck of ordinary playing cards.

There are 52 cards; hence the experiment has 52 outcomes. We reason that each of these 52 outcomes is equally likely. Also, only one card can be drawn on any draw, so the outcomes are mutually exclusive. The "event" in which we are interested is drawing a black card. There are 26 black cards in the deck, so the number of favorable outcomes of the event is 26. Thus, we have

$$P(\text{drawing a black card}) = \frac{\text{Favorable outcomes}}{\text{Total outcomes}} = \frac{26}{52} = \frac{1}{2}$$

Example:
Find the probability of drawing an ace from a deck of cards on a single draw.

There are four aces in the deck. Hence, four of the 52 possible outcomes of the experiment correspond to the event of drawing an ace. Therefore, we have

$$P(\text{drawing an ace}) = \frac{\text{Favorable outcomes}}{\text{Total outcomes}} = \frac{4}{52} = \frac{1}{13}$$

There are numerous other "ideal" situations involving dice, coins, balls of different colors, and so on that can be used to illustrate the finding of the probability of elementary events by application of the classical definition of probability.

A. Measures of Location

The Midrange

The midrange is the number halfway between the smallest and the largest observation. By definition:

$$\text{Midrange} = \frac{\text{Smallest observation} + \text{Largest observation}}{2}$$

Example:
A sample consists of the observations 51, 47, 62, 54, 58, 65, 48, 41. The smallest observation is 41, and the largest is 65. Thus we have

$$Midrange = \frac{41 + 65}{2} = \frac{106}{2} = 53$$

The Mode

The mode is defined as the observation in the sample that occurs most frequently. If each observation occurs the same number of times, there is no mode. If two or more observations occur the same number of times, there is more than one mode, and the sample is said to be *multimodal*. For example: If the sample is 14, 19, 16, 21, 18, 19, 24, 15, 19, the mode is 19. If the sample is 6, 7, 7, 3, 8, 5, 3, 9, there are two modes, 3 and 7.

The Median

If the sample observations are arranged in order from smallest to largest, the median is defined as the middle observation if the number of observations is *odd*, and as the number halfway between the two middle observations if the number of observations is *even*.

Example:

Given the observations 34, 29, 26, 37, 31. Arranging the observations in order, we have 26, 29, 31, 34, and 37. The number of observations is odd; the median is 31.

Given the observations 34, 29, 26, 37, 31, 34. Arranging the observations in order, we have 26, 29, 31, 34, 34, 37. The number of observations is even. The median is halfway between the third and fourth observations. Thus the median is 32.5.

The Arithmetic Mean

A commonly used quantitative measurement is the arithmetic mean or average. The definition is simple:

$$Mean = \frac{Sum\ of\ observations}{Number\ of\ observations}$$

The number of observations is usually denoted as n. Also, the first observation is denoted as x_1, the second observation as x_2, the third as x_3, and so on, with the last observation denoted as x_n. The mean of the sample is denoted by the symbol $\bar{x}$. Thus the definition can be rewritten as:

$$\bar{x} = \frac{x_1 + x_2 + x_3 + \ldots + x_n}{n}$$

Example:

If a sample consists of the observations 8, 7, 11, 8, 12, 14, what is the mean?

$$Mean = \bar{x} = \frac{8 + 7 + 11 + 8 + 12 + 14}{6} = \frac{60}{6} = 10$$

B. Measures of Variation

The variance and the standard deviation are measures of the spread of a set of measurements.

Sample Variance

The variance, like the mean, takes into account each value in a set of data. It is calculated by taking the average value of the squares of the deviation for each point from the mean. The sample variance formula is used when you have sample data and you are trying to estimate the population variance.

The variance (s^2) of a set of measurements $x_1, x_2, \ldots, x_n$ is defined as follows:

$$s^2 = \frac{\Sigma\ (x - \bar{x})^2}{n - 1}$$

$$= \frac{(x_1 - \bar{x})^2 + (x_2 - \bar{x})^2 + \ldots + (x_n - \bar{x})^2}{n - 1}$$

where $\bar{x}$ is the sample mean.

Standard Deviation

The variance and the standard deviation are intimately related. The standard deviation(s) is the square root of the variance.

$$s = \sqrt{s^2}$$

Example:

The number of kilometers, denoted as x_1, x_2, and x_3, that three cars traveled were 931, 972, and 935, respectively. Find the variance and the standard deviation for these data.

First, find the sample mean $(\bar{x})$:

$$\bar{x} = \frac{x_1 + x_2 + x_3 + \ldots + x_n}{n} = \frac{931 + 972 + 935}{3} = 946$$

Now find the sample variance:

$$s^2 = \frac{\Sigma (x - \bar{x})^2}{n - 1}$$

$$= \frac{(x_1 - \bar{x})^2 + (x_2 - \bar{x})^2 + \ldots + (x_n - \bar{x})^2}{n - 1}$$

$$= \frac{(931 - 946)^2 + (972 - 946)^2 + (935 - 946)^2}{3 - 1}$$

$$= \frac{225 + 676 + 121}{2} = \frac{1022}{2} = 511$$

Finally, use the sample variance to find the sample standard deviation:

$$s = \sqrt{s^2} = \sqrt{511} = 22.6$$

X. PLANE GEOMETRY CONCEPTS

A. Angles

An *angle* is formed by two lines or line segments intersecting at a point. The point of intersection is called the *vertex* of the angle. Angles are measured in degrees (°) or radians.

An *acute angle* is an angle whose degree measure is between 0° and 90°. A *right angle* is an angle whose degree measure is exactly 90°. An *obtuse angle* is an angle whose degree measure is between 90° and 180°. A *straight angle* is an angle whose degree measure is exactly 180°.

Two angles are *complementary* if together they make up a right angle (i.e., if the sum of their measures is 90°). Two angles are *supplementary* if together they make up a straight angle (i.e. if the sum of their measures is 180°).

B. Triangles

A *triangle* is a closed figure with three angles and three straight sides. The sum of the interior angles of any triangle is 180°.

The *altitude* (or height) of a triangle is the perpendicular distance from a vertex to the side opposite the vertex. The altitude may fall inside the triangle, outside the triangle, or on one of the sides.

The *perimeter* of a triangle is the distance around the triangle. In other words, the perimeter is equal to the sum of the lengths of the sides.

The *area* of a triangle can be found by using this formula:

$$Area = \frac{1}{2} \, Base \times Height$$

$$A = \frac{1}{2}bh$$

Similar and Congruent Triangles

Triangles are *similar* if they have the same shape, that is, if corresponding angles have the same measure. For instance, any two triangles whose angles measure 30°, 60°, and 90° are similar. In similar triangles, corresponding sides are in the same ratio.

Triangles are *congruent* if corresponding angles have the same measure and corresponding sides have the same length.

Example:
What is the perimeter of $\triangle ABC$ below?

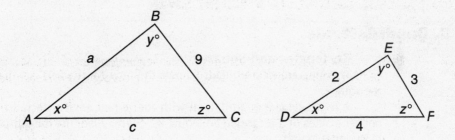

Each triangle, *ABC* and *DEF*, has an $x°$ angle, a $y°$ angle, and a $z°$ angle; therefore, triangles are similar, and corresponding sides are in the same ratio. *BC* and *EF* are corresponding sides; each is opposite the $x°$ angle. Since *BC* is three times the length of *EF*, each side of $\triangle ABC$ will be three times the length of the corresponding side of $\triangle DEF$. Therefore *AB* = 3(*DE*) or 6, and *AC* = 3(*DF*) or 12. The perimeter of $\triangle ABC$ is 6 + 12 + 9 = 27.

The ratio of the *areas* of two similar triangles is the *square* of the ratio of corresponding lengths. For instance, in the example above, since each side of $\triangle ABC$ is three times the length of the corresponding side of $\triangle DEF$, $\triangle ABC$ must have 3^2 or 9 times the area of $\triangle DEF$.

Right Triangles

A right triangle has one interior angle of 90°. The longest side, which lies opposite the right triangle, is called the *hypotenuse*. The other two sides are the *legs*.

The *Pythagorean theorem,* which holds for all right triangles, states that the square of the length of the hypotenuse is equal to the sum of the squares of the length of the legs.

$$(Leg_1)^2 + (Leg_2)^2 = (Hypotenuse)^2$$

Some sets of integers happen to satisfy the Pythagorean theorem and are commonly referred to as *Pythagorean triplets.* One very common set that you might remember is 3, 4, and 5. Since $3^2 + 4^2 = 5^2$, you can have a right triangle with legs of lengths 3 and 4 and hypotenuse of length 5. In addition, any multiple of these lengths makes another Pythagorean triplet; for instance, $6^2 + 8^2 = 10^2$, so 6, 8, and 10 also make a right triangle. One other triplet that appears occasionally is 5, 12, and 13.

The Pythagorean theorem is very useful whenever you are given the lengths of two sides of a right triangle; you can find the length of the third side with the Pythagorean theorem.

Example:

What is the length of the hypotenuse of a right triangle with legs of lengths 6 and 7?

Use the Pythagorean theorem: The square of the length of the hypotenuse equals the sum of the squares of the lengths of the legs. Here the legs are 6 and 7, so

$$\begin{aligned} Hypotenuse^2 &= 6^2 + 7^2 \\ &= 36 + 49 \\ &= 85 \\ &= \sqrt{85} \end{aligned}$$

C. Quadrilaterals

Rectangles and Squares

The most important quadrilaterals to know for the DAT are the rectangle and the square.

A *rectangle* is a quadrilateral with four equal angles, each a right angle. The opposite sides of a rectangle are equal in length. Also, the diagonals of a rectangle have equal lengths.

A *square* is a rectangle with four equal sides.

Areas of Quadrilaterals

To find the *area of a rectangle,* multiply the lengths of any two adjacent sides, called the length and width:

$$Area\ of\ rectangle = Length \times Width$$

$$A = lw$$

To find the *area of a square,* since the length and width are equal, square the length of the side:

$$Area\ of\ square = (side)^2$$

$$A = s^2$$

D. Circles

A circle is the set of all points in a plane at the same distance from a certain point. This point is called the *center* of the circle.

The *diameter* is a line segment that connects two points on the circle and passes through the center of the circle.

The *radius* is a line segment from the center of the circle to any point on the circle. The length of the radius of a circle is one-half the length of the diameter.

The *circumference* is the distance around the circle. The number π (pi) is the ratio of a circle's circumference to its diameter. The value of π is 3.1415926..., usually approximated as 3.14.

Since π equals the ratio of the circumference to the diameter, a formula for the circumference is:

$$Circumference = \pi \; (diameter) \qquad or \qquad Circumference = 2\pi \; (radius)$$

$$C = \pi d \qquad or \qquad C = 2\pi r$$

The *area of a circle* is given by the formula:

$$Area = \pi(radius)^2$$

$$A = \pi r^2$$

XI. TRIGONOMETRY

A. The Cartesian Coordinate System

In trigonometry, you will frequently find it necessary to describe the position of a point in a plane. You'll use the *Cartesian* or *rectangular* coordinate system to do this. For a point (x,y) in the Cartesian plane, the first, or x, coordinate determines the location of that point with respect to the horizontal, or x, axis, and the second, or y, coordinate determines the location of that point with respect to the vertical or y axis. The origin of the Cartesian coordinate system is point $(0,0)$.

The Distance Formula

If $A(x_1, y_1)$ and $B(x_2, y_2)$ are two points in a Cartesian plane, the *distance* between them, d_{AB}, is the length of the straight line segment joining the two points.

$$d_{AB} = \sqrt{(x_2 - x_1)^2 + (y_2 - y_1)^2}$$

Example:
Find the distance between points $(-2,3)$ and $(2,-3)$.

$$d = \sqrt{(-2 - 2)^2 + (3 - (-3))^2} = \sqrt{(-4)^2 + 6^2} = \sqrt{52} = 7.21$$

Example:
Find the lengths of the sides of the triangle whose vertices are at $A(9,4)$, $B(3,8)$, and $C(0,1)$.

$$d_{AB} = \sqrt{(9 - 3)^2 + (4 - 8)^2} = \sqrt{6^2 + (-4)^2} = \sqrt{52} = 7.21$$

$$d_{AC} = \sqrt{(9 - 0)^2 + (4 - 1)^2} = \sqrt{9^2 + 3^2} = \sqrt{90} = 9.49$$

$$d_{BC} = \sqrt{(3 - 0)^2 + (8 - 1)^2} = \sqrt{3^2 + 7^2} = \sqrt{58} = 7.62$$

Application of the Distance Formula to Circles

If (x,y) is a point on a circle with the center at the origin and radius r, the distance between (x,y) and $(0,0)$ is r.

Applying the distance formula to (x,y) and $(0,0)$ gives:

$$\sqrt{(x - 0)^2 + (y - 0)^2} = r$$

Simplifying and squaring both sides of the equation leads to the equation of a circle with radius r centered at the origin.

$$x^2 + y^2 = r^2$$

Example:
Find the equation for a circle with the center at the origin if $r = 2$.

Substituting into the simplified equation for a circle centered at the origin, the equation is:

$$x^2 + y^2 = 4$$

Example:
If the equation of a circle is as follows:

$$x^2 + y^2 = 25$$

What is the radius of the circle?

$$r^2 = 25$$
$$r = \sqrt{25} = 5$$

B. Trigonometry of the Right Triangle

A *right triangle* contains one 90° angle and two acute angles (less than 90°). By definition, y is the length of the leg opposite θ, x is the length of the leg adjacent to θ, where θ is one of the acute angles. The hypotenuse is the terminal side of θ, and its length is designated as h.

x = side adjacent

C. The Trigonometric Functions

The six trigonometric functions are the *sine, cosine, tangent, cosecant, secant,* and *cotangent* of an angle θ. They are defined as follows:

$$\sin \theta = \frac{\text{side opposite } \theta}{\text{hypotenuse}} = \frac{y}{h} \qquad \csc \theta = \frac{\text{hypotenuse}}{\text{side opposite } \theta} = \frac{h}{y}$$

$$\cos \theta = \frac{\text{side adjacent } \theta}{\text{hypotenuse}} = \frac{x}{h} \qquad \sec \theta = \frac{\text{hypotenuse}}{\text{side adjacent } \theta} = \frac{h}{x}$$

$$\tan \theta = \frac{\text{side opposite } \theta}{\text{side adjacent } \theta} = \frac{y}{x} \qquad \cot \theta = \frac{\text{side adjacent } \theta}{\text{side opposite } \theta} = \frac{x}{y}$$

Example:
Use the right triangle to find the six trigonometric functions of angle θ.
For θ:

$$\sin \theta = \frac{\text{side opposite } \theta}{\text{hypotenuse}} = \frac{3}{5} \qquad \csc \theta = \frac{\text{hypotenuse}}{\text{side opposite } \theta} = \frac{5}{3}$$

$$\cos \theta = \frac{\text{side adjacent } \theta}{\text{hypotenuse}} = \frac{4}{5} \qquad \sec \theta = \frac{\text{hypotenuse}}{\text{side adjacent } \theta} = \frac{5}{4}$$

$$\tan \theta = \frac{\text{side opposite } \theta}{\text{side adjacent } \theta} = \frac{3}{4} \qquad \cot \theta = \frac{\text{side adjacent } \theta}{\text{side opposite } \theta} = \frac{4}{3}$$

Numerical Range of the Trigonometric Functions

The length of the hypotenuse of any right angle is never less than the length of either of the other two legs; the values of the sine and cosine of an acute angle can never be greater than $+1$ or less than -1. Similarly, the values of the cosecant and secant, since they are reciprocals of the sine and cosine, can never take values between -1 and $+1$. Because the legs of a right triangle can be in any ratio to each other, however, the values of the tangent and cotangent can vary from arbitrarily large negative numbers to arbitrarily large positive values.

Complementary Angles

The two acute angles in a right triangle with a combined measure of 90° are *complementary angles*. The sine of an angle equals the cosine of its complementary angle. If $<A + <B = \frac{1}{2}\pi$, then:

$$\sin A = \frac{y}{h} = \cos B \qquad \csc A = \frac{h}{y} = \sec B$$

$$\cos A = \frac{x}{h} = \sin B \qquad \sec A = \frac{h}{x} = \csc B$$

$$\tan A = \frac{y}{x} = \cot B \qquad \cot A = \frac{y}{x} = \tan B$$

VALUES OF THE TRIGONOMETRIC FUNCTIONS FOR SELECTED ACUTE ANGLES

$\theta°$	(RADIANS)	SIN θ	COS θ	TAN θ	CSC θ	SEC θ	COT θ
0	(0)	0	1	0	Undefined	1	Undefined
30	$\left(\frac{\pi}{6}\right)$	$\frac{1}{2}$	$\frac{\sqrt{3}}{2}$	$\frac{\sqrt{3}}{3}$	2	$\frac{2\sqrt{3}}{3}$	$\sqrt{3}$
45	$\left(\frac{\pi}{4}\right)$	$\frac{\sqrt{2}}{2}$	$\frac{\sqrt{2}}{2}$	1	$\sqrt{2}$	$\sqrt{2}$	1
60	$\left(\frac{\pi}{3}\right)$	$\frac{\sqrt{3}}{2}$	$\frac{1}{2}$	$\sqrt{3}$	$\frac{2\sqrt{3}}{3}$	2	$\frac{\sqrt{3}}{3}$
90	$\left(\frac{\pi}{2}\right)$	1	0	Undefined	1	Undefined	0

Solving for Right Triangles

You can solve for right triangles by determining the two acute angles and the lengths of the three sides of the triangle. A trigonometric ratio of an acute angle involves three quantities: the length of two sides and an angle. Thus, given two of these quantities, either the length of one side and the measure of one angle, or the lengths of two sides, you can find the third.

Given the lengths of two sides of a right triangle, you can use the Pythagorean theorem to determine the length of the remaining side. You can then find any trigonometric function for either of the two unknown angles. Once you know one of the acute angles, you can find the other angle because the sum of the acute angles is 90°.

D. The Trigonometric Identities

The following trigonometric identities are consequences of the definitions of the six trigonometric functions given on page 298.

Reciprocal Identities

$$\frac{1}{\sin \theta} = \frac{1}{\frac{y}{h}} = \frac{h}{y} = \csc \theta \qquad \sin \theta \csc \theta = 1$$

$$\frac{1}{\cos \theta} = \frac{1}{\frac{x}{h}} = \frac{h}{x} = \sec \theta \qquad \cos \theta \sec \theta = 1$$

$$\frac{1}{\tan \theta} = \frac{1}{\frac{y}{x}} = \frac{x}{y} = \cot \theta \qquad \tan \theta \cot \theta = 1$$

Pythagorean Identities

$$\cos^2 \theta + \sin^2 \theta = 1$$

$$1 + \tan^2 \theta = \sec^2 \theta$$

$$1 + \cot^2 \theta = \csc^2 \theta$$

Ratio Identities

$$\tan \theta = \frac{y}{k} = \frac{\frac{y}{h}}{\frac{x}{h}} = \frac{\sin \theta}{\cos \theta}$$

$$\cot \theta = \frac{x}{y} = \frac{\frac{x}{h}}{\frac{y}{h}} = \frac{\cos \theta}{\sin \theta}$$

Verifying Trigonometric Identities

By applying algebraic processes such as factorization, addition, multiplication, and simplification of fractions to the fundamental identities, you can verify trigonometric identities.

Example:
Simplify $\sin^4 \theta - \cos^4 \theta$.

Factor as the difference of two squares, and use $\sin^2 \theta + \cos^2 \theta = 1$.

$$\sin^4 \theta - \cos^4 \theta = (\sin^2 \theta - \cos^2 \theta)(\sin^2 \theta + \cos^2 \theta)$$

$$= (\sin^2 \theta - \cos^2 \theta)(1)$$

$$= 1 - \cos^2 \theta - \cos^2 \theta$$

$$= 1 - 2\cos^2\theta$$

XII. APPLIED MATHEMATICAL PROBLEMS

Many people dislike word problems and not unreasonably. Turning a word problem into a straightforward question means that you must go to the trouble of translating the problem before you start working on it, but in some ways this actually makes the problem easier. The test makers figure that they have made the problem difficult enough by adding the extra step of translating from English to math. Once you have done this, however, you will generally find that the concepts and processes involved are rather simple, so that you stand an excellent chance of being able to solve the problem.

Here are a few general tips for solving word problems:

- Read through the whole problem first, without pausing for details, to get a sense of what is involved.
- Name the variables in a way that makes it easy to remember what they stand for. For example, denote the unknown quantity John's age as j, and the unknown quantity Brian's age as b.
- Be aware that, when you are asked to find numerical values for unknown quantities, the word problem will give you enough information to set up a sufficient number of equations to solve for those quantities.
- Be careful of the order in which you translate terms. For example, consider the following common mistranslation: 3 less than $4x$ equals 9. This translates as $4x - 3 = 9$, not $3 - 4x = 9$.

A. Percent Word Problems

Profit and Loss

The *profit* made on an item is the selling price minus the cost to the seller. If the cost is more than the selling price, there is a *loss*, not a profit.

Example:

If a camera priced at $360 represents a potential profit of 20% to a store if sold, what was the original cost of the camera to the store?

Let C represent the cost, then set up the equation to find the cost:

$$Cost\ +\ Profit\ =\ Selling\ price$$

$$C + (20\%)C = \$360$$

$$C + \frac{1}{5}C = \$360$$

$$\frac{6}{5}C = \$360$$

$$C = \$360 \times \frac{5}{6} = \$300$$

The cost of the camera to the store was $300.

Gross and Net

Gross is the total amount before any deductions are made; *net* is the amount after deductions are made. For instance, gross pay is the total amount of money earned, while net pay is gross pay minus any deductions, such as taxes.

Discount

The *discount* on an item is usually a percent of a previous price for the item.

Example:

What is the percent discount on a jacket marked down from $120 to $100?

The percent discount equals the amount of discount divided by the original price. The amount of discount is $120 – $100 or $20. The original price was $120. The percent discount equals:

$$Percent\ discount\ =\ \frac{Amount\ of\ discount}{Original\ price}$$

$$=\ \frac{\$120 - \$100}{\$120}\ =\ \frac{\$20}{\$120}\ =\ \frac{1}{6}\ =\ 16\frac{2}{3}\%$$

B. Ratio and Proportion Word Problems

A *ratio* is a comparison of two quantities by division. A ratio may be written with a fraction bar $\left(\dfrac{x}{y}\right)$, with a colon ($x$:$y$), or in words (ratio of x to y). In a ratio of two numbers, the numerator is often associated with the word *of*; the denominator with the word *to*.

We frequently deal with ratios by working with a *proportion*. A proportion is simply an equation in which two ratios are set equal to one another.

Example:

There are 32 marbles in a bag containing only blue and green marbles. If there are three green marbles for every blue marble, how many blue marbles are in the bag?

Translate from English into math. "Three green marbles for every blue marble" means the ratio of green to blue = 3:1.

Set up a proportion with a part to whole ratio to find the number of blue marbles. The ratio of the number of blue marbles to the total number of marbles is 1:[1 + 3] or 1:4.

Using b for the number of blue marbles, you have the proportion:

$$\frac{1}{4} = \frac{b}{32}$$

$$4b = 32$$

$$b = 8$$

There are eight blue marbles in the bag.

C. Word Problems Involving Distance, Rate, and Time

The solution of distance problems is based on this formula:

$$Distance = Rate \times Time$$

Example:

A car travels 60 kilometers in 1 hour before a piston breaks, then travels at 30 kilometers per hour for the remaining 60 kilometers to its destination. What is the average speed, in kilometers per hour for the entire trip?

The average speed equals the total distance the car travels divided by the total time. You are told that the car goes 60 kilometers in 1 hour before a piston breaks, and then travels another 60 kilometers at 30 kilometers per hour. The second part of the trip must take 2 hours, so the car travels a total of 120 kilometers and covers this distance in 3 hours. Its average speed equals

$$Rate = \frac{Distance}{Time}$$

$$= \frac{120 \text{ km}}{3\text{h}} = 40 \text{ km/h}$$

The average speed for the entire trip is 40 kilometers per hour.

D. Word Problems Involving Work Rates of Two Individuals

There is a general formula, the *work formula*, that can be used to find how long a number of people working together require to complete a task. Let's say that there are three people, the first takes t_1 units of time to complete the job, the second t_2 units of time, and the third t_3 units of time. If the time required for all three working together to complete the job is T, then

$$\frac{1}{t_1} + \frac{1}{t_2} + \frac{1}{t_3} = \frac{1}{T}$$

Example:

Cathy can finish a job in 5 hours, and Steve can finish the same job in 10 hours. How many minutes will it take both of them together to finish the job?

Call the amount of time Cathy takes to finish the job t_1 and the amount of time Steve takes t_2; that is, t_1 = 5 hours and t_2 = 10 hours. Then,

$$\frac{1}{5} + \frac{1}{10} = \frac{2}{10} + \frac{1}{10} = \frac{3}{10} = \frac{1}{T}$$
$$\frac{1}{T} = \frac{3}{10}$$
$$T = \frac{10}{3} \text{ hr}$$

Convert the hours to minutes:

$$\frac{10}{3}\text{hr} = \frac{10}{3} \times 60 \text{ min} = 200 \text{ min}$$

Working together, Cathy and Steve will take 200 minutes to finish the job.

E. Word Problems Using Odd and Even Integers

Integers are real numbers. They consist of negative numbers, zero, and positive numbers. The set of integers is $(\dots, -5, -4, -3, -2, -1, 0, 1, 2, 3, 4, 5, \dots)$. The set of even integers is $(\dots, -4, -2, 0, 2, 4, \dots)$. The set of odd integers is $(\dots, -3, -1, 0, 1, 3, \dots)$.

Consecutive integers are integers that are listed in consecutive order. If n is an even integer, three consecutive even integers are $n, n + 2, n + 4$. For example, if $n = 2$, the three consecutive even integers are 2, 4, and 6. If n is an odd integer, three consecutive odd integers are $n, n + 2, n + 4$. For example, if $n = 3$, the three consecutive odd integers are 3, 5, and 7.

Example:

Find five consecutive even integers that have a sum equal to 40.

Let n represent the smallest even integer. The four other even integers will be expressed in terms of n.

Let n = 1st even integer,
$n + 2$ = 2nd even integer,
$n + 4$ = 3rd even integer,
$n + 6$ = 4th even integer,
$n + 8$ = 5th even integer.

$$n + (n + 2) + (n + 4) + (n + 6) + (n + 8) = 40$$
$$5n + 20 = 40$$
$$5n = 40 - 20$$
$$= 20$$
$$n = 4$$

The five consecutive even integers that have a sum of 40 are 4, 6, 8, 10, and 12.

F. Word Problems Involving Ages

Age problems are solved by comparing ages at the present, in the future, and in the past. If the present age is represented by x, a future age is found by adding years to x, and a past age is found by subtracting years from x.

Example:

Philip is now five times as old as Ed was 5 years ago. If the sum of Philip's and Ed's ages is 35, in how many years will Philip be twice as old as Ed?

Let p = Philip's current age

and e = Ed's current age

Translate the first sentence to get the first equation:

Philip's current age is five times Ed's age 5 years ago.

$$p = 5(e - 5)$$

Translate the first part of the second sentence to get the second equation:

The sum of Philip's and Ed's ages is 35.

$$p + e = 35$$

Now you are ready to solve for the two unknowns. Solve for e in terms of p in the second equation.

$$p + e = 35$$
$$e = 35 - p$$

Now plug this value for e into the first equation and solve for p:

$$p = 5(e - 5)$$
$$= 5(35 - p - 5)$$
$$= 5(30 - p)$$
$$= 150 - 5p$$
$$6p = 150 - 5p$$
$$p = 25$$

Plug this value for p into either equation to solve for e:

$$e = 35 - p$$
$$= 35 - 25 = 10$$

Philip is currently 25 and Ed is currently 10. You still haven't answered the question asked, though; you need to set up an equation to find the number of years after which Philip will be twice as old as Ed.

Let x be the number of years from now in which Philip will be twice as old as Ed. Set up the equation and solve for x.

$$25 + x = 2(10 + x)$$
$$25 + x = 20 + 2x$$
$$x = 5$$

So Philip will be twice as old as Ed in 5 years.

Model Examination A

Answer Sheet

DIRECTIONS: Locate the question number to which you are responding, then fill in the circle containing the letter of the answer you have chosen. (Note: This answer sheet and the additional sheets provided on pages 433–436 are for practice purposes *only*. The actual DAT is given in a computer test format. It is highly recommended that you obtain a copy of the DAT tutorial disk to familiarize yourself with the format. See page 416 for information on how to obtain a copy of the disk.)

SURVEY OF THE NATURAL SCIENCES

1. Ⓐ Ⓑ Ⓒ Ⓓ Ⓔ
2. Ⓐ Ⓑ Ⓒ Ⓓ Ⓔ
3. Ⓐ Ⓑ Ⓒ Ⓓ Ⓔ
4. Ⓐ Ⓑ Ⓒ Ⓓ Ⓔ
5. Ⓐ Ⓑ Ⓒ Ⓓ Ⓔ
6. Ⓐ Ⓑ Ⓒ Ⓓ Ⓔ
7. Ⓐ Ⓑ Ⓒ Ⓓ Ⓔ
8. Ⓐ Ⓑ Ⓒ Ⓓ Ⓔ
9. Ⓐ Ⓑ Ⓒ Ⓓ Ⓔ
10. Ⓐ Ⓑ Ⓒ Ⓓ Ⓔ
11. Ⓐ Ⓑ Ⓒ Ⓓ Ⓔ
12. Ⓐ Ⓑ Ⓒ Ⓓ Ⓔ
13. Ⓐ Ⓑ Ⓒ Ⓓ Ⓔ
14. Ⓐ Ⓑ Ⓒ Ⓓ Ⓔ
15. Ⓐ Ⓑ Ⓒ Ⓓ Ⓔ
16. Ⓐ Ⓑ Ⓒ Ⓓ Ⓔ
17. Ⓐ Ⓑ Ⓒ Ⓓ Ⓔ
18. Ⓐ Ⓑ Ⓒ Ⓓ Ⓔ
19. Ⓐ Ⓑ Ⓒ Ⓓ Ⓔ
20. Ⓐ Ⓑ Ⓒ Ⓓ Ⓔ
21. Ⓐ Ⓑ Ⓒ Ⓓ Ⓔ
22. Ⓐ Ⓑ Ⓒ Ⓓ Ⓔ
23. Ⓐ Ⓑ Ⓒ Ⓓ Ⓔ
24. Ⓐ Ⓑ Ⓒ Ⓓ Ⓔ
25. Ⓐ Ⓑ Ⓒ Ⓓ Ⓔ
26. Ⓐ Ⓑ Ⓒ Ⓓ Ⓔ
27. Ⓐ Ⓑ Ⓒ Ⓓ Ⓔ

28. Ⓐ Ⓑ Ⓒ Ⓓ Ⓔ
29. Ⓐ Ⓑ Ⓒ Ⓓ Ⓔ
30. Ⓐ Ⓑ Ⓒ Ⓓ Ⓔ
31. Ⓐ Ⓑ Ⓒ Ⓓ Ⓔ
32. Ⓐ Ⓑ Ⓒ Ⓓ Ⓔ
33. Ⓐ Ⓑ Ⓒ Ⓓ Ⓔ
34. Ⓐ Ⓑ Ⓒ Ⓓ Ⓔ
35. Ⓐ Ⓑ Ⓒ Ⓓ Ⓔ
36. Ⓐ Ⓑ Ⓒ Ⓓ Ⓔ
37. Ⓐ Ⓑ Ⓒ Ⓓ Ⓔ
38. Ⓐ Ⓑ Ⓒ Ⓓ Ⓔ
39. Ⓐ Ⓑ Ⓒ Ⓓ Ⓔ
40. Ⓐ Ⓑ Ⓒ Ⓓ Ⓔ
41. Ⓐ Ⓑ Ⓒ Ⓓ Ⓔ
42. Ⓐ Ⓑ Ⓒ Ⓓ Ⓔ
43. Ⓐ Ⓑ Ⓒ Ⓓ Ⓔ
44. Ⓐ Ⓑ Ⓒ Ⓓ Ⓔ
45. Ⓐ Ⓑ Ⓒ Ⓓ Ⓔ
46. Ⓐ Ⓑ Ⓒ Ⓓ Ⓔ
47. Ⓐ Ⓑ Ⓒ Ⓓ Ⓔ
48. Ⓐ Ⓑ Ⓒ Ⓓ Ⓔ
49. Ⓐ Ⓑ Ⓒ Ⓓ Ⓔ
50. Ⓐ Ⓑ Ⓒ Ⓓ Ⓔ
51. Ⓐ Ⓑ Ⓒ Ⓓ Ⓔ
52. Ⓐ Ⓑ Ⓒ Ⓓ Ⓔ
53. Ⓐ Ⓑ Ⓒ Ⓓ Ⓔ
54. Ⓐ Ⓑ Ⓒ Ⓓ Ⓔ
55. Ⓐ Ⓑ Ⓒ Ⓓ Ⓔ
56. Ⓐ Ⓑ Ⓒ Ⓓ Ⓔ
57. Ⓐ Ⓑ Ⓒ Ⓓ Ⓔ

58. Ⓐ Ⓑ Ⓒ Ⓓ Ⓔ
59. Ⓐ Ⓑ Ⓒ Ⓓ Ⓔ
60. Ⓐ Ⓑ Ⓒ Ⓓ Ⓔ
61. Ⓐ Ⓑ Ⓒ Ⓓ Ⓔ
62. Ⓐ Ⓑ Ⓒ Ⓓ Ⓔ
63. Ⓐ Ⓑ Ⓒ Ⓓ Ⓔ
64. Ⓐ Ⓑ Ⓒ Ⓓ Ⓔ
65. Ⓐ Ⓑ Ⓒ Ⓓ Ⓔ
66. Ⓐ Ⓑ Ⓒ Ⓓ Ⓔ
67. Ⓐ Ⓑ Ⓒ Ⓓ Ⓔ
68. Ⓐ Ⓑ Ⓒ Ⓓ Ⓔ
69. Ⓐ Ⓑ Ⓒ Ⓓ Ⓔ
70. Ⓐ Ⓑ Ⓒ Ⓓ Ⓔ
71. Ⓐ Ⓑ Ⓒ Ⓓ Ⓔ
72. Ⓐ Ⓑ Ⓒ Ⓓ Ⓔ
73. Ⓐ Ⓑ Ⓒ Ⓓ Ⓔ
74. Ⓐ Ⓑ Ⓒ Ⓓ Ⓔ
75. Ⓐ Ⓑ Ⓒ Ⓓ Ⓔ
76. Ⓐ Ⓑ Ⓒ Ⓓ Ⓔ
77. Ⓐ Ⓑ Ⓒ Ⓓ Ⓔ
78. Ⓐ Ⓑ Ⓒ Ⓓ Ⓔ
79. Ⓐ Ⓑ Ⓒ Ⓓ Ⓔ
80. Ⓐ Ⓑ Ⓒ Ⓓ Ⓔ
81. Ⓐ Ⓑ Ⓒ Ⓓ Ⓔ
82. Ⓐ Ⓑ Ⓒ Ⓓ Ⓔ
83. Ⓐ Ⓑ Ⓒ Ⓓ Ⓔ
84. Ⓐ Ⓑ Ⓒ Ⓓ Ⓔ
85. Ⓐ Ⓑ Ⓒ Ⓓ Ⓔ
86. Ⓐ Ⓑ Ⓒ Ⓓ Ⓔ
87. Ⓐ Ⓑ Ⓒ Ⓓ Ⓔ

88. Ⓐ Ⓑ Ⓒ Ⓓ Ⓔ
89. Ⓐ Ⓑ Ⓒ Ⓓ Ⓔ
90. Ⓐ Ⓑ Ⓒ Ⓓ Ⓔ
91. Ⓐ Ⓑ Ⓒ Ⓓ Ⓔ
92. Ⓐ Ⓑ Ⓒ Ⓓ Ⓔ
93. Ⓐ Ⓑ Ⓒ Ⓓ Ⓔ
94. Ⓐ Ⓑ Ⓒ Ⓓ Ⓔ
95. Ⓐ Ⓑ Ⓒ Ⓓ Ⓔ
96. Ⓐ Ⓑ Ⓒ Ⓓ Ⓔ
97. Ⓐ Ⓑ Ⓒ Ⓓ Ⓔ
98. Ⓐ Ⓑ Ⓒ Ⓓ Ⓔ
99. Ⓐ Ⓑ Ⓒ Ⓓ Ⓔ
100. Ⓐ Ⓑ Ⓒ Ⓓ Ⓔ

PERCEPTUAL ABILITY TEST

1. Ⓐ Ⓑ Ⓒ Ⓓ Ⓔ
2. Ⓐ Ⓑ Ⓒ Ⓓ Ⓔ
3. Ⓐ Ⓑ Ⓒ Ⓓ Ⓔ
4. Ⓐ Ⓑ Ⓒ Ⓓ Ⓔ
5. Ⓐ Ⓑ Ⓒ Ⓓ Ⓔ
6. Ⓐ Ⓑ Ⓒ Ⓓ Ⓔ
7. Ⓐ Ⓑ Ⓒ Ⓓ Ⓔ
8. Ⓐ Ⓑ Ⓒ Ⓓ Ⓔ
9. Ⓐ Ⓑ Ⓒ Ⓓ Ⓔ
10. Ⓐ Ⓑ Ⓒ Ⓓ Ⓔ
11. Ⓐ Ⓑ Ⓒ Ⓓ Ⓔ
12. Ⓐ Ⓑ Ⓒ Ⓓ Ⓔ
13. Ⓐ Ⓑ Ⓒ Ⓓ Ⓔ
14. Ⓐ Ⓑ Ⓒ Ⓓ Ⓔ

15. Ⓐ Ⓑ Ⓒ Ⓓ Ⓔ
16. Ⓐ Ⓑ Ⓒ Ⓓ Ⓔ
17. Ⓐ Ⓑ Ⓒ Ⓓ Ⓔ
18. Ⓐ Ⓑ Ⓒ Ⓓ Ⓔ
19. Ⓐ Ⓑ Ⓒ Ⓓ Ⓔ
20. Ⓐ Ⓑ Ⓒ Ⓓ Ⓔ
21. Ⓐ Ⓑ Ⓒ Ⓓ Ⓔ
22. Ⓐ Ⓑ Ⓒ Ⓓ Ⓔ
23. Ⓐ Ⓑ Ⓒ Ⓓ Ⓔ
24. Ⓐ Ⓑ Ⓒ Ⓓ Ⓔ
25. Ⓐ Ⓑ Ⓒ Ⓓ Ⓔ
26. Ⓐ Ⓑ Ⓒ Ⓓ Ⓔ
27. Ⓐ Ⓑ Ⓒ Ⓓ Ⓔ
28. Ⓐ Ⓑ Ⓒ Ⓓ Ⓔ
29. Ⓐ Ⓑ Ⓒ Ⓓ Ⓔ
30. Ⓐ Ⓑ Ⓒ Ⓓ Ⓔ
31. Ⓐ Ⓑ Ⓒ Ⓓ Ⓔ
32. Ⓐ Ⓑ Ⓒ Ⓓ Ⓔ
33. Ⓐ Ⓑ Ⓒ Ⓓ Ⓔ
34. Ⓐ Ⓑ Ⓒ Ⓓ Ⓔ
35. Ⓐ Ⓑ Ⓒ Ⓓ Ⓔ
36. Ⓐ Ⓑ Ⓒ Ⓓ Ⓔ
37. Ⓐ Ⓑ Ⓒ Ⓓ Ⓔ
38. Ⓐ Ⓑ Ⓒ Ⓓ Ⓔ
39. Ⓐ Ⓑ Ⓒ Ⓓ Ⓔ
40. Ⓐ Ⓑ Ⓒ Ⓓ Ⓔ
41. Ⓐ Ⓑ Ⓒ Ⓓ Ⓔ
42. Ⓐ Ⓑ Ⓒ Ⓓ Ⓔ
43. Ⓐ Ⓑ Ⓒ Ⓓ Ⓔ
44. Ⓐ Ⓑ Ⓒ Ⓓ Ⓔ
45. Ⓐ Ⓑ Ⓒ Ⓓ Ⓔ
46. Ⓐ Ⓑ Ⓒ Ⓓ Ⓔ
47. Ⓐ Ⓑ Ⓒ Ⓓ Ⓔ
48. Ⓐ Ⓑ Ⓒ Ⓓ Ⓔ
49. Ⓐ Ⓑ Ⓒ Ⓓ Ⓔ
50. Ⓐ Ⓑ Ⓒ Ⓓ Ⓔ
51. Ⓐ Ⓑ Ⓒ Ⓓ Ⓔ
52. Ⓐ Ⓑ Ⓒ Ⓓ Ⓔ
53. Ⓐ Ⓑ Ⓒ Ⓓ Ⓔ
54. Ⓐ Ⓑ Ⓒ Ⓓ Ⓔ
55. Ⓐ Ⓑ Ⓒ Ⓓ Ⓔ
56. Ⓐ Ⓑ Ⓒ Ⓓ Ⓔ
57. Ⓐ Ⓑ Ⓒ Ⓓ Ⓔ
58. Ⓐ Ⓑ Ⓒ Ⓓ Ⓔ

59. Ⓐ Ⓑ Ⓒ Ⓓ Ⓔ
60. Ⓐ Ⓑ Ⓒ Ⓓ Ⓔ
61. Ⓐ Ⓑ Ⓒ Ⓓ Ⓔ
62. Ⓐ Ⓑ Ⓒ Ⓓ Ⓔ
63. Ⓐ Ⓑ Ⓒ Ⓓ Ⓔ
64. Ⓐ Ⓑ Ⓒ Ⓓ Ⓔ
65. Ⓐ Ⓑ Ⓒ Ⓓ Ⓔ
66. Ⓐ Ⓑ Ⓒ Ⓓ Ⓔ
67. Ⓐ Ⓑ Ⓒ Ⓓ Ⓔ
68. Ⓐ Ⓑ Ⓒ Ⓓ Ⓔ
69. Ⓐ Ⓑ Ⓒ Ⓓ Ⓔ
70. Ⓐ Ⓑ Ⓒ Ⓓ Ⓔ
71. Ⓐ Ⓑ Ⓒ Ⓓ Ⓔ
72. Ⓐ Ⓑ Ⓒ Ⓓ Ⓔ
73. Ⓐ Ⓑ Ⓒ Ⓓ Ⓔ
74. Ⓐ Ⓑ Ⓒ Ⓓ Ⓔ
75. Ⓐ Ⓑ Ⓒ Ⓓ Ⓔ
76. Ⓐ Ⓑ Ⓒ Ⓓ Ⓔ
77. Ⓐ Ⓑ Ⓒ Ⓓ Ⓔ
78. Ⓐ Ⓑ Ⓒ Ⓓ Ⓔ
79. Ⓐ Ⓑ Ⓒ Ⓓ Ⓔ
80. Ⓐ Ⓑ Ⓒ Ⓓ Ⓔ
81. Ⓐ Ⓑ Ⓒ Ⓓ Ⓔ
82. Ⓐ Ⓑ Ⓒ Ⓓ Ⓔ
83. Ⓐ Ⓑ Ⓒ Ⓓ Ⓔ
84. Ⓐ Ⓑ Ⓒ Ⓓ Ⓔ
85. Ⓐ Ⓑ Ⓒ Ⓓ Ⓔ
86. Ⓐ Ⓑ Ⓒ Ⓓ Ⓔ
87. Ⓐ Ⓑ Ⓒ Ⓓ Ⓔ
88. Ⓐ Ⓑ Ⓒ Ⓓ Ⓔ
89. Ⓐ Ⓑ Ⓒ Ⓓ Ⓔ
90. Ⓐ Ⓑ Ⓒ Ⓓ Ⓔ

READING COMPREHENSION TEST

1. Ⓐ Ⓑ Ⓒ Ⓓ Ⓔ
2. Ⓐ Ⓑ Ⓒ Ⓓ Ⓔ
3. Ⓐ Ⓑ Ⓒ Ⓓ Ⓔ
4. Ⓐ Ⓑ Ⓒ Ⓓ Ⓔ
5. Ⓐ Ⓑ Ⓒ Ⓓ Ⓔ
6. Ⓐ Ⓑ Ⓒ Ⓓ Ⓔ
7. Ⓐ Ⓑ Ⓒ Ⓓ Ⓔ

8. Ⓐ Ⓑ Ⓒ Ⓓ Ⓔ
9. Ⓐ Ⓑ Ⓒ Ⓓ Ⓔ
10. Ⓐ Ⓑ Ⓒ Ⓓ Ⓔ
11. Ⓐ Ⓑ Ⓒ Ⓓ Ⓔ
12. Ⓐ Ⓑ Ⓒ Ⓓ Ⓔ
13. Ⓐ Ⓑ Ⓒ Ⓓ Ⓔ
14. Ⓐ Ⓑ Ⓒ Ⓓ Ⓔ
15. Ⓐ Ⓑ Ⓒ Ⓓ Ⓔ
16. Ⓐ Ⓑ Ⓒ Ⓓ Ⓔ
17. Ⓐ Ⓑ Ⓒ Ⓓ Ⓔ
18. Ⓐ Ⓑ Ⓒ Ⓓ Ⓔ
19. Ⓐ Ⓑ Ⓒ Ⓓ Ⓔ
20. Ⓐ Ⓑ Ⓒ Ⓓ Ⓔ
21. Ⓐ Ⓑ Ⓒ Ⓓ Ⓔ
22. Ⓐ Ⓑ Ⓒ Ⓓ Ⓔ
23. Ⓐ Ⓑ Ⓒ Ⓓ Ⓔ
24. Ⓐ Ⓑ Ⓒ Ⓓ Ⓔ
25. Ⓐ Ⓑ Ⓒ Ⓓ Ⓔ
26. Ⓐ Ⓑ Ⓒ Ⓓ Ⓔ
27. Ⓐ Ⓑ Ⓒ Ⓓ Ⓔ
28. Ⓐ Ⓑ Ⓒ Ⓓ Ⓔ
29. Ⓐ Ⓑ Ⓒ Ⓓ Ⓔ
30. Ⓐ Ⓑ Ⓒ Ⓓ Ⓔ
31. Ⓐ Ⓑ Ⓒ Ⓓ Ⓔ
32. Ⓐ Ⓑ Ⓒ Ⓓ Ⓔ
33. Ⓐ Ⓑ Ⓒ Ⓓ Ⓔ
34. Ⓐ Ⓑ Ⓒ Ⓓ Ⓔ
35. Ⓐ Ⓑ Ⓒ Ⓓ Ⓔ
36. Ⓐ Ⓑ Ⓒ Ⓓ Ⓔ
37. Ⓐ Ⓑ Ⓒ Ⓓ Ⓔ
38. Ⓐ Ⓑ Ⓒ Ⓓ Ⓔ
39. Ⓐ Ⓑ Ⓒ Ⓓ Ⓔ
40. Ⓐ Ⓑ Ⓒ Ⓓ Ⓔ
41. Ⓐ Ⓑ Ⓒ Ⓓ Ⓔ
42. Ⓐ Ⓑ Ⓒ Ⓓ Ⓔ
43. Ⓐ Ⓑ Ⓒ Ⓓ Ⓔ
44. Ⓐ Ⓑ Ⓒ Ⓓ Ⓔ
45. Ⓐ Ⓑ Ⓒ Ⓓ Ⓔ
46. Ⓐ Ⓑ Ⓒ Ⓓ Ⓔ
47. Ⓐ Ⓑ Ⓒ Ⓓ Ⓔ
48. Ⓐ Ⓑ Ⓒ Ⓓ Ⓔ
49. Ⓐ Ⓑ Ⓒ Ⓓ Ⓔ
50. Ⓐ Ⓑ Ⓒ Ⓓ Ⓔ

QUANTITATIVE REASONING TEST

1. Ⓐ Ⓑ Ⓒ Ⓓ Ⓔ
2. Ⓐ Ⓑ Ⓒ Ⓓ Ⓔ
3. Ⓐ Ⓑ Ⓒ Ⓓ Ⓔ
4. Ⓐ Ⓑ Ⓒ Ⓓ Ⓔ
5. Ⓐ Ⓑ Ⓒ Ⓓ Ⓔ
6. Ⓐ Ⓑ Ⓒ Ⓓ Ⓔ
7. Ⓐ Ⓑ Ⓒ Ⓓ Ⓔ
8. Ⓐ Ⓑ Ⓒ Ⓓ Ⓔ
9. Ⓐ Ⓑ Ⓒ Ⓓ Ⓔ
10. Ⓐ Ⓑ Ⓒ Ⓓ Ⓔ
11. Ⓐ Ⓑ Ⓒ Ⓓ Ⓔ
12. Ⓐ Ⓑ Ⓒ Ⓓ Ⓔ
13. Ⓐ Ⓑ Ⓒ Ⓓ Ⓔ
14. Ⓐ Ⓑ Ⓒ Ⓓ Ⓔ
15. Ⓐ Ⓑ Ⓒ Ⓓ Ⓔ
16. Ⓐ Ⓑ Ⓒ Ⓓ Ⓔ
17. Ⓐ Ⓑ Ⓒ Ⓓ Ⓔ
18. Ⓐ Ⓑ Ⓒ Ⓓ Ⓔ
19. Ⓐ Ⓑ Ⓒ Ⓓ Ⓔ
20. Ⓐ Ⓑ Ⓒ Ⓓ Ⓔ
21. Ⓐ Ⓑ Ⓒ Ⓓ Ⓔ
22. Ⓐ Ⓑ Ⓒ Ⓓ Ⓔ
23. Ⓐ Ⓑ Ⓒ Ⓓ Ⓔ
24. Ⓐ Ⓑ Ⓒ Ⓓ Ⓔ
25. Ⓐ Ⓑ Ⓒ Ⓓ Ⓔ
26. Ⓐ Ⓑ Ⓒ Ⓓ Ⓔ
27. Ⓐ Ⓑ Ⓒ Ⓓ Ⓔ
28. Ⓐ Ⓑ Ⓒ Ⓓ Ⓔ
29. Ⓐ Ⓑ Ⓒ Ⓓ Ⓔ
30. Ⓐ Ⓑ Ⓒ Ⓓ Ⓔ
31. Ⓐ Ⓑ Ⓒ Ⓓ Ⓔ
32. Ⓐ Ⓑ Ⓒ Ⓓ Ⓔ
33. Ⓐ Ⓑ Ⓒ Ⓓ Ⓔ
34. Ⓐ Ⓑ Ⓒ Ⓓ Ⓔ
35. Ⓐ Ⓑ Ⓒ Ⓓ Ⓔ
36. Ⓐ Ⓑ Ⓒ Ⓓ Ⓔ
37. Ⓐ Ⓑ Ⓒ Ⓓ Ⓔ
38. Ⓐ Ⓑ Ⓒ Ⓓ Ⓔ
39. Ⓐ Ⓑ Ⓒ Ⓓ Ⓔ
40. Ⓐ Ⓑ Ⓒ Ⓓ Ⓔ

SURVEY OF THE NATURAL SCIENCES

Directions: The following items are questions or incomplete statements. Read each item carefully, then choose the best answer. Blacken the corresponding space on the answer sheet. **This section contains 100 items: Biology (1–40), General Chemistry (41–70), and Organic Chemistry (71–100).**

Time Limit: 90 minutes

1. In the process of exocytosis, the plasma membrane and the membrane of which organelle come together?
   A. mitochondria
   B. peroxisome
   C. nucleus
   D. secretory vesicle
   E. ribosome

2. In comparison to the passage of polar solvents through a cell membrane, the passage of nonpolar solvents through a cell membrane occurs much more rapidly. This is indicative of
   A. the presence of more than a single layer of cells in the membrane
   B. the random distribution of the molecules of the membrane
   C. the "fluidity" of the membrane under normal conditions
   D. a significant proportion of lipid in the composition of the membrane
   E. an organized and layered arrangement of molecules within the membrane

3. When energy is expended to move molecules up a concentration gradient, the process is termed
   A. passive transport
   B. active transport
   C. simple diffusion
   D. facilitated diffusion
   E. osmosis

4. Which of the following organelles is NOT encapsulated within a membrane?
   A. nucleus
   B. mitochondrion
   C. Golgi apparatus
   D. peroxisome
   E. centriole

5. The addition of an enzyme to a solution yields glucose. The enzyme may have acted on which of the following components of the original solution to produce the glucose?
   A. lipids
   B. RNA
   C. DNA
   D. glycogen
   E. albumin

6. NAD and FAD are important to biochemical pathways because of their role as
   A. oxidation-reduction coenzymes
   B. regulators of O_2 levels
   C. enzymes to reduce the activation energy needed for essential reactions
   D. glycolytic ATP
   E. regulators of acetyl Co-A levels

7. Organisms that use respiration in conjunction with glycolysis are _____ organisms that use anaerobic means of obtaining energy from the degradation of food.
   A. half as efficient as
   B. twice as efficient as
   C. many more times as efficient as
   D. equally as efficient as
   E. not as efficient as

8. The accessory pigments involved in photosynthesis, chlorophyll b, xanthophylls, anthocyanins, and carotenoids, have importance because they
   A. can go from a ground state to an excited state without any form of electromagnetic radiation
   B. absorb different wavelengths and pass them on to chlorophyll a
   C. receive photons from chlorophyll a
   D. are responsible for the absorption of O_2 and nutrients
   E. are primarily responsible for the absorption of X rays and gamma rays

9. Which of the following invertebrates share the most similarities with primitive vertebrates?
   A. Arthropoda
   B. Annelida
   C. Cnidaria
   D. Nematoda
   E. Echinodermata

10. Of the following, which is (are) considered to be a true cell (true cells)?

    I. Erythrocytes
    II. Leukocytes
    III. Platelets

    A. I only
    B. II only
    C. III only
    D. I and II
    E. I and III

11. When referring to the propagation of an impulse within the heart, the _____ is referred to as the "pacemaker" because it has the _____ rate of spontaneous depolarization.
    A. atrioventricular node; slowest
    B. atrioventricular node; fastest
    C. sinoatrial node; fastest
    D. sinoatrial node; slowest
    E. moderator band; fastest

12. A coma may result from an excessive amount of insulin. This excess is due to
    A. a depletion of norepinephrine
    B. a depletion of epinephrine
    C. a depletion of blood sugar
    D. an excessivly high blood sugar level
    E. an exceeesively high level of both norepinephrine and epinephrine

13. Which of the following are globular proteins?

    I. Antibodies
    II. Actin and myosin
    III. Collagen
    IV. Hemoglobin

    A. I and IV
    B. II and III
    C. I and III
    D. II and IV

14. Tropomyosin
    A. blocks the binding sites on actin, preventing myosin cross-bridge attachment at low Ca^{2+} levels
    B. blocks the binding sites on myosin preventing actin cross-bridge attachment at high Ca^{2+} levels
    C. blocks the binding sites on actin preventing myosin cross-bridge attachment at high Ca^{2+} levels
    D. blocks the binding sites on myosin preventing actin cross-bridge attachment at low Ca^{2+} levels
    E. assists the binding of actin to myosin at low Ca^{2+} levels

15. A cell undergoing mitosis that has lost its nuclear membrane but in which chromosomes are aligned before separation and migration to opposite poles is in which stage?
    A. anaphase
    B. prophase
    C. telophase
    D. metaphase
    E. between anaphase and telophase

16. In contrast to electrical synapses, chemical synapses are
    A. the site of bidirectional communication between neurons
    B. the site of unidirectional communication between neurons
    C. gap junctions that contain protein channels
    D. far more common in embryonic nervous tissue
    E. more abundant in cardiac muscle fibers to permit rhythmic excitation

17. Assuming independent assortment, the possible number of different gamete types from three homologous pairs is
    A. 3
    B. 4
    C. 8
    D. 9
    E. 16

18. The final electron acceptor in the electron transport chain is
    A. FAD
    B. NAD+
    C. molecular oxygen
    D. pyruvate
    E. oxaloacetate

19. Unequal distribution of cytoplasm from the germ cell is found in
    A. oogenesis
    B. spermatogenesis
    C. both oogenesis and spermatogenesis during the primary cytokinesis
    D. both oogenesis and spermatogenesis during the secondary cytokinesis
    E. neither oogenesis nor spermatogenesis

20. Gastrulation refers to
    A. the formation of the cardiac, fundic, and pyloric divisions of the stomach
    B. the body's natural defense to parasitic attack on the musculature of the digestive system
    C. the formation of gastrin and HCL
    D. the division of the gastrointestinal tract into regions with specialized tasks of digestion
    E. the developmental process that produces the three primary germ layers

21. A "zinger" denotes an abnormal phenotype. When zingers are interbred, a phenotypic ratio of two zingers to one normal occurs; $\frac{1}{4}$ of the offspring die. When a zinger is crossed with a mate having a normal phenotype, $\frac{1}{2}$ of the offspring are zingers, $\frac{1}{2}$ are normal, and none dies. The most probable explanation is that zingers
    A. have recessive traits that are lethal when homozygous
    B. have dominant traits that are lethal when homozygous
    C. are recessive traits that are lethal when heterozygous
    D. are dominant traits that are lethal when heterozygous
    E. have weak immune systems when young

22. _____ polymerizes to form the fibrous portion of a clot.
    A. Fibrinogen
    B. Prothrombin
    C. Fibrin
    D. Thrombin
    E. Platelets

23. Which of the following vessels carries oxygenated blood?
    A. pulmonary artery
    B. umbilical artery
    C. thoracic duct
    D. umbilical vein
    E. hepatic vein

24. Lymph from the small intestines travels directly to the
    A. cisterna chyli
    B. blood capillaries
    C. thoracic duct
    D. left bronchomediastinal trunk
    E. right bronchomediastinal trunk

25. Most homeostatic control mechanisms function via
  A. biological control centers that respond primarily to changes in blood pH
  B. positive feedback causing an increase in the original stimulus
  C. negative feedback causing an increase in the original stimulus
  D. positive feedback causing an increase in the original stimulus
  E. negative feedback causing a decrease in the original stimulus

26. When members of two species are neither benefited nor harmed by an association, the relationship is termed
  A. parasitism
  B. mutualism
  C. commensalism
  D. behavioral adaptation
  E. symbiosis

27. The level of taxonomic classification that includes the greatest number of organisms is the
  A. genus
  B. class
  C. order
  D. species
  E. family

28. Meat is cured with large amounts of salt to retard spoilage. The salt causes the cells of bacteria and fungi to
  A. hemolyze
  B. crenate
  C. form ionic bonds with the myofilaments
  D. form ionic bonds with each other
  E. reach an isotonic state

29. Which of the following is INCORRECTLY associated with its description?
  A. vitamin A: retinol, fat soluble, required for synthesis of photoreceptor pigments
  B. vitamin B_2: thiamine, large amounts stored in body, part of coenzyme cocarboxylase
  C. vitamin C: excess excreted by kidneys, important in collagen synthesis, antioxidant
  D. vitamin D: produced in skin by irradiation of 7-dehydrocholesterol by ultraviolet light
  E. niacin: deprivation can cause pellagra, very limited amount stored in body

30. The primary difference between eukaryotes and prokaryotes is that prokaryotes lack
  A. a nuclear envelope
  B. a cell wall
  C. a plasma membrane
  D. cytoplasm
  E. chlorophyll

31. A cell is found to have ribosomes, lysosomes, and chromosomes, but no cell wall. This cell is from
  A. an animal, but not a protozoan
  B. either an animal or protozoan
  C. a plant
  D. a protozoan
  E. a plant or a protozoan

32. Two different DNA molecules are described below.

  DNA molecule #1 has a greater proportion of adenine-thyamine (A–T) bonds than guanine-cytosine (G–C) bonds.

  DNA molecule #2 has a greater proportion of guanine-cytosine (G–C) bonds than adenine-thyamine (A–T) bonds.

  It can be concluded that

  A. DNA #1 will be more stable
  B. DNA #2 will be more stable
  C. DNA #1 and #2 will exhibit equal stability
  D. DNA #1 will be altered during mitosis
  E. DNA #2 will be altered during meiosis

33. _____(1707–1778) developed the binomial system of taxonomy that is still used today to group organisms into hierarchical categories. He is known as the father of taxonomy.
  A. Charles Darwin
  B. Marshall Nirenberg
  C. Jean Baptiste Lamarck
  D. Georges Cuvier
  E. Carolus Linnaeus

34. The following are all forms of prezygotic reproduction isolation mechanisms EXCEPT
  A. gametic
  B. mechanical
  C. reduced hybrid viability
  D. ecological
  E. temporal

35. During transcription
    A. the information contained within RNA is transferred to a polypeptide
    B. the information contained within the polypeptide sequence is transferred to RNA
    C. information from nucleic acids is moved to proteins
    D. RNA molecules are formed from DNA templates by a process not unlike DNA replication
    E. tRNA functions as an important interpreter

36. Which of the following statements is FALSE regarding the process of protein synthesis?
    A. The A site holds the tRNA attached to the growing polypeptide chain, while the P site holds the next amino acid to be added.
    B. If the reading frame is shifted, a completely different set of amino acids will result.
    C. The start codon is usually AUG.
    D. There are three steps: chain initiation, chain elongation, and chain termination.
    E. Peptidyl transferase is the enzyme involved in the formation of the peptide bond between the polypeptide in the P site and the amino acid in the A site.

37. Which of the statements below is (are) true in regard to the following pedigree?

    The father has the genotype *rr* and the mother has the genotype *Rr*.

    I.   The recessive homozygotes are phenotypically normal.
    II. The genotype for the male grandchildren is *rr*.
    III. The probability that the first generation will inherit the trait is $\frac{1}{2}$.
    A. I
    B. II
    C. II and III
    D. I and II
    E. I and III

38. Which of the following hormones is produced in the posterior pituitary?
    A. prolactin
    B. leutinizing hormone
    C. growth hormone
    D. corticosteroid hormone
    E. oxytocin

39. Which of the following is a mode (are modes) of asexual reproduction?
    A. Fragmentation
    B. Regeneration
    C. Budding
    D. A and C
    E. A, B, and C

40. Which of the following describes the characteristics of a savanna?
    A. tropical or semitropical grassland; low precipitation; found in the interiors of continents
    B. among the harshest of biomes; temperatures can reach 54°C; low precipitation
    C. midaltitude; mild, rainy winters and long, dry, hot summers; found along coastlines
    D. little variation in mean annual temperature; 25°C; rainfall more than 250 cm annually; harbors the most complex communities; found near the Equator
    E. characterized by coniferous or boreal forests; harsh winters and short summers

41. The characteristics of metals can be best explained by their property of
    A. brittleness
    B. dipole moments
    C. molecular crystals
    D. highly mobile electrons
    E. ionic bonding

42. Which of the following is expected to be tetrahedral?
    A. H_2O
    B. NH_3
    C. HCN
    D. NH_4^+
    E. CO_3

43. The diffusion rate of methane gas compared to that of helium is
    A. twice as fast
    B. 4 times as slow
    C. 4 times as fast
    D. half as fast
    E. 12 times as fast

44. Which of the following shows atoms and ions in order of increasing size?
    A. $Ar > Cl^- > S^{2-} > K^+$
    B. $K^+ > S^{2-} > Cl^- > Ar$
    C. $S^{2-} > Cl^- > Ar > K^+$
    D. $S^{2-} > Ar > Cl^- > K^+$
    E. $K^+ > Ar > S^{2-} > Cl^-$

45. Which ion is isoelectronic with Ba^{2+}?
    A. Xe
    B. Cs
    C. Rb
    D. Hf
    E. I

46. What is the mass, in grams, of 245 milliliters of SO_2 at STP?
    A. 7.01
    B. 0.694
    C. 0.651
    D. 0.732
    E. 6.51

47. In the following reaction,

    $$N_2\ (g) + 3\ H_2\ (g) \leftrightarrow 2\ NH_3\ (g),$$

    an increase in pressure would cause the reaction to

    A. shift to the right
    B. shift to the left
    C. shut down
    D. do nothing, it is at equilibrium
    E. Not enough information is given.

48. Which of the following is NOT a colligative property?
    A. freezing point depression
    B. osmotic pressure
    C. melting point depression
    D. boiling point elevation
    E. vapor pressure lowering

49. Which of the following will produce an increase in the entropy of a system?

    I.   Increase in temperature
    II. Formation of gaseous products from solid reactants
    III. Formation of a precipitate in a liquid solution
    IV. Increase in the volume of a system
    V.   Formation of a solid from a gas

    A. I, II, III
    B. I, V
    C. I, II, IV, V
    D. I, II, IV
    E. I, II, III, IV

50. To balance the following equation:

    $$ZnS + HCl \rightarrow ZnCl_2 + H_2S$$

    the correct order of coefficients is

    A. 1, 2, 2, 1
    B. 1, 2, 1, 1
    C. 1, 1, 2, 2
    D. 2, 4, 2, 2
    E. 1, 4, 2, 1

51. How many mole of sulfur are in 1 mole of As_2S_3?
   A. 3
   B. 2.4
   C. 1
   D. 0.1
   E. 5

52. How many moles are in 50 grams of aluminum?
   A. 0.669
   B. 2.3
   C. 1.85
   D. 2.43
   E. 1.2

53. For the reaction $A + B \rightarrow C$, the rate of formation of C is given by the formula

   Rate $= k[A][B]^2$.

   Doubling the concentration of A will

   A. quadruple the initial rate
   B. double the initial rate
   C. have no effect on the initial rate
   D. reduce the rate to $\frac{1}{4}$ of its value
   E. reduce the rate to $\frac{1}{2}$ of its value

54. In which reaction is H_2O acting like an acid?
   A. $Zn(s) + 2H_3O^+ \rightarrow Zn^{++} + H_2O\ (g) + 2H_2O$
   B. $HCl\ (g) + H_2O \rightarrow H_3O^+ + Cl^-$
   C. $HC_2H_3O_2 + H_2O \leftrightarrow H_3O^+ + C_2H_3O_2^-$
   D. $NH_3 + H_2O \leftrightarrow NH_4^+ + OH^-$
   E. $NH_3 + H_2O^+ \leftrightarrow NH_4^+ + H_2O$

55. Catalysts have which of the following effects on a chemical reaction?
   A. They lower the activation energy.
   B. They increase the free energy.
   C. They cause the reaction to proceed spontaneously.
   D. They increase the rate at which the product is formed.
   E. They shift the equilibrium so the reverse reaction proceeds more easily.

56. Which of the following has the LOWEST percent of carbon by mass?
   A. CH_4
   B. C_2H_4
   C. $Na_2C_2O_2$
   D. $C_6H_{12}O_6$
   E. CH_3CO_2H

57. The data shown below were obtained from the following reaction:

   $$A + 2B \rightarrow 2C + D$$

TRIAL	INITIAL [A] (M) (10^{-4})	INITIAL [B] (M) (10^{-2})	RATE (M min^{-1})
1	1.0	1.0	0.65
2	2.0	1.0	1.30
3	2.0	0.50	0.65
4	0.50	2.0	0.65

   What is the rate law for this system?

   A. $k\,[C]^2\,[D]/[A]\,[B]^2$
   B. $k\,[A]\,[B]$
   C. $k\,[A]\,[B]^2$
   D. $k\,[B]^2$
   E. $k\,[A]$

58. If 14 grams of NaF are dissoloved in 400 milligrams of water, what is the resulting molality of the solution?
   A. 0.4 m
   B. 0.83 m
   C. 0.93 m
   D. 0.54 m
   E. 0.32 m

59. How much 4 M $Ca(OH)_2$ is needed to neutralize 300 milliliters of 3 M HNO_3?
   A. 234 mL
   B. 655 mL
   C. 623 mL
   D. 723 mL
   E. 112.5 mL

60. How many atoms of carbon are in 4.00×10^{-8} grams of C_3H_8?
   A. 1.64×10^{15}
   B. 2.34×10^{11}
   C. 1.89×10^{14}
   D. 4.66×10^2
   E. 4.00×10^4

61. In an experiment, 3.4 grams of a carbon-oxygen containing compound was obtained in a test tube. The weight of oxygen was found to be 0.65 gram. What was the percentage of carbon in the compound?
    A. $(1 - (0.65/3.4))(100)$
    B. $((1 + 0.65)/3.4)(100)$
    C. $(0.65)(1/100 \times 3.4)$
    D. $(3.4/0.65)(100)$
    E. $(3.4 \times 0.65)(100)$

62. An alloy contains atoms of
    A. one element and has the properties of a metal
    B. more than one element and has the properties of a nonmetal
    C. one element and has the properties of a nonmetal
    D. more than one element and has the properties of a metal
    E. one element and has the properties of a semiconductor

63. Which of the following is the definition of an Arrhenius base?
    A. a substance that donates a proton to another substance
    B. a substance that accepts a proton from another substance
    C. a substance that produces a hydroxy ion in the presence of an aqueous solution
    D. a substance that donates a pair of electrons
    E. a substance that donates a hydrogen ion in the presence of an aqueous solution

64. Which of the following, if any, is FALSE?

    Chemical reactions are accelerated by . . .

    A. increasing the concentrations of reactants
    B. adding a catalyst
    C. decreasing the surface area available for the reaction
    D. increasing the temperature
    E. All of the above are correct.

65. If all of the chloride in a 5.0-gram sample of an unknown metal chloride is precipitated as AgCl with 70.9 milliliters of 0.201 M $AgNO_3$, what is the percentage of chloride in the sample?
    A. 50.55%
    B. 20.22%
    C. 1.43%
    D. 10.10%
    E. none of the above

66. In which of the following are the atoms arranged by increasing atomic size?
    A. Be < Na < Mg
    B. Be < Mg < Na
    C. Mg < Na < Be
    D. Mg < Be < Na
    E. Na < Be < Mg

67. As one moves across the periodic table in a leftward and descending direction, which of the following properties increases?
    A. ionization energy
    B. electron affinity
    C. electronegativity
    D. electron affinity
    E. atomic radius

68. Which of the following is an example of a halogen?
    A. F
    B. Ba
    C. O
    D. C
    E. He

69. The geometric configuration of CO_2 is
    A. linear
    B. bent
    C. tetrahedral
    D. trigonal planar
    E. trigonal pyramidal

70. Isotopes have
    A. the same number of protons and electrons
    B. the same atomic number and equal numbers of protons
    C. the same mass number and equal numbers of protons
    D. the same atomic number and equal numbers of neutrons
    E. the same mass number and equal numbers of neutrons

71. The breaking of an O–H bond in water is an example of _____ cleavage. The breaking of the O–O bond in hydrogen peroxide is an example of _____ cleavage.
    A. homolytic, heterolytic
    B. heterolytic, homolytic
    C. homolytic, homolytic
    D. heterolytic, heterolytic
    E. none of the above

72. The orientation of the bond between the two sp^2 hybridized carbons in the molecule ethene can best be described as _____ in relation to the orientation of its pi bond.
    A. parallel
    B. perpendicular
    C. at a 109.5° angle
    D. at a 120° angle
    E. at a 180° angle

73. The correct name for the following compound is

$$CH_3 - CH - \overset{\overset{\displaystyle O}{\|}}{C} - CH - CH_2 - CH_3$$
$$\underset{CH_3}{|} \qquad \underset{CH_3}{|}$$

    A. 3,5-dimethyl-4-hexanone
    B. 2,4-dione-3-hexane
    C. 2-ethyl-4-methyl-3-pentanone
    D. 2-methyl-4-ethyl-3-pentanone
    E. 2,4-dimethyl-3-hexanone

74. Which of the following compounds is NOT aromatic?

    A.
    D.
    B.
    E.
    C.

75. Which of the following will be produced when an oxidizing agent reacts with a 2° alcohol?
    A. esters
    B. ethers
    C. aldehydes
    D. ketones
    E. caroxylic acids

76. Which is the best description of the propagation step in free-radical halogenation?
    A. Two radicals bond to create a nonradical.
    B. Two radicals react to form a third radical.
    C. A halogen radical is formed from the presence of light or heat.
    D. A radical causes the homolytic cleavage of an alkane. The reaction proceeds with an alkyl radical that splits an X_2.
    E. None of the above

77. Which of the following has an effect on the strength of an acid?
    A. the number of resonance forms possible for the conjugate base
    B. the electronegativity of the conjugate base
    C. inductive effects that cause a shift in electron density
    D. all of the above
    E. none of the above

78. All of the following are oxidizing agents EXCEPT
    A. $KMnO_4$
    B. CrO_3
    C. $LiAlH_4$
    D. H_2CrO_4
    E. OsO_4

79. Of the following, the most stable radical is

    A.

    B. $^\bullet CH_3$

    C. $CH_3 \diagdown \overset{\bullet}{C}H \diagup CH_3$

    D.

    E. $CH_3 - C\overset{\bullet}{H}_2$

80. Which is the most basic?
   A. $C_6H_5NH_2$
   B. $BrCH_2NH_2$
   C. FCH_2NH_2
   D. CH_3NH_2
   E. $ClCH_2NH_2$

81. The correct IUPAC name for the following compound is

   A. N-propyl-N-ethyl-1-methanamine
   B. N-ethyl-N-methyl-1-propanamine
   C. N,N-propylethylamine
   D. N,N,N-propylethylmethylamine
   E. N-ethyl-N-propyl-1-methanamine

82. The correct ranking of the following in order of increasing acid strength is

   A. 1, 2, 4, 3
   B. 4, 1, 3, 2
   C. 4, 3, 1, 2
   D. 1, 2, 3, 4
   E. 3, 2, 4, 1

83. Carboxylic acids are more acidic than alcohols primarily because of the
   A. resonance of the carboxylate ion
   B. electron donating effect of carbonyl oxygen
   C. electron-donating effect of the hydroxyl group
   D. inductive effects of an extra oxygen atom
   E. electron-donating effect of the carbonyl group

84. All of the following are characteristics of which nucleophilic reaction(s)?

   One step;
   bimolecular-second order;
   prefers smaller, less sterically hindered reactants;
   results in an inversion of configuration;
   nucleophile replaces leaving group.

   A. S_N1
   B. S_N2
   C. $E1$
   D. $E2$
   E. B and D

85. The following NMR and IR spectroscopy information is characteristic of which group?

A. alcohol
B. phenyl
C. double bond
D. ketone
E. aldehyde

86. What is the IUPAC name of the following compound?

A. 4-hydroxy-2,5-dimethylheptane
B. 2-ethyl-3-hydroxy-5-methylhexane
C. 4-hydroxy-3,6-dimethylheptane
D. 5-ethyl-4-hydroxy-2-methylhexane
E. either A or C

87. What is the structure of 5-ethyl-2,2-dimethyl octane?

A.

B.

C.

D.

E. none of the above

88. What is the IUPAC name of the following compound?

$$CH_2 - C = CH - CH_3$$
$$\quad | \qquad |$$
$$\quad Cl \quad\ CH_3$$

A. 4-chloro-3-methyl-2-butene
B. 2-chloromethyl-2-butene
C. 1-chloro-2-methyl-2-butene
D. 1-chloromethyl-1-methylpropene
E. none of the above

89. Which of the following pairs of compounds would be considered tautomers?

I. $CH_2 = \underset{\underset{OH}{|}}{C} - CH_3 \;\rightleftharpoons\; CH_3 - \underset{\underset{\|}{O}}{C} - CH_3$

II. $^-CH_2 - \underset{\underset{OH}{|}}{C} - CH_3 \;\rightleftharpoons\; {}^-CH_2 - \underset{\underset{O^-}{|}}{C} - CH_3$

III. $CH_2 = \underset{\underset{OH}{|}}{C} - CH_3 \;\rightleftharpoons\; CH_3 - \underset{\underset{OH}{|}}{C} = CH_2$

A. I only
B. II only
C. I and II only
D. I and III only
E. I, II, and III

90. Which of the following is (are) considered terminal functional groups?

I. Aldehydes
II. Ketones
III. Carboxylic acids
IV. Esters

A. III only
B. I and III only
C. II and III only
D. I, III, and IV only
E. I, II, III, and IV

91. Which is the IUPAC name for the following compound?

$$CH_3 - \underset{\underset{CH_3}{|}}{CH} - CH_2 - CH = CH_2$$

A. 4-methyl-1-pentene
B. 1-methyl-4-pentene
C. 1-isopropyl-2-propene
D. 3-isopropyl-1-propene
E. none of the above

92. Which of the following reactions is an example of a free-radical chain termination step?
A. $Cl\bullet + CH_4 \rightarrow HCl + CH_3\bullet$
B. $Cl_2 \rightarrow 2Cl\bullet$
C. $Cl\bullet + CH_3\bullet \rightarrow CH_3Cl$
D. $CH_3\bullet + Cl_2 \rightarrow CH_3Cl + Cl\bullet$
E. $Cl\bullet + CH_2=CH_2 \rightarrow CH_2Cl-CH_2\bullet$

93. Which of the following conformations of cyclohexane is (are) most stable?

I.

II.

III.

A. I
B. II
C. III
D. I and II exhibit identical stability.
E. II and III exhibit identical stability.

94. Which of the following conformations of butane is (are) most stable?

A.

B.

C.

D.

E. A and B are equally stable.

95. Which of the following compounds, if any, is NOT optically active?

A.

B.

C.

D.

$$Br - \overset{\overset{\displaystyle OH}{|}}{\underset{\underset{\displaystyle Cl}{|}}{C}} - H$$

E. All of the above compounds contain chiral centers, hence all are optically active.

96. The molecule below contains how many chiral centers?

A. 1
B. 2
C. 3
D. 4
E. 5

97. How many isomers exist for the following aldehyde?

$$
\underset{O}{\overset{H}{\diagdown}} C - \underset{\underset{H}{|}}{\overset{\overset{OH}{|}}{C}} - \underset{\underset{H}{|}}{\overset{\overset{OH}{|}}{C}} - \underset{\underset{H}{|}}{\overset{\overset{OH}{|}}{C}} - H
$$

A. 2
B. 3
C. 4
D. 8
E. 16

98. Which of the following orbitals is (are) contained in the outer energy level of the carbon atom in CH_4?

I. s
II. p
III. sp
IV. sp^2
V. sp^3

A. I, II, and V only
B. I, II, and IV only
C. I and II only
D. II and V only
E. V only

99. Which of the following compounds, if any, does NOT possess at least one σ bond?
A. CH_4
B. C_2H_2
C. C_2H_4
D. N_2
E. All of these compounds have at least one sigma bond.

100. The hybridizations of the carbon atom and the nitrogen atom in the CN^- ion are
A. sp^3 and sp^3, respectively
B. sp^3 and sp, respectively
C. sp and sp^3, respectively
D. sp and sp, respectively
E. none of the above

PERCEPTUAL ABILITY TEST

Time Limit: 60 Minutes

Part 1

For questions 1 through 15:

This section of the exam consists of 15 items similar to the example below. In each item, a three-dimensional object is shown on the left, followed by outlines of five apertures to its right.

The task is the same for each item. Conceptualize how the three-dimensional object looks from each possible side (in addition to the side shown). Then, pick the outline in which the three-dimensional object could pass if the proper side were inserted. Choose the letter corresponding to the correct aperture.

Here are rules for Part 1, the aperture section:

1. The irregular solid three-dimensional object on the left can be rotated in any direction prior to passing through the aperture.
2. The object may not be twisted or rotated in any way once it has started to be passed through the aperture. The correct answer is the exact representation of the external outline of the object viewed from the appropriate side.
3. The objects and the outlines are drawn to the same scale.
4. There are no irregularities in hidden portions of the objects. If the figure has symmetric indentations, it is assumed that the hidden portion is symmetric with the portion shown.
5. There is only one correct answer.

Example:

The correct answer is C.

Proceed to the questions.

1.

2.

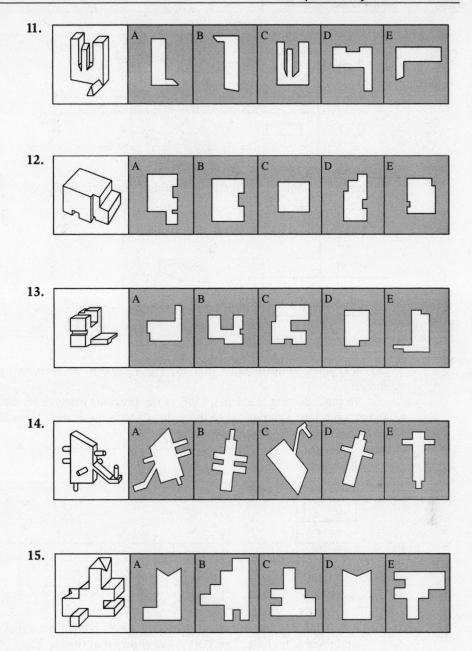

Part 2

For questions 16 through 30:

The pictures that follow are representations of solid objects from three different views: top, front, and end views. The pictures are views drawn without perspective: the surface viewed is along parallel lines of vision. The projection that is labeled TOP VIEW is shown looking DOWN on its top surface and is pictured in the upper-left corner. The projection labeled FRONT VIEW is shown looking at the object from the FRONT and is pictured in the lower-left corner. The projection labeled END VIEW is shown looking at the object from the END (or side) and is pictured in the lower-right corner. These three views are always in their respective corners and labeled accordingly.

If there were a hole in the figure, it would be represented like this:

DOTTED lines indicate lines that exist but cannot be seen in the perspective shown.

In the following problems, TWO of the previous three views discussed will be shown with four alternatives to the right. Choose the correct letter that represents the correct view that completes the set.

Example:

The FRONT VIEW shows that there is a smaller block on top of a larger block and there is no hole. The TOP VIEW shows that the top block is round and is centered on a rectangular block. From this information gathered in the two views given, the correct answer must be B.

In the following problems, one of the three views will be omitted, it is not always the END VIEW as shown in the example.

Proceed to the questions.

16. Choose the correct FRONT VIEW.

17. Choose the correct FRONT VIEW.

18. Choose the correct TOP VIEW.

19. Choose the correct END VIEW.

20. Choose the correct FRONT VIEW.

21. Choose the correct END VIEW.

22. Choose the correct TOP VIEW.

23. Choose the correct END VIEW.

24. Choose the correct FRONT VIEW.

25. Choose the correct FRONT VIEW.

26. Choose the correct TOP VIEW.

27.　Choose the correct END VIEW.

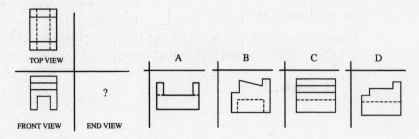

28.　Choose the correct END VIEW.

29.　Choose the correct TOP VIEW.

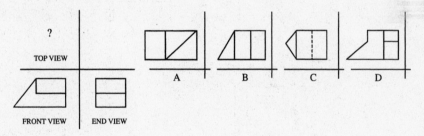

30.　Choose the correct TOP VIEW.

Part 3

For questions 31 through 45:

Examine the INTERNAL ANGLES and rank them in terms of degrees from SMALL to LARGE. Select the alternative that represents the correct ranking.

Example:

A. 1 – 2 – 4 – 3
B. 2 – 1 – 4 – 3
C. 3 – 4 – 2 – 1
D. 3 – 4 – 1 – 2

1   2   3   4

The correct ranking is 2–1–4–3. Therefore, the correct answer is B.

Proceed to the questions.

31.

A. 2 – 4 – 3 – 1
B. 4 – 2 – 3 – 1
C. 4 – 2 – 1 – 3
D. 2 – 3 – 4 – 1

32.

A. 3 – 4 – 1 – 2
B. 1 – 3 – 2 – 4
C. 3 – 1 – 4 – 2
D. 1 – 3 – 4 – 2

33.

A. 1 – 2 – 4 – 3
B. 2 – 4 – 1 – 3
C. 4 – 1 – 2 – 3
D. 1 – 4 – 2 – 3

34.

A. 2 – 1 – 3 – 4
B. 2 – 1 – 4 – 3
C. 2 – 4 – 1 – 3
D. 2 – 4 – 3 – 1

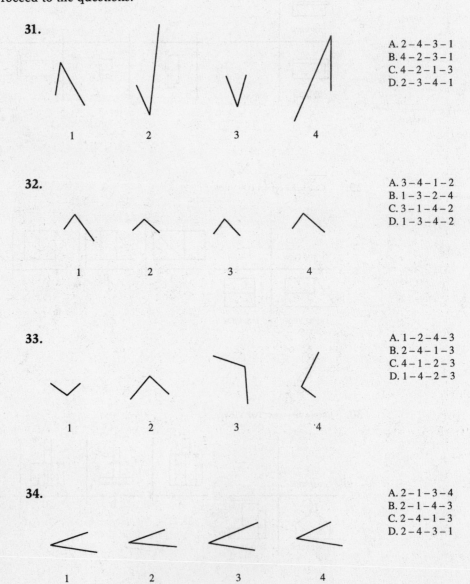

35.

A. 2 – 3 – 4 – 1
B. 1 – 3 – 4 – 2
C. 4 – 3 – 2 – 1
D. 3 – 4 – 1 – 2

1   2   3   4

36.

A. 3 – 2 – 1 – 4
B. 4 – 3 – 2 – 1
C. 3 – 1 – 2 – 4
D. 2 – 3 – 1 – 4

1   2   3   4

37.

A. 4 – 2 – 1 – 3
B. 2 – 1 – 3 – 4
C. 3 – 1 – 2 – 4
D. 1 – 2 – 4 – 3

1   2   3   4

38.

A. 4 – 3 – 1 – 2
B. 3 – 4 – 2 – 1
C. 1 – 3 – 4 – 2
D. 3 – 2 – 4 – 1

1   2   3   4

39.

A. 1 – 2 – 4 – 3
B. 2 – 1 – 4 – 3
C. 2 – 1 – 3 – 4
D. 1 – 2 – 3 – 4

1   2   3   4

40.

A. 1 – 2 – 3 – 4
B. 2 – 1 – 4 – 3
C. 4 – 2 – 3 – 1
D. 2 – 4 – 1 – 3

1   2   3   4

41.

A. 2 – 1 – 4 – 3
B. 2 – 4 – 1 – 3
C. 4 – 2 – 1 – 3
D. 4 – 1 – 2 – 3

42.

A. 3 – 2 – 1 – 4
B. 1 – 2 – 4 – 3
C. 1 – 3 – 4 – 2
D. 2 – 3 – 1 – 4

43.

A. 1 – 2 – 4 – 3
B. 2 – 1 – 3 – 4
C. 1 – 2 – 3 – 4
D. 1 – 2 – 4 – 3

44.

A. 4 – 1 – 2 – 3
B. 2 – 4 – 3 – 1
C. 4 – 1 – 3 – 2
D. 4 – 2 – 3 – 1

45.

A. 3 – 2 – 4 – 1
B. 4 – 3 – 2 – 1
C. 4 – 3 – 1 – 2
D. 3 – 4 – 2 – 1

Part 4

For questions 46 through 60:

A flat, square piece of paper is folded one or more times starting from the left, proceeding stepwise, to the illustrations to the right. The original position of the paper is represented by broken lines. The solid line indicates edges of the folded paper. The piece of paper is never twisted or turned and always remains within the outline of the original square. There may be ONE FOLD, TWO FOLDS, or THREE FOLDS in each item. After the last fold, a hole is punched in the paper. Your task is to unfold the paper in your mind and determine the placement of the holes on the original flat, square piece of paper. There is only one correct pattern of hole punches for each item. The black circles indicate hole punches. Choose the pattern that indicates the correct pattern of hole punches in the unfolded paper.

Practice Illustrations:

Figure 1   Figure 2   Figure 3   Figure 4

In this example Figure 1 shows the original flat, square piece of paper. Figure 2 shows the first fold. Figure 3 shows the location of the hole punch in the folded paper. The black circles in Figure 4 show the pattern of the hole punches on the unfolded paper. The answer has two holes since the paper was two layers thick in the position where the hole was punched.

Example:

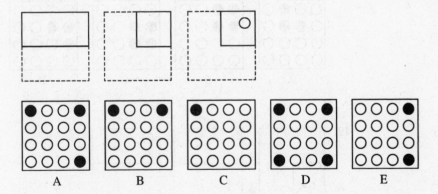

     A   B   C   D   E

The correct answer is D. The paper was four thicknesses and therefore has four hole punches. The punch was made in the corner, so the four hole punches in the four corners are shown in black in the correct pattern.

Proceed to the questions.

46.

47.

48.

49.

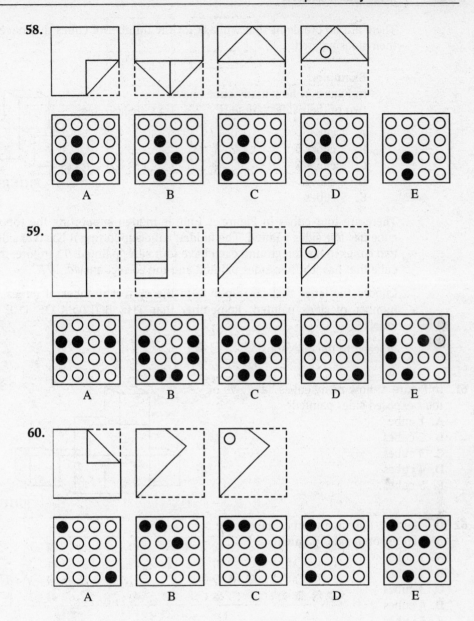

Part 5

For questions 61 through 75:

Each of the figures in this section is representative of cubes of the same size that have been cemented together. After the cubes were cemented, the group of cubes were painted on each of the exposed sides WITH EXCEPTION TO THE BOTTOM SIDE ON WHICH THE FIGURE IS RESTING. Some illustrations contain hidden cubes. The only hidden cubes are cubes that are necessary to support other cubes.

In each item you are to determine how many cubes have

- ONE side painted,
- TWO sides painted,
- THREE sides painted,
- FOUR sides painted, or
- FIVE sides painted.

There are no problems that will ask for the number of cubes that have none (zero) of their sides painted.

Example:

In Figure A, how many cubes have two of their sides painted?

hidden cube

FIGURE A

A. 1 cube
B. 2 cubes
C. 3 cubes
D. 4 cubes
E. 5 cubes

There are four cubes in Figure A (one is hidden supporting the top cube). The top cube has five sides painted. The hidden cube supporting it has two sides painted. The two cubes in the foreground each have four sides painted. Therefore, there is only one cube that has just two sides painted and the correct answer is A.

Choose the letter that corresponds to the correct number of cubes with the given number of sides painted. Remember that THE BOTTOM OF THE CUBE IS NOT PAINTED.

Proceed to the questions.

61. In Figure A, how many cubes have two of their exposed sides painted?
   A. 1 cube
   B. 2 cubes
   C. 3 cubes
   D. 4 cubes
   E. 5 cubes

FIGURE A

62. In Figure A, how many cubes have three of their exposed sides painted?
   A. 1 cube
   B. 2 cubes
   C. 3 cubes
   D. 4 cubes
   E. 5 cubes

63. In Figure A, how many cubes have four of their exposed sides painted?
   A. 1 cube
   B. 2 cubes
   C. 3 cubes
   D. 4 cubes
   E. 5 cubes

64. In Figure A, how many cubes have five of their exposed sides painted?
   A. 1 cube
   B. 2 cubes
   C. 3 cubes
   D. 4 cubes
   E. 5 cubes

65. In Figure B, how many cubes have two of
their exposed sides painted?
   A. 1 cube
   B. 2 cubes
   C. 3 cubes
   D. 4 cubes
   E. 5 cubes

FIGURE B

66. In Figure B, how many cubes have five of
their exposed sides painted?
   A. 1 cube
   B. 2 cubes
   C. 3 cubes
   D. 4 cubes
   E. 5 cubes

67. In Figure C, how many cubes have two of
their exposed sides painted?
   A. 1 cube
   B. 2 cubes
   C. 3 cubes
   D. 4 cubes
   E. 5 cubes

FIGURE C

68. In Figure C, how many cubes have three
of their exposed sides painted?
   A. 1 cube
   B. 2 cubes
   C. 3 cubes
   D. 4 cubes
   E. 5 cubes

69. In Figure C, how many cubes have five of
their exposed sides painted?
   A. 1 cube
   B. 2 cubes
   C. 3 cubes
   D. 4 cubes
   E. 5 cubes

70. In Figure D, how many cubes have two of
their exposed sides painted?
   A. 1 cube
   B. 2 cubes
   C. 3 cubes
   D. 4 cubes
   E. 5 cubes

FIGURE D

71. In Figure D, how many cubes have three
of their exposed sides painted?
   A. 1 cube
   B. 2 cubes
   C. 3 cubes
   D. 4 cubes
   E. 5 cubes

72. In Figure D, how many cubes have four of
    their exposed sides painted?
    A. 1 cube
    B. 2 cubes
    C. 3 cubes
    D. 4 cubes
    E. 5 cubes

FIGURE D

73. In Figure E, how many cubes have one of
    their exposed sides painted?
    A. 1 cube
    B. 2 cubes
    C. 3 cubes
    D. 4 cubes
    E. 5 cubes

74. In Figure E, how many cubes have two of
    their exposed sides painted?
    A. 2 cubes
    B. 3 cubes
    C. 4 cubes
    D. 5 cubes
    E. 6 cubes

FIGURE E

75. In Figure E, how many cubes have four of
    their exposed sides painted?
    A. 1 cube
    B. 2 cubes
    C. 3 cubes
    D. 4 cubes
    E. 5 cubes

Part 6

For questions 76 through 90:

A flat pattern will be presented in the box to the left. Your task is to mentally fold this
pattern into a three-dimensional figure and choose the correct representation from the
choices to the right. There is only one correct choice for each item.

Example:

Folding the pattern in the left-most box can form only one of the figures to the
right. The only figure that accurately represents the shaded areas once the pattern is folded is D.

Choose the letter that represents the three-dimensional object that correctly represents the folded pattern.

Proceed to the questions.

76.

77.

78.

79.

80.

81.

82.

83.

84.

85.

86.

87.

88.

89.

90.

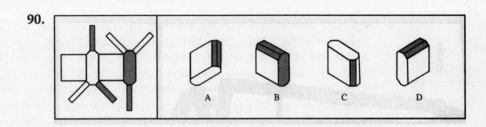

READING COMPREHENSION TEST

Directions: This section consists of three passages, with questions and/or incomplete statements following each passage. Read each passage; then read the questions and/or incomplete statements and answer choices carefully. For each question and/or incomplete statement choose the best answer and blacken the corresponding space on the answer sheet. This section contains 50 items.

Time Limit: 60 minutes

Vitamin A Deficiency

Although tissues of ectodermal origin—that is, the epidermis—are primarily affected in vitamin A deficiency, bones and teeth also record this deficiency. Vitaminosis A is evinced by marked metaplasia of the enamel organ, which results in defective enamel and dentin formation. Likewise, bone is laid down in abnormal locations, and its remodeling sequences seem to be affected. Both osteoclasts and osteoblasts have been shown to be affected by this disease process. Dentinal irregularities associated with vitamin A deficiency in developing teeth appear as areas characterized by either excessive osteodentin deposition (bonelike, with cell inclusions) or insufficient dentin depositions. Alterations of the differentiated odontoblasts appear to be associated with these conditions. Some investigators, however, ascribe the primary effects of vitamin A deficiency to oral epithelial cells. This view originates from histological changes seen initially in the oral mucosa and extending to the degeneration of the epithelial-derived ameloblasts, which results in a hypoplastic enamel matrix. If the vitamin A deficiency is severe, ameloblast cells will become completely atrophied, resulting in an absence of enamel formation. In less severe cases, the columnar ameloblasts apparently shorten, and adjacent enamel exhibits hypoplasia. Several authors have described bone defects due to vitamin A deficiency. Most have noted that the defects are attributable to impaired endochondral ossification and faulty bone modeling. The normal appositional rhythm of dentin deposition may be altered. Vascular inclusions sometimes are seen in the dentin. If the vitamin A deficiency is relieved during subsequent tooth development, normal dentin and enamel are produced, although defective tissue is not repaired.

Vitamin C Deficiency

Ascorbic acid deficiency has been described in guinea pigs, monkeys, and humans. Because none of these species synthesizes vitamin C, they must depend on a dietary supply to maintain health. Scurvy, the disease resulting from vitamin C deficiency, causes bone, dentin, and cementum deposition to cease and formative cells to atrophy, if severe. Vitamin C is required for collagen formation. It is necessary for the hydroxylation of the amino acids proline and lysine; an absence or deficiency of vitamin C during dentinogenesis results in defective dentinal tissue development. Dentinal tubules become irregular and reduced in number, vascular inclusions become apparent, and those odontoblasts present are short, with some taking on a spindle-shaped, fibroblast-like appearance. Embryologically, vitamin C is essential for proper development of all mesenchymally derived structures, including bone, dentin, and cementum. Clinically, vitamin C deficiency is manifested by gingival bleeding and loosening of the teeth due to bone resorption. Weakness, anemia, and susceptibility to hemorrhage also may be evident. Administration of vitamin C results in rapid elimination of the symptoms associated with this deficiency.

Tetracycline and Fluoride

Tetracycline and fluoride, if available during the mineralization phases, may be incorporated in dentin, enamel, cementum, and bone. They are very different compounds. Fluoride is a binary compound of fluorine useful as an anticaries substance. Tetracycline, on the other hand, is used as an antibacterial agent. Both are deposited along with minerals in developing hard tissues. Tetracycline is derived from a yellow-gold fungus whose color is maintained in the purified antibiotic and transferred to the hard tissues in which it is incorporated. On prolonged exposure to light, tetracycline-stained dental tissue will change in color to brown and then to gray (i.e., these shades of discoloration are eventually seen in the teeth). Other effects of tetracyclines include hypoplasia or absence of enamel. Staining is most notable in the dentin, especially in the first-formed dentin at the dentinoenamel junction. Notable staining of the crown results primarily from discolored dentin being seen through the translucent and relatively unaffected enamel. Tetracycline staining is more notable under ultraviolet (UV) light. The amount of damage is directly related to the magnitude and duration of the dosage; any defects caused by the tetracycline may be compounded by the effects of the illness for which it was prescribed. The precise mechanism of tetracycline incorporation into mineralizing tissue is not yet known, but it is believed that a chelate of calcium and tetracycline forms. At higher concentrations, cells may be altered. In both ameloblasts and odontoblasts, the cisternae of the endoplasmic reticulum become dilated, and protein synthesis is impaired. This, in turn, will result in hypoplasia of the enamel and dentin matrix.

Tetracycline and, to a limited extent, sodium fluoride cross the placental barrier and are available to the human fetus. If a pregnant female consumes fluoridated water during mineralization of the fetal teeth, the teeth will incorporate this compound. Such teeth exhibit higher resistance to dental caries. Compared with fluoride blood levels in the maternal circulation, fluoride blood levels in the fetus are relatively low. If, on the other hand, tetracycline antibiotics are administered to the mother during the period of tooth mineralization, the deciduous teeth may later be stained. Tetracycline staining of teeth is permanent; staining of bone is not permanent because bone is remodeled continuously. The period marked by mineralization of crowns extends from approximately 5 months *in utero* to 12 years of age and includes the mineralization of both primary and permanent dentitions. Sodium fluoride when taken into the body in concentrations of 5 parts per million (ppm) (which occurs in some naturally fluoridated areas in this country) is anticariogenic but often causes mottled enamel. The mottled areas may or may not be mineralized. The enamel rods follow an irregular course through these areas. Despite their unsightly appearance, these teeth are completely free of caries. Fluoride is most beneficial to the teeth in concentrations of approximately 0.5 to 1 ppm of water. Concentrations of 0.5 ppm may not prevent caries. Higher concentrations, such as 5 ppm, cause mottling and hypoplasia of the enamel and hypomineralized dentin, with increased interglobular spaces.

As hydroxyapatite crystals form, they may incorporate fluoride either by an exchange with the hydroxyl groups or by simple adsorption. The hydroxyl group exchange is slower and less reversible than adsorption. In the latter process, the fluoride may be adsorbed to the surface of hydroxyapatite crystals. This adsorptive process involves weak electrostatic bonding. Adsorption is believed to be rapid although reversible. It is believed that fluoride found in inner enamel is taken up mainly during the secretory stage of amelogenesis and that fluoride found in the outer 30 to 50 μm of enamel is deposited during the maturative stage. Because the latter stage lasts longer, there is time for more fluoride to be deposited in the outer enamel. The maturative stage lasts from 1 to 2 years in primary teeth and from 4 to 5 years in permanent teeth. This may be the reason why less fluoride is found in primary teeth than in permanent teeth.

When histological examination is conducted on teeth from areas of high fluoride concentration, the enamel is found to be altered more than is the dentin. Enamel rod formation is affected, and zones of hypoplasia are commonly found. Tetracycline was first discovered to be present in human teeth and bones when traces were detected in bones being viewed under UV light. This observation provided a new method of marking bones and teeth in order to follow their development. Tetracycline compound initially is deposited in the predentin as it mineralizes into dentin. Evidence of this marking is demonstrated in the increasing distance between new predentin formed and the area of fluorescent dentin. Because the therapeutic dosage level and visual tissue-labeling levels coincide, tetracycline has been widely used to visually record growth in experimental animals. The daily deposition rate of dentin can thus be recorded by measuring the width of dentin between each two fluorescent dines. Some tetracycline is deposited in the dentinal tubules. Tetracycline may be used also to evaluate tooth movement by revealing bone and dentin formation.

1. What will happen if ascorbic acid is withheld during dentinogenesis?
   A. Dentinal tissue formation will not be affected.
   B. Enamel will be metaplastic.
   C. Scurvy will result.
   D. Enamel tissue development will be defective.
   E. Dentinal tissue development will be affected.

2. When does mineralization of the crowns take place?
   A. 5 months to 12 years of age
   B. 5 years to 12 years of age
   C. 5 months to 12 months of age
   D. 5 days *in utero* to 12 years of age
   E. 5 months *in utero* to 12 years of age

3. Which of the following is an antibacterial agent?
   A. fluoride
   B. ascorbic acid
   C. tetracycline
   D. vitamin A
   E. ameloblast

4. What may be seen with severe vitamin A deficiency?
   A. atrophy of ameloblast cells
   B. thinning of enamel
   C. vitamin C deficiency
   D. tetracycline staining
   E. excessive enamel deposition

5. Vitamin C is essential for which of the following?
   A. development of bone
   B. development of dentin
   C. hydroxylation of lysine
   D. development of cementum
   E. all of the above

6. Marked metaplasia of enamel may be due to which of the following?
   A. ascorbic acid deficiency
   B. high fluoride levels
   C. vitaminosis A
   D. fluoride deficiency
   E. high levels of vitamin A

7. What experimental function does tetracycline serve?
   A. to mark the boundary between dentin and enamel
   B. to measure pulp growth
   C. to record the deposition rate of dentin
   D. to record the deposition rate of enamel
   E. Tetracycline is not used experimentally because of its toxicity.

Reading Comprehension Test

8. Where is tetracycline staining most evident?
   A. in the dentin at the dentinoenamel junction
   B. in the enamel at the dentinoenamel junction
   C. in the pulp
   D. Tetracycline does not stain teeth.
   E. Tetracycline stains the whole tooth evenly.

9. Vitamin A deficiency may result in which of the following?
   A. excessive osteodentin deposition
   B. excessive enamel deposition
   C. insufficient dentin deposition
   D. B and C
   E. A and C

10. Fluoride has the greatest effect on which of the following?
    A. dentin
    B. pulp
    C. dentinoenamel junction
    D. enamel
    E. root

11. Why would monkeys be used to study vitamin C deficiency?
    A. Monkeys can synthesize vitamin C.
    B. The effects are seen soon after the withdrawal of vitamin C.
    C. The effects are pronounced.
    D. Monkeys do not synthesize vitamin C.
    E. Only guinea pigs are used for this purpose.

12. Vitamin C is necessary for which of the following?
    A. hydroxylation of leucine
    B. collagen formation
    C. hydroxylation of purine
    D. the onset of scurvy
    E. all of the above

13. Tetracycline forms a chelate with what substance?
    A. fluoride
    B. sodium fluoride
    C. calcium
    D. vitamin A
    E. ascorbic acid

14. When is the fluoride found in the inner enamel introduced?
    A. throughout enamel formation
    B. during dentin formation
    C. during pulp formation
    D. in the maturative stage of amelogenesis
    E. in the secretory stage of amelogenesis

15. What will happen if vitamin A deficiency is relieved during tooth development?
    A. Defective tissue will be repaired.
    B. Normal dentin and enamel will be produced.
    C. Normal dentin will be produced, but enamel will still be defective.
    D. Normal enamel will be produced, but dentin will still be defective.
    E. A and B

16. At what concentration is fluoride most beneficial to teeth?
    A. 5 ppm
    B. 0.5–1 ppm
    C. 1–5 ppm
    D. 0.1–0.5 ppm
    E. 30–50 ppm

17. Scurvy is a result of what?
    A. ascorbic acid deficiency
    B. vitamin A deficiency
    C. tetracycline deficiency
    D. fluoride deficiency
    E. excessive fluoride intake

Effect of Organic Peroxide Additives on Wear Resistance of Composite Resin

Composite resin plays a major role in the esthetic restoration of anterior teeth. Caries preparations for Classes III, IV, and V are routinely restored with this type of agent. However, composite resin is used much less often in posterior teeth. The problems associated with posterior composite resins commonly relate to technique sensitivity, time required for placement, and inadequate wear resistance. Although manipulation techniques remain complex and relatively difficult to master, the problem of wear has been reduced appreciably with several newer composite resin systems.

Recent clinical studies at the University of Alabama have identified a number of formulations that exhibit annual wear values slightly better than those for amalgam. Although wear rates of earlier composite systems have an annual average ranging from 40 µm to 50 µm, the values for most current formulations are 10 µm or less.

Almost all composite resin manufacturers currently require the use of visible-light energy to cause polymerization. One exception is the Marathon® system. Although this system can be light-cured, it can also be converted into a dual-cure type of system by adding Marathon® Initiator with Infinite Cure®. This organic peroxide not only permits autocuring but also extends the depth of cure to all areas of the restoration, regardless of how the composite resin is polymerized.

In the last several years, an *in vitro* wear-testing device has been developed that generates wear rates closely resembling those obtained with clinical restorations. Designed as a three-body wear system, the device is capable of predicting 3-year clinical wear rates in fewer than 100 hours of *in vitro* testing. Such a test has great potential for manufacturers who may be considering several formulations for clinical trial.

The purpose of the *in vitro* study at the University of Alabama was to determine the potential for increasing the wear resistance of a composite resin by using a special organic peroxide additive, Marathon® Infinite Cure®. Another purpose was to evaluate the wear rate.

Materials and Methods

The *in vitro* device used in this study measures the wear of posterior composite resins. It can best be described as a three-body wear system. All the restorative systems evaluated are presented. They included Marathon® and TrueVitality™, with and without organic peroxide (Marathon® Infinite Cure® paste). Three other proprietary posterior composite resins were included for the purpose of comparison: P-50™ Posterior Restorative, Heliomolar®, and Tetric®. An amalgam, Dispersalloy®, was used as a control.

Sample Preparation

Sound, caries-free, extracted human molars were selected and mounted in a brass specimen holder. The occlusal surface was ground flat within enamel, using a series of metallographic papers to a 600 grit. After surfacing, a well-defined cylindrical-shaped cavity preparation was developed in the center of the tooth specimen. The preparation was 4 mm in diameter and 3 mm in depth. All cavosurface margins were carefully finished with a sharp No. 245 carbide bur. The taper of the preparation closely resembled that of the cutting instrument.

Next, the entire preparation was acid-conditioned, and an enamel or dentin bonding agent was placed according to the manufacturer's recommendations. For the Marathon® composite resin, the entire cavity was etched with Etch-N-Seal™ (37% phosphoric acid) for 20 seconds, rinsed thoroughly with tap water, and then gently air-dried. Then, Tenure® Quick™ with fluoride bonding agent was applied to the entire cavity three times and air-dispersed. For specimens without organic peroxide, Marathon® shade paste was used directly. The composite was inserted in three segments. Each increment was photo-cured for 40 seconds. The last segment, however, was cured for 60 seconds.

For specimens to which the additive was included, an equal amount of Marathon® Infinite Cure® paste was hand-mixed with the Marathon® Shade paste. The composite paste was bulk-filled into the cavity with a Centrix™ syringe and light-cured for 60 seconds.

The surface of the tooth/restoration specimen was ground carefully to a flat plane using a series of silicon carbide papers, and the final surface was completed with a 600-grit paper. This was all accomplished by using a special hand-held device to ensure that the flat occlusal surface was parallel to the flat surface of the energy-generating stylus.

For the inlay preparation, the walls of the cavity were tapered slightly to the occlusal margin. The inlay restoration was first prepared directly as an inlay. This was accomplished by generating the inlay in the cavity preparation after applying a separating medium. The composite resin was light-cured in the same manner as the direct restoration. The inlay restoration was removed and then heat-treated in a specially made tubular at 110°C for 10 minutes (as recommended by the manufacturer). At this point, the inlay was cemented into the preparation using a composite resin luting agent (Infinity® cement). Cementation was performed in strict accordance with the manufacturer's instruction. Equal amounts of base and catalyst paste were mixed thoroughly for 30 seconds and applied to the inlay, as well as to the walls of the preparation. The luting cement was light-cured for 60 seconds and maintained at room temperature for 30 minutes to achieve maximum polymerization. The tooth/restoration specimen was resurfaced with a 600-grit metallographic paper.

Specimens for the other composite materials were fabricated according to their respective manufacturers' instructions. All specimens for both the direct and indirect restorations were stored in 37°C water for 24 hours before wear testing.

In Vitro Wear Test

Using a specially designed aligning device, the mounted specimen was inserted in the wear-testing apparatus. The mounted tooth was then surrounded by a tight-fitting cylinder or ring. Next, a water slurry of unplasticized polymethylmethacrylate (PMMA) beads, averaging 44 µm, was poured on the surface of the restored teeth. The small acrylic resin beads served as an artificial food bolus. This assembly, along with a bank of three other specimens, was submerged in a water bath at room temperature. A flat-planed stylus, machined from polyacetal, was then positioned over the restored area. The diameter of the flat stylus, approximately 8 mm, was appropriately centered so that it covered the entire restoration, as well as 2 mm beyond the margins. At a rate of 1.2 times per second, the stylus was vertically loaded on the restored surface under a load of 17 lbs. or 75.6 Newtons (N). As the stylus initiated contact with the particles of PMMA lying over the restored surface, it automatically began to rotate clockwise 30 degrees. After counterrotating, the stylus moved upward vertically to its original position. The entire cycling procedure was repeated 400,000 times and took approximately 90 hours. After the wear test, the surface was replicated twice with a polyvinylsiloxane impression (Reprosil® light body). The first impression was discarded because it served to debride the surface. The second one was converted into epoxy replicas with an epoxy die model (Epoxy Die) and used for wear determinations using a profilometric stylus (Surfanalyzer®). Procedurally, the profilometric stylus was traversed across the specimen surface in single planes, each 45 degrees away from the next. This procedure produced eight different wear-measurement readings. Five different specimens were tested for each experiment. The vertical distance between the cavo-surface margin and the worn occlusal surface of the composite resin was used to express the amount of material loss or wear in microns. This procedure generated eight readings, which were averaged to express the wear value for each resin composite. The accuracy of the profilometer was 0.15 µm, and the data were statistically analyzed by analysis of variance.

Results

The Marathon® formulation without the organic peroxide additive exhibited the highest wear among the materials tested. Also, it was significantly different ($p < .05$) from the other materials. The addition of the peroxide modifier to Marathon® increased the wear resistance dramatically. The wear value of the modified material dropped from 17.2 μm to 8.6 μm, nearly a 50% reduction. There were no statistically significant differences among the values for Marathon® with Infinite Cure®, Tetric®, P-50™ Posterior Restorative, and Heliomolar®.

The heat-treated composite inlay (TrueVitality™) had minimal wear values compared to the other composite resins tested. A comparison of the values for the two groups of inlays with and without the Marathon® Infinite Cure® demonstrated again that the peroxide additive resulted in a lower wear rate. Specifically, the wear rate for the Marathon® Infinite Cure®-free TrueVitality™ averaged 4.9 μm, whereas TrueVitality™ with the additive revealed a 1.8 μm rate. (The differences between the two values are statistically significant.) Interestingly, this heat-treated composite inlay system with the peroxide additive exhibited a wear value that was significantly lower than the amalgam control wear value (1.8 μm vs. 3 μm).

18. Before wear testing, all specimens were
    A. stored in 37°K water for 24 hr
    B. stored in 37°C water for 24 days
    C. stored in 47°C water for 24 hr
    D. stored in 37°C water for 24 hr
    E. stored in 37°C water for 24 min

19. The resulting wear values in this experiment are
    A. averages of 5 readings
    B. averages of 5 specimens
    C. averages of 8 readings
    D. averages of 8 readings on 5 specimens
    E. approximately 0.15 μm

20. What is meant by surfacing?
    A. finishing of cavo-surface margins
    B. tapering the preparation
    C. formation of a cylindrical-shaped cavity preparation
    D. placing acid on the preparation
    E. grinding down the occlusal surface

21. Recent studies show that composite resins may be better than amalgam because of
    A. lower annual wear values for composites
    B. the fact that composites are visible-light-cured
    C. an annual wear of 40–50 μm for amalgam
    D. the inability to use amalgam for Classes III, IV, and V
    E. the Marathon® system

22. What type of inlay, based on the experiment, will most likely last the longest?
    A. True Vitality™ with peroxide
    B. True Vitality™ without peroxide
    C. amalgam
    D. P-50
    E. light-cured composite

23. How was the composite with organic peroxide placed?
    A. in three segments
    B. in two segments
    C. in bulk
    D. in four segments
    E. This information is not provided in the passage.

24. What was the purpose of using PMMA beads?
    A. to aid in polymerization
    B. to simulate a food bolus
    C. to surface the tooth
    D. to cure the composite resin
    E. to aid in storage

25. How many restorative materials were included in the trial?
    A. 3
    B. 4
    C. 5
    D. 6
    E. 7

26. How long did the actual wear test take?
    A. 90 min
    B. 100 hr
    C. 100 min
    D. 45 hr
    E. 90 hr

27. Based on the results, which composite resin would the experimenter be LEAST likely to endorse?
    A. Tetric®
    B. Marathon® with peroxide additive
    C. Heliomolar®
    D. Marathon® without Infinite Cure®
    E. All are basically the same.

28. The passage suggests that autocuring may be better than light curing because
    A. light curing takes longer
    B. autocuring is more reliable
    C. autocuring extends the cure depth to all areas of the preparation
    D. autocuring allows the composite resin to polymerize
    E. all of the above

29. The polyacetal stylus was used to
    A. load the restoration
    B. pack the restoration
    C. place the composite resin
    D. place the inlay
    E. cure the composite resin

30. What was done after each of the first two segments of composite resin was placed?
    A. Marathon® shade paste was added.
    B. The specimen was light-cured for 40 sec.
    C. Etch-N-Seal™ was added.
    D. The specimen was light-cured for 60 sec.
    E. The specimen was air-dried.

31. The purpose(s) of taking two impressions after the wear test was (were)
    A. to ensure at least one accurate impression
    B. to determine wear
    C. to debride the surface
    D. to make it possible to run two tests simultaneously
    E. B and C

32. Why is the new *in vitro* wear-testing device such an important advancement?
    A. It allows composite resin durability to be tested.
    B. It allows amalgam durability to be tested.
    C. It is more accurate than previous devices.
    D. Long-term results can be determined in a matter of days.
    E. A and C

33. Composite resin luting agent was used to
    A. cement the inlay to the restoration
    B. prepare the restoration for the inlay
    C. surface the tooth
    D. cure the composite resin
    E. test wear on the composite

34. Composite resin is generally used for_____
    A. Class III
    B. Class V
    C. Class VI
    D. Posterior teeth
    E. A and B

Bone Implant Interfaces

In 1952, Branemark embarked on studies that resulted in the introduction of a treatment concept and implant design in the early 1980s after an extensive examination of cylindrical, threaded endosteal implants. A variety of implant models and surgical techniques have led to the development of our present concepts of fibro-osseous integration, osseointegration, and biointegration. Fibro-osseous integration is defined as a connective tissue-encapsulated implant within bone. This type of integration was an early histological finding in implant development and resulted from early types of implant materials, possibly because of a lack of primary stability, premature loading of the implant, and/or a traumatic surgical procedure causing heat-induced bone necrosis. A long-term clinical study has demonstrated a success rate of approximately 50% over a 10-year period for this type of implant integration. Materials that stimulate this type of reaction are nonprecious metals, acrylates, polymers, and vitreous carbon. With the newer materials, fibro-osseous integration makes up a much smaller percentage of the interface to the implant, while osseointegration or biointegration comprises the majority of the interface.

Osseointegration was defined by Branemark as a direct structural and functional connection between ordered, living bone and the surface of a load-carrying implant without soft tissue intervention at the light microscopic level. This type of integration has been shown to yield the most predictable success for long-term implant stability. Factors that enhance osseointegration include (1) atraumatic surgical procedures with minimal heat generated, and (2) close fit of the implant fixture to the formed socket. Present implant surgical research indicates that the best result is achieved with a low drilling speed (under 800 rpm) and abundant irrigation with chilled saline, which minimizes bone tissue injury. Use of a precision drilling system increases the initial implant-bone contact. The implant materials, surface characteristics of the implant, and type of recipient bone are factors that help determine the final implant-tissue interface. In addition, the appropriate timing of placing the implant in function supporting a prosthesis is an essential element in maintaining osseointegration.

Biointegration is a form of implant interface that is achieved with bioactive materials such as hydroxylapatite (HA) and bioglass that bond directly to bone, similar to ankylosis of natural teeth. The bone matrix is deposited on the HA layer as the result of a physiochemical interaction between the collagen of bone and the HA crystals of the implant. HA-coated implants appear to develop bone contact faster than do noncoated implants. However, after a year, there seems to be little difference in bone contact between coated and noncoated implants. The HA-coated implants continue to be improved in their purity and manufacturing processes. Dental implants differ significantly from natural teeth in their interface with the alveolar bone and connective tissue fibers. The junctional epithelium, however, appears to have the same interface characteristics with implants as with natural teeth. Because implants do not have a cemental surface for the insertion of the periodontal ligament and gingival connective tissue fibers, successful implants depend on direct contact with the alveolar bone and connective tissue adhesion coronal to the alveolar housing. A histologically successful implant would be defined as having 35 to 90% direct bone contact, a connective tissue adhesion above the bone, and an intact noninflamed junctional epithelium. Clinically, the implant should be nonmobile and free of discomfort in function. An implant can be considered successful if (1) mucosal health is substantiated by clinical parameters such as a lack of redness, of bleeding on probing, or of suppuration. Soft tissue inflammation, when present, should be amenable to treatment; (2) there is no significant or progressive loss of supporting bone; (3) there is no persistent infection; (4) the implant functions in the absence of discomfort; (5) there is no increasing mobility of the implant on evaluation when the prosthesis is removed; and (6) the implant is prosthetically useful.

Bone is a specialized, calcified connective tissue. Alveolar bone is a combination of both cortical and cancellous bone. Both forms of bone have been shown to osseointegrate with the implant surface. In addition, blood vessels within the bone have been shown to proliferate in contact with the implant surface. To date, the implant materials that have demonstrated the most rapid ability for osseointegration are titanium (commercially pure, alloy, and plasma-sprayed) and the calcium phosphate ceramic material, HA. The biologically active surface on titanium is a dense protective oxide layer 15 to 50 µm thick. This layer forms quickly after processing and is relatively resistant to further corrosion by proteolytic enzymes or chemical attack. Titanium plasma-spraying of the implant increases the surface area for osseointegration almost sixfold. The HA-coated implants appear to osseointegrate more rapidly and to have a higher percentage of bone contact than titanium. However, within a year's time, the difference does not appear to be clinically significant. The HA coating is used because it is manufactured with a commercially pure material that has proved to be nontoxic and has a resemblance to the inorganic phase of the human skeleton. The percentage of cortical bone in contact with implants appears to increase because of the remodeling of the bone associated with functional adaptation.

Epithelium Tissue Interface

The interface of epithelium with an implant is similar to that found with the natural tooth. The sulcus and the junctional epithelium are both in contact with the implant. The healthy sulcus consists of a 5- to 15-cell layer of nonkeratinized epithelium with wide intercellular spaces. The junctional epithelium is approximately 2 mm in length and 2 to 5 cell layers thick, with basal and suprabasal cells in direct contact with the implant surface. These cells are attached to the implant surface by a basal lamina and hemidesmosomes. The epithelial interface is similar to that with the natural tooth, whereas the connective tissue interface is significantly different.

Connective Tissue Interface

The initial success of dental implants is determined by the ability of the implant material to integrate with the alveolar bone. With the placement of the implant abutment through the oral mucosa, the long-term success is dependent on the "transmucosal seal" that forms between the implant abutment's polished or machined surface and the mucosa's connective tissue and epithelium. In the peri-implant tissue, the vast majority of large collagen fiber bundles are attached to the marginal alveolar bone and insert into the marginal gingiva, not onto the titanium. These fiber bundles are highly organized and are oriented parallel to the surface of the machined titanium surface. The connective tissues adjacent to a tooth above the crestal bone are normally arranged into three different fiber groups: (1) dentogingival fibers extending from their insertion into cementum to the marginal connective tissue; (2) dentoperiosteal fibers extending from the cementum to the alveolar bone crest; and (3) circular fibers present in the connective tissue of the marginal gingiva and supra-alveolar connective tissue. All these fiber groups are functionally oriented (perpendicular) to the tooth. One research group has observed collagen fibers appearing to insert into the neck of a plasma-sprayed implant surface in monkeys. These collagen fibers were arranged in a perpendicular arrangement similar to the connective tissue fibers in cementum, as in a normal functioning tooth. The results of this research are not well understood. The width of supracrestal connective tissue around the neck of a healthy implant is approximately 1 to 1.5 mm. This width may vary based on the initial thickness of the mucosa and the degree of adaptation of the mucosa at the time the transmucosal abutment is placed. If the direct bone-implant contact is broken, connective tissue will fill the space between the alveolar crest and implant. These fiber bundles run parallel to the implant surface. Both the connective tissue and the epithelial interfaces have proved to provide adequate resistance to oral function and marginal irritation.

35. Why might biointegration be preferable to osseointegration?
    A. With biointegration more bone is deposited.
    B. With biointegration bone contact occurs more rapidly.
    C. With biointegration less connective tissue is deposited.
    D. With biointegration the bone-implant interface is stronger.
    E. With biointegration higher drill speeds can be used.

36. Over the long term the success of an implant depends on
    A. the epithelium tissue interface
    B. the amount of osseointegration
    C. the ability of the implant to integrate with alveolar bone
    D. the transmucosal seal
    E. all of the above

37. What term describes an implant that is within bone and encapsulated by connective tissue?
    A. fibro-osseous integration
    B. biointegration
    C. osseointegration
    D. bone-implant interface
    E. implant fixture

38. For rapid osseointegration to occur, what type of material should be used?
    A. vitreous carbon
    B. acrylates
    C. titanium
    D. polymer
    E. nonprecious metal

39. The width of supracrestal connective tissue around the neck of a healthy implant
    A. may vary based on initial mucosal thickness
    B. is approximately 1–1.5 μm
    C. is approximately 1–1.5 cm
    D. may vary with time
    E. A and B

40. If vitreous carbon implants are used, what percent can be expected to fail?
    A. 40%
    B. 35%
    C. 60%
    D. 50%
    E. This information is not provided in the passage.

41. After 1 year what difference can be noted between a plasma-sprayed titanium implant and an HA-coated implant?
    A. Little to no difference is apparent.
    B. The plasma-sprayed implant has a six-fold increase in osseointegration.
    C. The HA-coated implant has a higher percentage of bone contact.
    D. The HA-coated implant has less bone contact.
    E. The plasma-sprayed implant has less bone contact.

42. An implant coated with bioglass will result in
    A. osseointegration
    B. fibro-osseous integration
    C. reduced bone deposition
    D. biointegration
    E. C and D

43. Alveolar bone is made up of
    A. fibrous connective tissue
    B. cancellous bone
    C. cortical bone
    D. junctional epithelium
    E. B and C

44. What reason is (reasons are) given to explain why fibro-osseous integration occurs?
    A. premature loading of the implant
    B. heat-induced bone necrosis
    C. lack of primary stability
    D. A and B
    E. all of the above

45. Suprabasal cells are attached to the implant by
    A. junctional epithelium
    B. nonkeratinized epithelium
    C. hemidesmosomes
    D. connective tissue
    E. transmucosal seal

46. The best results are achieved with osseointegration when
    A. space is left around the implant for bone growth
    B. heat is kept to a minimum
    C. drill speed is kept above 800 rpm
    D. warm saline is used
    E. A and B

47. What biologically active surface is added to titanium implants?
    A. oxide layer 25–30 µm thick
    B. oxide layer 15–50 µm thick
    C. peroxide layer 15–50 µm thick
    D. plasma
    E. none

48. Osseointegration differs from fibro-osseous integration in that with osseointegration
    A. soft tissue intervenes at the microscopic level
    B. bone contacts the implant except at the microscopic level
    C. bone directly contacts the implant
    D. the implant ankyloses to the bone
    E. the implant is encapsulated in connective tissue

49. In peri-implant tissue most large collagen fiber bundles are attached at the
    A. marginal gingiva
    B. marginal alveolar bone
    C. titanium
    D. HA
    E. A and B

50. For an implant to be deemed histologically successful what requirement must be met?
    A. 35–90% connective tissue adhesion
    B. no connective tissue adhesion
    C. connective tissue adhesion within the bone
    D. biointegration
    E. 35–90% direct bone contact

QUANTITATIVE REASONING TEST

Directions: The following items are questions or incomplete statements. Read each item carefully, then choose the best answer or completion. Blacken the corresponding space on the answer sheet. This section contains 40 items.

Time Limit: 45 minutes

1. Since 1 meter = 3.28 feet, $\frac{2}{3}$ foot equals approximately what fraction of a meter?
   A. $\frac{1}{5}$
   B. $\frac{1}{4}$
   C. $\frac{1}{3}$
   D. $\frac{1}{2}$
   E. $\frac{3}{4}$

2. If $y = \frac{x + 4}{x - 1}$, which of the following represents x?
   A. $\frac{3y}{y + 1}$
   B. $\frac{3y + 2}{y - 1}$
   C. $\frac{3y + 2}{y}$
   D. $\frac{4 + y}{y - 1}$
   E. $\frac{4y - 2}{y - 1}$

3. If $\sqrt{6 + \frac{1}{x}} = 8$, $x = ?$
   A. $\frac{1}{2}$
   B. 2
   C. 58
   D. $\sqrt{\frac{1}{28}}$
   E. $\frac{1}{58}$

4. A train covers 150 yards in 12.5 seconds. What is the average speed, in feet per second, of the train?
   A. 18
   B. 34
   C. 24
   D. 36
   E. 12

5. If $4x - 6 > 5x + 4$, which of the following must be true?
   A. $x > -10$
   B. $x > \frac{4}{5}$
   C. $x < -4$
   D. $x < 10$
   E. $x < -10$

6. Evaluate the expression $(4 \times 10^{-5}) \times (2 \times 10^8)$.
   A. 6×10^{-3}
   B. 8×10^3
   C. 8×10^{13}
   D. 8×10^{-3}
   E. 6×10^3

7. The perimeter of a square is 40. Which of the following represents the area?
   A. 100
   B. 10
   C. 40
   D. 80
   E. 20

8. If $F(x) = 4x^2 - 5x$, then $F(-1)$ equals which of the following?
   A. -9
   B. -1
   C. 9
   D. 1
   E. 6

9. A salesperson receives a 15% commission on all sales. If he receives $300 in commissions in a week, what is the value of his sales?
   A. $45
   B. $20
   C. $4,500
   D. $20,000
   E. $2,000

10. The slope of the line $10 - 2y = -4x$ is
    A. -5
    B. -2
    C. 2
    D. 5
    E. 4

11. The value of sec t is equal to
    A. $\dfrac{1}{\cos t}$
    B. $\dfrac{1}{\tan t}$
    C. $\dfrac{\cos t}{\sin t}$
    D. $\dfrac{1}{\sin t}$
    E. $\dfrac{\sin t}{\cos t}$

12. If the side length of a square is increased by 50%, the area increases by what percent?
    A. 125
    B. 225
    C. 25
    D. 50
    E. 75

13. Which of the following is the largest?
    A. $\dfrac{23}{25}$
    B. $\dfrac{27}{30}$
    C. $\dfrac{15}{16}$
    D. $\dfrac{14}{15}$
    E. $\dfrac{7}{8}$

14. Which line is parallel to the y-axis?
    A. $x = 4y$
    B. $x = (\dfrac{2}{y°})b$
    C. $x = y + 6$
    D. $xy = 2$
    E. $xy = 2 + 4y^{-1}$

15. A fly sits at the edge of a 12-inch-diameter phonograph record that is playing at $33\dfrac{1}{3}$ revolutions per minute. Approximately how fast, in feet per minute, is the fly moving?
    A. 3
    B. 33
    C. 50
    D. 100
    E. 396

16. Rich is $\dfrac{1}{6}$ of his father's age. In 20 years he will be $\dfrac{1}{2}$ of his father's age at that time. How old is his father now?
    A. 24 yr.
    B. 36 yr.
    C. 30 yr.
    D. 42 yr.
    E. 38 yr.

17. If $3x + y = 5$ and $5x + y = 6$, then $y = ?$
    A. 1
    B. 3.5
    C. $\dfrac{5}{6}$
    D. 2
    E. 3

18. What is the distance on a two-dimensional graph between points (7,6) and (2,-6)?
    A. 9
    B. 5
    C. 17
    D. 13
    E. $\sqrt{153}$

19. Kate has six different books. Assuming the order of selection doesn't matter, how many ways can Kate select, from these six books, two different books?
    A. 18
    B. 15
    C. 30
    D. 36
    E. 12

20. If $z = 2$, $y = \frac{1}{2}$, and $\frac{1}{x} = 1$, what is the value of $x + \frac{1y}{z}$?

A. $\frac{5}{4}$

B. 2

C. 7

D. $1\frac{1}{2}$

E. $1\frac{2}{3}$

21. Sales reductions force a factory to cut back its output by 20%. By what percentage must the reduced sales be increased to allow production to be brought back to normal?

A. 40

B. 30

C. 35

D. 20

E. 25

22. The current sales price of a power drill is $117.00. This is $30.00 more than half the list price. At what discount is the drill being sold?

A. 32.8%

B. 25.6%

C. 74.4%

D. 67.2%

E. 48.7%

23. The set of numbers (1, 2, 3, 6) has an average arithmetic mean (average) of 3 and a variance of 3.5. What are the arithmetic mean and the variance of the set of numbers (2, 8, 10, 16)?

A. 12; 7.5

B. 9; 25

C. 6; 9

D. 6; 25

E. 9; 10.5

24. A bowl contains 7 blue and 3 red marbles. What is the probability that 2 marbles selected at random from this bowl without replacement are both red?

A. $\frac{9}{100}$

B. $\frac{1}{15}$

C. $\frac{6}{10}$

D. $\frac{47}{90}$

E. $\frac{21}{100}$

25 Which of the following represents 5% of 2% of 0.6?

A. 6

B. 0.06

C. 0.006

D. 0.0006

E. 0.00006

26. One pump can fill a pool in 10 minutes. Another pump can fill the pool in 15 minutes. How many minutes are required to fill the pool if both pumps are operating at the same time?

A. 12

B. 12.5

C. 6

D. 25

E. $\frac{1}{6}$

27. If Bob must have a mark of 70% to pass a test of 30 items, the number of items he may miss and still pass the test is

A. 8

B. 10

C. 9

D. 28

E. 21

28. A 25-foot ladder is placed against a building at a point 20 feet from the ground. The distance from the base of the building to the base of the ladder is

A. 12 ft.

B. 25 ft.

C. 18 ft.

D. 30 ft.

E. 15 ft.

29. Two committees are formed with seven people on one committee and eight on the other. If three people are in both groups, how many people belong to only one group?
    A. 7
    B. 9
    C. 12
    D. 8
    E. 6

30. If $5 - 2x = 13$, what is the value of y if $10 - y = x^2$?
    A. −6
    B. 30
    C. 2
    D. 22
    E. 4

31. Right triangle ABC has the right angle at C, and $AB = 12$, $BC = 6$. Find AC.
    A. 3
    B. $3\sqrt{3}$
    C. 6
    D. 12
    E. $6\sqrt{3}$

32. 20 is to $4y$ as $25x$ is to which of the following?
    A. $\dfrac{5x}{y}$
    B. $5x$
    C. $\dfrac{5y}{x}$
    D. $5xy$
    E. $\dfrac{x}{5y}$

33. If 0.04 is 25% of x, x is
    A. 0.01
    B. 0.16
    C. 0.1
    D. 1.0
    E. 1.6

34. If $(a^3b^{-2})^{-2}$ is simplified to a form in which the exponents are positive, the result is
    A. $\dfrac{a^6}{b^4}$
    B. a^2b
    C. $\dfrac{a}{b^4}$
    D. $\dfrac{b^4}{a^6}$
    E. $\dfrac{1}{a^2b}$

35. The distance a train travels varies directly according to its rate times the time it takes to complete the trip. If the rate and one time are both quadrupled, the distance
    A. becomes 16 times greater
    B. becomes 8 times greater
    C. stays the same
    D. is doubled
    E. is quadrupled

36. The value of $\sin\left(\dfrac{\pi}{3}\right)$ equals the value of
    A. $\sin\left(\dfrac{2\pi}{3}\right)$
    B. $\sin\left(\dfrac{-\pi}{3}\right)$
    C. $\sin\left(\dfrac{-5}{6}\right)$
    D. $\sin\left(\dfrac{5\pi}{6}\right)$
    E. $\sin\left(\dfrac{-2\pi}{3}\right)$

37. David weighs $1\frac{1}{4}$ times what Mark weighs and twice what Susan weighs. If Mark weighs 176 pounds, how much does Susan weigh?
    A. 110 lb.
    B. 70 lb.
    C. 88 lb.
    D. 141 lb.
    E. 220 lb.

38. A gift of $180 is to be shared by Brett and Andrew in such a way that Andrew gets 25% more than Brett. How much does Brett get?
A. $100
B. $72
C. $108
D. $144
E. $80

39. Which of the following is the equation of the line that contains point $(3,-1)$ and is perpendicular to the line $y = 3x + 3$?
A. $y = \left(\dfrac{-1}{3}\right)x$
B. $y = 3x - 10$
C. $y = 3 - 8$
D. $y = \left(\dfrac{-1}{3}\right)x + 2$
E. $y = \left(\dfrac{-1}{3}\right)x - 2$

40. Simplify: $\dfrac{-7}{8} + \dfrac{1}{6} - \dfrac{3}{4}$
A. $\dfrac{1}{4}$
B. $1\dfrac{11}{24}$
C. $\dfrac{5}{12}$
D. $\dfrac{-5}{12}$
E. $-1\dfrac{11}{24}$

MODEL EXAMINATION A ANSWER KEY

Survey of the Natural Sciences

1. D	11. C	21. A	31. B	41. D	51. A	61. A	71. B	81. B	91. A
2. D	12. C	22. C	32. B	42. D	52. C	62. A	72. A	82. B	92. C
3. B	13. A	23. B	33. E	43. D	53. B	63. C	73. E	83. A	93. A
4. E	14. A	24. A	34. C	44. C	54. D	64. C	74. C	84. B	94. B
5. D	15. D	25. E	35. C	45. A	55. B	65. E	75. D	85. D	95. C
6. A	16. B	26. C	36. A	46. B	56. C	66. A	76. D	86. A	96. C
7. C	17. C	27. B	37. C	47. A	57. A	67. E	77. D	87. A	97. C
8. B	18. C	28. B	38. E	48. C	58. B	68. A	78. C	88. C	98. E
9. E	19. A	29. C	39. E	49. D	59. E	69. A	79. A	89. A	99. E
10. D	20. E	30. A	40. A	50. B	60. E	70. B	80. D	90. B	100. D

Perceptual Ability Test

1. C	10. D	19. B	28. B	37. B	46. C	55. B	64. B	73. A	82. B
2. B	11. E	20. B	29. A	38. A	47. E	56. A	65. A	74. E	83. B
3. C	12. C	21. C	30. B	39. D	48. B	57. C	66. C	75. E	84. A
4. E	13. A	22. A	31. B	40. D	49. E	58. C	67. C	76. B	85. D
5. E	14. D	23. D	32. D	41. C	50. D	59. C	68. B	77. C	86. B
6. B	15. E	24. D	33. B	42. D	51. B	60. A	69. A	78. C	87. A
7. A	16. D	25. C	34. A	43. B	52. D	61. B	70. C	79. D	88. A
8. B	17. B	26. C	35. C	44. A	53. D	62. B	71. D	80. D	89. B
9. B	18. D	27. D	36. C	45. D	54. E	63. C	72. D	81. B	90. A

Reading Comprehension Test

1. E	6. C	11. D	16. B	21. A	26. E	31. E	36. D	41. A	46. B
2. E	7. C	12. B	17. A	22. A	27. D	32. D	37. A	42. D	47. E
3. C	8. A	13. C	18. D	23. C	28. C	33. A	38. C	43. E	48. C
4. A	9. E	14. E	19. C	24. B	29. A	34. E	39. E	44. E	49. B
5. E	10. D	15. B	20. E	25. D	30. B	35. B	40. D	45. C	50. E

Quantitative Reasoning Test

1. A	5. E	9. E	13. C	17. B	21. E	25. D	29. B	33. B	37. A
2. D	6. B	10. C	14. B	18. D	22. A	26. C	30. A	34. D	38. E
3. E	7. A	11. A	15. D	19. B	23. B	27. C	31. E	35. A	39. A
4. D	8. C	12. A	16. C	20. A	24. B	28. E	32. D	36. A	40. E

STANDARD SCORE TO RAW SCORE CONVERSION CHART

STANDARD SCORE	QRT	RCT	BIOLOGY	GENERAL CHEMISTRY	ORGANIC CHEMISTRY	SNS (TOTAL SCIENCE)	PAT
30	40	50	–	–	30	100	90
29	39	–	40	–	–	99	89
28	–	49	–	30	29	98	88
27	–	–	–	–	–	97	–
26	38	48	39	–	–	96	87
25	37	47	–	29	28	95	85-86
24	36	–	38	–	–	94	84
23	35	46	–	28	27	92-93	81-83
22	33-34	43-45	37	–	–	89-91	78-80
21	31-32	40-42	35-36	27	26	86-88	74-77
20	29-30	37-39	34	26	25	81-85	70-73
19	27-28	34-36	32-33	24-25	23-24	76-80	68-69
18	24-26	31-33	30-31	22-23	21-22	70-75	59-64
17	22-23	26-30	27-29	20-21	19-20	63-69	52-58
16	19-21	24-25	24-26	18-19	17-18	56-62	46-51
15	16-18	20-23	21-23	16-17	15-16	48-55	39-45
14	14-15	18-19	18-20	13-15	13-14	41-47	32-38
13	11-13	16-17	15-17	11-12	11-12	33-40	26-31
12	9-10	13-15	12-14	9-10	8-10	27-32	21-25
11	7-8	10-12	10-11	7-8	7	21-26	17-20
10	6	9	8-9	6	5-6	17-20	13-16
9	5	7-8	6-7	4-5	4	13-16	10-12
8	4	–	5	3	3	10-12	7-9
7	3	6	4			7-9	6
6	2	4-5	3	2	2	5-6	4-5
5	–	–	2	–	–	4	3
4	–	3	–	1	1	3	2
3	1	2	1	–	–	2	–
2	–	–	–	–	–	–	–
1	0	1	0	0	0	0-1	0-1

Model Examination B

Answer Sheet

DIRECTIONS: Locate the question number to which you are responding, then fill in the circle containing the letter of the answer you have chosen. (Note: This answer sheet and the additional sheets provided on pages 433–436 are for practice purposes *only*. The actual DAT is given in a computer test format. It is highly recommended that you obtain a copy of the DAT tutorial disk to familiarize yourself with the format. See page 416 for information on how to obtain a copy of the disk.)

SURVEY OF THE NATURAL SCIENCES

1. Ⓐ Ⓑ Ⓒ Ⓓ Ⓔ
2. Ⓐ Ⓑ Ⓒ Ⓓ Ⓔ
3. Ⓐ Ⓑ Ⓒ Ⓓ Ⓔ
4. Ⓐ Ⓑ Ⓒ Ⓓ Ⓔ
5. Ⓐ Ⓑ Ⓒ Ⓓ Ⓔ
6. Ⓐ Ⓑ Ⓒ Ⓓ Ⓔ
7. Ⓐ Ⓑ Ⓒ Ⓓ Ⓔ
8. Ⓐ Ⓑ Ⓒ Ⓓ Ⓔ
9. Ⓐ Ⓑ Ⓒ Ⓓ Ⓔ
10. Ⓐ Ⓑ Ⓒ Ⓓ Ⓔ
11. Ⓐ Ⓑ Ⓒ Ⓓ Ⓔ
12. Ⓐ Ⓑ Ⓒ Ⓓ Ⓔ
13. Ⓐ Ⓑ Ⓒ Ⓓ Ⓔ
14. Ⓐ Ⓑ Ⓒ Ⓓ Ⓔ
15. Ⓐ Ⓑ Ⓒ Ⓓ Ⓔ
16. Ⓐ Ⓑ Ⓒ Ⓓ Ⓔ
17. Ⓐ Ⓑ Ⓒ Ⓓ Ⓔ
18. Ⓐ Ⓑ Ⓒ Ⓓ Ⓔ
19. Ⓐ Ⓑ Ⓒ Ⓓ Ⓔ
20. Ⓐ Ⓑ Ⓒ Ⓓ Ⓔ
21. Ⓐ Ⓑ Ⓒ Ⓓ Ⓔ
22. Ⓐ Ⓑ Ⓒ Ⓓ Ⓔ
23. Ⓐ Ⓑ Ⓒ Ⓓ Ⓔ
24. Ⓐ Ⓑ Ⓒ Ⓓ Ⓔ
25. Ⓐ Ⓑ Ⓒ Ⓓ Ⓔ
26. Ⓐ Ⓑ Ⓒ Ⓓ Ⓔ
27. Ⓐ Ⓑ Ⓒ Ⓓ Ⓔ
28. Ⓐ Ⓑ Ⓒ Ⓓ Ⓔ
29. Ⓐ Ⓑ Ⓒ Ⓓ Ⓔ
30. Ⓐ Ⓑ Ⓒ Ⓓ Ⓔ
31. Ⓐ Ⓑ Ⓒ Ⓓ Ⓔ
32. Ⓐ Ⓑ Ⓒ Ⓓ Ⓔ
33. Ⓐ Ⓑ Ⓒ Ⓓ Ⓔ
34. Ⓐ Ⓑ Ⓒ Ⓓ Ⓔ
35. Ⓐ Ⓑ Ⓒ Ⓓ Ⓔ
36. Ⓐ Ⓑ Ⓒ Ⓓ Ⓔ
37. Ⓐ Ⓑ Ⓒ Ⓓ Ⓔ
38. Ⓐ Ⓑ Ⓒ Ⓓ Ⓔ
39. Ⓐ Ⓑ Ⓒ Ⓓ Ⓔ
40. Ⓐ Ⓑ Ⓒ Ⓓ Ⓔ
41. Ⓐ Ⓑ Ⓒ Ⓓ Ⓔ
42. Ⓐ Ⓑ Ⓒ Ⓓ Ⓔ
43. Ⓐ Ⓑ Ⓒ Ⓓ Ⓔ
44. Ⓐ Ⓑ Ⓒ Ⓓ Ⓔ
45. Ⓐ Ⓑ Ⓒ Ⓓ Ⓔ
46. Ⓐ Ⓑ Ⓒ Ⓓ Ⓔ
47. Ⓐ Ⓑ Ⓒ Ⓓ Ⓔ
48. Ⓐ Ⓑ Ⓒ Ⓓ Ⓔ
49. Ⓐ Ⓑ Ⓒ Ⓓ Ⓔ
50. Ⓐ Ⓑ Ⓒ Ⓓ Ⓔ
51. Ⓐ Ⓑ Ⓒ Ⓓ Ⓔ
52. Ⓐ Ⓑ Ⓒ Ⓓ Ⓔ
53. Ⓐ Ⓑ Ⓒ Ⓓ Ⓔ
54. Ⓐ Ⓑ Ⓒ Ⓓ Ⓔ
55. Ⓐ Ⓑ Ⓒ Ⓓ Ⓔ
56. Ⓐ Ⓑ Ⓒ Ⓓ Ⓔ
57. Ⓐ Ⓑ Ⓒ Ⓓ Ⓔ
58. Ⓐ Ⓑ Ⓒ Ⓓ Ⓔ
59. Ⓐ Ⓑ Ⓒ Ⓓ Ⓔ
60. Ⓐ Ⓑ Ⓒ Ⓓ Ⓔ
61. Ⓐ Ⓑ Ⓒ Ⓓ Ⓔ
62. Ⓐ Ⓑ Ⓒ Ⓓ Ⓔ
63. Ⓐ Ⓑ Ⓒ Ⓓ Ⓔ
64. Ⓐ Ⓑ Ⓒ Ⓓ Ⓔ
65. Ⓐ Ⓑ Ⓒ Ⓓ Ⓔ
66. Ⓐ Ⓑ Ⓒ Ⓓ Ⓔ
67. Ⓐ Ⓑ Ⓒ Ⓓ Ⓔ
68. Ⓐ Ⓑ Ⓒ Ⓓ Ⓔ
69. Ⓐ Ⓑ Ⓒ Ⓓ Ⓔ
70. Ⓐ Ⓑ Ⓒ Ⓓ Ⓔ
71. Ⓐ Ⓑ Ⓒ Ⓓ Ⓔ
72. Ⓐ Ⓑ Ⓒ Ⓓ Ⓔ
73. Ⓐ Ⓑ Ⓒ Ⓓ Ⓔ
74. Ⓐ Ⓑ Ⓒ Ⓓ Ⓔ
75. Ⓐ Ⓑ Ⓒ Ⓓ Ⓔ
76. Ⓐ Ⓑ Ⓒ Ⓓ Ⓔ
77. Ⓐ Ⓑ Ⓒ Ⓓ Ⓔ
78. Ⓐ Ⓑ Ⓒ Ⓓ Ⓔ
79. Ⓐ Ⓑ Ⓒ Ⓓ Ⓔ
80. Ⓐ Ⓑ Ⓒ Ⓓ Ⓔ
81. Ⓐ Ⓑ Ⓒ Ⓓ Ⓔ
82. Ⓐ Ⓑ Ⓒ Ⓓ Ⓔ
83. Ⓐ Ⓑ Ⓒ Ⓓ Ⓔ
84. Ⓐ Ⓑ Ⓒ Ⓓ Ⓔ
85. Ⓐ Ⓑ Ⓒ Ⓓ Ⓔ
86. Ⓐ Ⓑ Ⓒ Ⓓ Ⓔ
87. Ⓐ Ⓑ Ⓒ Ⓓ Ⓔ
88. Ⓐ Ⓑ Ⓒ Ⓓ Ⓔ
89. Ⓐ Ⓑ Ⓒ Ⓓ Ⓔ
90. Ⓐ Ⓑ Ⓒ Ⓓ Ⓔ
91. Ⓐ Ⓑ Ⓒ Ⓓ Ⓔ
92. Ⓐ Ⓑ Ⓒ Ⓓ Ⓔ
93. Ⓐ Ⓑ Ⓒ Ⓓ Ⓔ
94. Ⓐ Ⓑ Ⓒ Ⓓ Ⓔ
95. Ⓐ Ⓑ Ⓒ Ⓓ Ⓔ
96. Ⓐ Ⓑ Ⓒ Ⓓ Ⓔ
97. Ⓐ Ⓑ Ⓒ Ⓓ Ⓔ
98. Ⓐ Ⓑ Ⓒ Ⓓ Ⓔ
99. Ⓐ Ⓑ Ⓒ Ⓓ Ⓔ
100. Ⓐ Ⓑ Ⓒ Ⓓ Ⓔ

PERCEPTUAL ABILITY TEST

1. Ⓐ Ⓑ Ⓒ Ⓓ Ⓔ
2. Ⓐ Ⓑ Ⓒ Ⓓ Ⓔ
3. Ⓐ Ⓑ Ⓒ Ⓓ Ⓔ
4. Ⓐ Ⓑ Ⓒ Ⓓ Ⓔ
5. Ⓐ Ⓑ Ⓒ Ⓓ Ⓔ
6. Ⓐ Ⓑ Ⓒ Ⓓ Ⓔ
7. Ⓐ Ⓑ Ⓒ Ⓓ Ⓔ
8. Ⓐ Ⓑ Ⓒ Ⓓ Ⓔ
9. Ⓐ Ⓑ Ⓒ Ⓓ Ⓔ
10. Ⓐ Ⓑ Ⓒ Ⓓ Ⓔ
11. Ⓐ Ⓑ Ⓒ Ⓓ Ⓔ
12. Ⓐ Ⓑ Ⓒ Ⓓ Ⓔ
13. Ⓐ Ⓑ Ⓒ Ⓓ Ⓔ
14. Ⓐ Ⓑ Ⓒ Ⓓ Ⓔ

15. Ⓐ Ⓑ Ⓒ Ⓓ Ⓔ
16. Ⓐ Ⓑ Ⓒ Ⓓ Ⓔ
17. Ⓐ Ⓑ Ⓒ Ⓓ Ⓔ
18. Ⓐ Ⓑ Ⓒ Ⓓ Ⓔ
19. Ⓐ Ⓑ Ⓒ Ⓓ Ⓔ
20. Ⓐ Ⓑ Ⓒ Ⓓ Ⓔ
21. Ⓐ Ⓑ Ⓒ Ⓓ Ⓔ
22. Ⓐ Ⓑ Ⓒ Ⓓ Ⓔ
23. Ⓐ Ⓑ Ⓒ Ⓓ Ⓔ
24. Ⓐ Ⓑ Ⓒ Ⓓ Ⓔ
25. Ⓐ Ⓑ Ⓒ Ⓓ Ⓔ
26. Ⓐ Ⓑ Ⓒ Ⓓ Ⓔ
27. Ⓐ Ⓑ Ⓒ Ⓓ Ⓔ
28. Ⓐ Ⓑ Ⓒ Ⓓ Ⓔ
29. Ⓐ Ⓑ Ⓒ Ⓓ Ⓔ
30. Ⓐ Ⓑ Ⓒ Ⓓ Ⓔ
31. Ⓐ Ⓑ Ⓒ Ⓓ Ⓔ
32. Ⓐ Ⓑ Ⓒ Ⓓ Ⓔ
33. Ⓐ Ⓑ Ⓒ Ⓓ Ⓔ
34. Ⓐ Ⓑ Ⓒ Ⓓ Ⓔ
35. Ⓐ Ⓑ Ⓒ Ⓓ Ⓔ
36. Ⓐ Ⓑ Ⓒ Ⓓ Ⓔ
37. Ⓐ Ⓑ Ⓒ Ⓓ Ⓔ
38. Ⓐ Ⓑ Ⓒ Ⓓ Ⓔ
39. Ⓐ Ⓑ Ⓒ Ⓓ Ⓔ
40. Ⓐ Ⓑ Ⓒ Ⓓ Ⓔ
41. Ⓐ Ⓑ Ⓒ Ⓓ Ⓔ
42. Ⓐ Ⓑ Ⓒ Ⓓ Ⓔ
43. Ⓐ Ⓑ Ⓒ Ⓓ Ⓔ
44. Ⓐ Ⓑ Ⓒ Ⓓ Ⓔ
45. Ⓐ Ⓑ Ⓒ Ⓓ Ⓔ
46. Ⓐ Ⓑ Ⓒ Ⓓ Ⓔ
47. Ⓐ Ⓑ Ⓒ Ⓓ Ⓔ
48. Ⓐ Ⓑ Ⓒ Ⓓ Ⓔ
49. Ⓐ Ⓑ Ⓒ Ⓓ Ⓔ
50. Ⓐ Ⓑ Ⓒ Ⓓ Ⓔ
51. Ⓐ Ⓑ Ⓒ Ⓓ Ⓔ
52. Ⓐ Ⓑ Ⓒ Ⓓ Ⓔ
53. Ⓐ Ⓑ Ⓒ Ⓓ Ⓔ
54. Ⓐ Ⓑ Ⓒ Ⓓ Ⓔ
55. Ⓐ Ⓑ Ⓒ Ⓓ Ⓔ
56. Ⓐ Ⓑ Ⓒ Ⓓ Ⓔ
57. Ⓐ Ⓑ Ⓒ Ⓓ Ⓔ
58. Ⓐ Ⓑ Ⓒ Ⓓ Ⓔ

59. Ⓐ Ⓑ Ⓒ Ⓓ Ⓔ
60. Ⓐ Ⓑ Ⓒ Ⓓ Ⓔ
61. Ⓐ Ⓑ Ⓒ Ⓓ Ⓔ
62. Ⓐ Ⓑ Ⓒ Ⓓ Ⓔ
63. Ⓐ Ⓑ Ⓒ Ⓓ Ⓔ
64. Ⓐ Ⓑ Ⓒ Ⓓ Ⓔ
65. Ⓐ Ⓑ Ⓒ Ⓓ Ⓔ
66. Ⓐ Ⓑ Ⓒ Ⓓ Ⓔ
67. Ⓐ Ⓑ Ⓒ Ⓓ Ⓔ
68. Ⓐ Ⓑ Ⓒ Ⓓ Ⓔ
69. Ⓐ Ⓑ Ⓒ Ⓓ Ⓔ
70. Ⓐ Ⓑ Ⓒ Ⓓ Ⓔ
71. Ⓐ Ⓑ Ⓒ Ⓓ Ⓔ
72. Ⓐ Ⓑ Ⓒ Ⓓ Ⓔ
73. Ⓐ Ⓑ Ⓒ Ⓓ Ⓔ
74. Ⓐ Ⓑ Ⓒ Ⓓ Ⓔ
75. Ⓐ Ⓑ Ⓒ Ⓓ Ⓔ
76. Ⓐ Ⓑ Ⓒ Ⓓ Ⓔ
77. Ⓐ Ⓑ Ⓒ Ⓓ Ⓔ
78. Ⓐ Ⓑ Ⓒ Ⓓ Ⓔ
79. Ⓐ Ⓑ Ⓒ Ⓓ Ⓔ
80. Ⓐ Ⓑ Ⓒ Ⓓ Ⓔ
81. Ⓐ Ⓑ Ⓒ Ⓓ Ⓔ
82. Ⓐ Ⓑ Ⓒ Ⓓ Ⓔ
83. Ⓐ Ⓑ Ⓒ Ⓓ Ⓔ
84. Ⓐ Ⓑ Ⓒ Ⓓ Ⓔ
85. Ⓐ Ⓑ Ⓒ Ⓓ Ⓔ
86. Ⓐ Ⓑ Ⓒ Ⓓ Ⓔ
87. Ⓐ Ⓑ Ⓒ Ⓓ Ⓔ
88. Ⓐ Ⓑ Ⓒ Ⓓ Ⓔ
89. Ⓐ Ⓑ Ⓒ Ⓓ Ⓔ
90. Ⓐ Ⓑ Ⓒ Ⓓ Ⓔ

READING COMPREHENSION TEST

1. Ⓐ Ⓑ Ⓒ Ⓓ Ⓔ
2. Ⓐ Ⓑ Ⓒ Ⓓ Ⓔ
3. Ⓐ Ⓑ Ⓒ Ⓓ Ⓔ
4. Ⓐ Ⓑ Ⓒ Ⓓ Ⓔ
5. Ⓐ Ⓑ Ⓒ Ⓓ Ⓔ
6. Ⓐ Ⓑ Ⓒ Ⓓ Ⓔ
7. Ⓐ Ⓑ Ⓒ Ⓓ Ⓔ

8. Ⓐ Ⓑ Ⓒ Ⓓ Ⓔ
9. Ⓐ Ⓑ Ⓒ Ⓓ Ⓔ
10. Ⓐ Ⓑ Ⓒ Ⓓ Ⓔ
11. Ⓐ Ⓑ Ⓒ Ⓓ Ⓔ
12. Ⓐ Ⓑ Ⓒ Ⓓ Ⓔ
13. Ⓐ Ⓑ Ⓒ Ⓓ Ⓔ
14. Ⓐ Ⓑ Ⓒ Ⓓ Ⓔ
15. Ⓐ Ⓑ Ⓒ Ⓓ Ⓔ
16. Ⓐ Ⓑ Ⓒ Ⓓ Ⓔ
17. Ⓐ Ⓑ Ⓒ Ⓓ Ⓔ
18. Ⓐ Ⓑ Ⓒ Ⓓ Ⓔ
19. Ⓐ Ⓑ Ⓒ Ⓓ Ⓔ
20. Ⓐ Ⓑ Ⓒ Ⓓ Ⓔ
21. Ⓐ Ⓑ Ⓒ Ⓓ Ⓔ
22. Ⓐ Ⓑ Ⓒ Ⓓ Ⓔ
23. Ⓐ Ⓑ Ⓒ Ⓓ Ⓔ
24. Ⓐ Ⓑ Ⓒ Ⓓ Ⓔ
25. Ⓐ Ⓑ Ⓒ Ⓓ Ⓔ
26. Ⓐ Ⓑ Ⓒ Ⓓ Ⓔ
27. Ⓐ Ⓑ Ⓒ Ⓓ Ⓔ
28. Ⓐ Ⓑ Ⓒ Ⓓ Ⓔ
29. Ⓐ Ⓑ Ⓒ Ⓓ Ⓔ
30. Ⓐ Ⓑ Ⓒ Ⓓ Ⓔ
31. Ⓐ Ⓑ Ⓒ Ⓓ Ⓔ
32. Ⓐ Ⓑ Ⓒ Ⓓ Ⓔ
33. Ⓐ Ⓑ Ⓒ Ⓓ Ⓔ
34. Ⓐ Ⓑ Ⓒ Ⓓ Ⓔ
35. Ⓐ Ⓑ Ⓒ Ⓓ Ⓔ
36. Ⓐ Ⓑ Ⓒ Ⓓ Ⓔ
37. Ⓐ Ⓑ Ⓒ Ⓓ Ⓔ
38. Ⓐ Ⓑ Ⓒ Ⓓ Ⓔ
39. Ⓐ Ⓑ Ⓒ Ⓓ Ⓔ
40. Ⓐ Ⓑ Ⓒ Ⓓ Ⓔ
41. Ⓐ Ⓑ Ⓒ Ⓓ Ⓔ
42. Ⓐ Ⓑ Ⓒ Ⓓ Ⓔ
43. Ⓐ Ⓑ Ⓒ Ⓓ Ⓔ
44. Ⓐ Ⓑ Ⓒ Ⓓ Ⓔ
45. Ⓐ Ⓑ Ⓒ Ⓓ Ⓔ
46. Ⓐ Ⓑ Ⓒ Ⓓ Ⓔ
47. Ⓐ Ⓑ Ⓒ Ⓓ Ⓔ
48. Ⓐ Ⓑ Ⓒ Ⓓ Ⓔ
49. Ⓐ Ⓑ Ⓒ Ⓓ Ⓔ
50. Ⓐ Ⓑ Ⓒ Ⓓ Ⓔ

QUANTITATIVE REASONING TEST

1. Ⓐ Ⓑ Ⓒ Ⓓ Ⓔ
2. Ⓐ Ⓑ Ⓒ Ⓓ Ⓔ
3. Ⓐ Ⓑ Ⓒ Ⓓ Ⓔ
4. Ⓐ Ⓑ Ⓒ Ⓓ Ⓔ
5. Ⓐ Ⓑ Ⓒ Ⓓ Ⓔ
6. Ⓐ Ⓑ Ⓒ Ⓓ Ⓔ
7. Ⓐ Ⓑ Ⓒ Ⓓ Ⓔ
8. Ⓐ Ⓑ Ⓒ Ⓓ Ⓔ
9. Ⓐ Ⓑ Ⓒ Ⓓ Ⓔ
10. Ⓐ Ⓑ Ⓒ Ⓓ Ⓔ
11. Ⓐ Ⓑ Ⓒ Ⓓ Ⓔ
12. Ⓐ Ⓑ Ⓒ Ⓓ Ⓔ
13. Ⓐ Ⓑ Ⓒ Ⓓ Ⓔ
14. Ⓐ Ⓑ Ⓒ Ⓓ Ⓔ
15. Ⓐ Ⓑ Ⓒ Ⓓ Ⓔ
16. Ⓐ Ⓑ Ⓒ Ⓓ Ⓔ
17. Ⓐ Ⓑ Ⓒ Ⓓ Ⓔ
18. Ⓐ Ⓑ Ⓒ Ⓓ Ⓔ
19. Ⓐ Ⓑ Ⓒ Ⓓ Ⓔ
20. Ⓐ Ⓑ Ⓒ Ⓓ Ⓔ
21. Ⓐ Ⓑ Ⓒ Ⓓ Ⓔ
22. Ⓐ Ⓑ Ⓒ Ⓓ Ⓔ
23. Ⓐ Ⓑ Ⓒ Ⓓ Ⓔ
24. Ⓐ Ⓑ Ⓒ Ⓓ Ⓔ
25. Ⓐ Ⓑ Ⓒ Ⓓ Ⓔ
26. Ⓐ Ⓑ Ⓒ Ⓓ Ⓔ
27. Ⓐ Ⓑ Ⓒ Ⓓ Ⓔ
28. Ⓐ Ⓑ Ⓒ Ⓓ Ⓔ
29. Ⓐ Ⓑ Ⓒ Ⓓ Ⓔ
30. Ⓐ Ⓑ Ⓒ Ⓓ Ⓔ
31. Ⓐ Ⓑ Ⓒ Ⓓ Ⓔ
32. Ⓐ Ⓑ Ⓒ Ⓓ Ⓔ
33. Ⓐ Ⓑ Ⓒ Ⓓ Ⓔ
34. Ⓐ Ⓑ Ⓒ Ⓓ Ⓔ
35. Ⓐ Ⓑ Ⓒ Ⓓ Ⓔ
36. Ⓐ Ⓑ Ⓒ Ⓓ Ⓔ
37. Ⓐ Ⓑ Ⓒ Ⓓ Ⓔ
38. Ⓐ Ⓑ Ⓒ Ⓓ Ⓔ
39. Ⓐ Ⓑ Ⓒ Ⓓ Ⓔ
40. Ⓐ Ⓑ Ⓒ Ⓓ Ⓔ

SURVEY OF THE NATURAL SCIENCES

Directions: The following items are questions or incomplete statements. Read each item carefully, then choose the best answer. Blacken the corresponding space on the answer sheet. **This section contains 100 items: Biology (1–40), General Chemistry (41–70), and Organic Chemistry (71–100).**

Time Limit: 90 minutes

1. If 120 amino acids form a protein, the gene for that protein contains _____ nucleotides.
   A. 60
   B. 40
   C. 240
   D. 360
   E. 120

2. In the process of respiration, oxygen
   A. combines with carbon to form CO^2
   B. produces energy in the form of ATP as it passes through the respiratory chain
   C. acts as the final electron acceptor
   D. is a cofactor for glycolytic enzymes
   E. bonds to lactic acid to form pyruvic acid

3. Mitosis and meiosis share several characteristics. Which of the following processes occurs in mitosis but does NOT occur in meiosis?
   A. Genetically identical daughter cells are produced.
   B. Spindle fibers form.
   C. Centromeres divide.
   D. Sex chromosomes segregate.
   E. Homologous pairs come together to form tetrads.

4. Organisms that obtain energy from light are
   A. heterotrophic
   B. lytic
   C. hydrophilic
   D. heliotrophic
   E. autotrophic

5. In association with reproductive organs, the follicle
   A. secretes androgen to the testes
   B. is a sac that protects and nourishes the egg
   C. fuses to the yolk sac to form the umbilical cord
   D. later becomes the digestive tract
   E. has the same function as the zygote

6. The process of fermentation
   A. converts ethanol into fructose
   B. yields glucose as an endproduct
   C. occurs only if oxygen is present
   D. takes place in the endoplasmic reticulum
   E. is less efficient than aerobic respiration in producing energy

7. Which of the following organelles is absent from fungi?
   A. secretory vesicles
   B. mitochondria
   C. chloroplasts
   D. Golgi bodies
   E. ribosomes

8. The liver has several functions. One of those functions is to
   A. convert ammonia into urea
   B. remove salts from filtrates
   C. return filtered blood to the circulatory system
   D. secrete antidiuretic hormone
   E. return sugars and amino acids to the blood

9. In the testes, the _____ respond to the leutinizing hormone by producing steroids.
   A. gametes
   B. germ cells
   C. interstitial cells
   D. tubules
   E. endometrial cells

10. Which of the following terms best describes a bacteriophage?
    A. prokaryote
    B. virus
    C. organelle
    D. bacterium
    E. eukaryote

11. In the absence of oxygen, aerobic organisms obtain their energy from
    A. oxidative phosphorylation
    B. the Krebs cycle
    C. glycolysis
    D. respiration
    E. photosynthesis

12. Eukaryotic cell membranes
    A. invaginate to form cristae, on which are arranged the electron transport systems
    B. are single layers of molecules approximately 75 angstroms in thickness
    C. are composed exclusively of phospholipids
    D. form rigid layers that prevent the cell from expanding
    E. are selectively permeable

13. Research into a new drug reveals that one of its side effects is to destroy the ectodermal germ layer of developing embryos. If this drug were administered to a pregnant woman, which of the following would be absent in the fetus?
    A. adrenal medulla
    B. femur
    C. stomach
    D. heart
    E. iliac vein

14. _____ synthesizes complementary nucleic acid strands in a process called transcription.
    A. DNA polymerase
    B. DNA ligase
    C. RNA polymerase
    D. Helicase
    E. Toposiomerase

15. An example of a group of prokaryotic cells is
    A. fungus
    B. yeast
    C. slime mold
    D. moss
    E. cyanobacterium

16. The part of the brain that regulates heart rate is the
    A. hypothalamus
    B. cerebral cortex
    C. cerebellum
    D. pons
    E. thalamus

17. The plasma molecules that help in regulating blood pressure are called
    A. albumins
    B. globulins
    C. fibrinogens
    D. platelets
    E. leukocytes

18. When a gene is sex-linked,
    A. the X-linked characters are always passed on from mother to daughter
    B. normal males always possess a Y-chromosome
    C. recessive autosomal characters are expressed in the father and expressed in his son
    D. the sex of the offspring is determined by the X-linked traits
    E. the X-linked characters are never passed on from mother to daughter

19. A population of rabbits is in Hardy-Weinberg equilibrium, with 9 percent of the population homozygous recessive for the albino trait. The percent of the population that is heterozygous for the albino trait is
    A. 3
    B. 21
    C. 18
    D. 27
    E. 36

20. Corals are in the same phylum as
    A. sponges
    B. giant squid
    C. starfish
    D. jellyfish
    E. tapeworms

21. Darwin's theory of natural selection states that evolution "selects" for traits that
    A. increase an organism's ability to survive in an environment
    B. decrease the number of deleterious genes
    C. increase the number of viable offspring for an individual
    D. result in longer life spans
    E. lead to improved social behavior

22. The term *saltatory conduction* describes
    A. the process by which neurotransmitters are inhibited in a chemical synapse
    B. the transmission of impulses between the dendrites of a gap junction
    C. changes in the sodium concentrations of axon
    D. the processing of information by a nerve cell
    E. the propagation of an impulse along an insulated axon

23. Albinism is inherited as an autosomal recessive trait. If a man and a woman are both heterozygous for albinism, what is the probability that their child will also be heterozygous for this trait?
    A. 0
    B. .25
    C. .5
    D. .75
    E. 1

24. During the process of neurulation,
    A. the ectoderm begins to develop into the notochord
    B. three distinct germ layers develop
    C. organogenesis begins
    D. the neural tube opens and begins to develop into the spinal column
    E. the third and fourth cleavages take place

25. Within a eukaryotic cell, the site for chemical modification of proteins is the
    A. secretory vesicles
    B. Golgi apparatus
    C. mitochondria
    D. ribosomes
    E. nucleolus

26. Cholesterol is an example of
    A. a steroid
    B. a carbohydrate
    C. a polysaccharide
    D. an amino acid
    E. a protein

27. The following statements describe different aspects of a cell's cytoskeleton. Which statement is FALSE?
    A. The cytoskeleton is associated with three different classes of filaments.
    B. Cilia and flagella terminate in structures known as basal bodies.
    C. Intermediate filaments are about 10 nm in diameter.
    D. Microtubules are composed of two types of lipids.
    E. One function of the cytoskeleton is to maintain the shape of the cell.

28. Which of the following does (do) NOT belong to the peripheral nervous system?
    A. afferent neurons
    B. efferent neurons
    C. optic nerve
    D. spinal cord
    E. olfactory bulbs

29. During a menstrual cycle, hormone levels vary according to a programmed sequence. Which of the following describes the correct sequence of events?
    A. increase in FSH, decrease in LH, increase in estrogen
    B. increase in estrogen, increase in FSH, decrease in progesterone
    C. decrease in LH, increase in FSH, increase in progesterone
    D. increase in FSH, increase in estrogen, decrease in progesterone
    E. increase in FSH, increase in estrogen, increase in progesterone

30. If an individual is heterozygous for five independently assorting genes, how many genetically different gametes can he produce?
    A. 5
    B. 10
    C. 50
    D. 5^2
    E. 2^5

31. Measles, herpes, and smallpox are caused by the activity of viruses. Yet the debate continues as to whether viruses are even alive. Which statement best supports the argument that viruses are NOT alive?
    A. Viruses are not eukaryotic cells.
    B. Viruses are primitive and extremely small.
    C. Viruses need other cells in order to reproduce.
    D. Viruses are parasitic.
    E. Viruses can lie dormant for long periods of time.

32. Sucrose is a
    A. subunit of starch
    B. subunit of cellulose
    C. trisaccaharide of fructose, galactose, and glucose
    D. disaccharide of glucose and fructose
    E. sugar produced in glycolysis

33. Muscle contractions are triggered by
    A. calcium
    B. phosphorus
    C. sodium
    D. potassium
    E. myofibrils

34. Which of the following is NOT consistent with a humoral immune response?
    A. B-cell production of antibodies
    B. T-cell destruction of foreign cells
    C. decrease in B-cell production after infection is controlled
    D. storage of memory cells in the spleen
    E. removed by phagocytic cells of complexes of antigen

35. Which of the following glands has both an endocrine and an exocrine function?
    A. adrenal
    B. pancreas
    C. pituitary
    D. pinneal
    E. thyroid

36. In which of the following phyla are only bilaterally symmetrical animals found?
    A. Chordata
    B. Echinodermata
    C. Mollusca
    D. Ctenophora
    E. Platyhelminthes

37. In an experiment to better understand bird speciation, a researcher placed a mesh fence in the middle of a large bird cage. The fence prevented birds on one side from mating with birds on the other side. This experiment simulates
    A. parapatric speciation
    B. genetic drift
    C. sympatric speciation
    D. allopatric speciation
    E. Hardy-Weinberg equilibrium

38. On a remote island, a new spider species is discovered. The spider strongly resembles a well-known poisonous species, but is harmless. The spider is an example of
    A. mutualism
    B. parasitism
    C. Batesian mimicry
    D. Mullerian mimicry
    E. intraspecific competition

39. If a segment of a DNA base sequence is CAT, what is the complementary portion of mRNA?
    A. CAT
    B. TAC
    C. ATC
    D. GTU
    E. GUA

40. Which of the following characteristics does NOT describe an r-selected species?
    A. occurs more often in stable environments
    B. has a high birth rate
    C. has a short life span
    D. tends to stay below carrying capacity
    E. maximizes population growth

41. In which of the following compounds is the oxidation number of Sulfur equal to +2?
    A. H_2S
    B. S_8
    C. SCl_2
    D. Na_2SO_3
    E. SO_4^{2-}

42. Which of the following molecular species is trigonal pyramidal?
    A. SO_2
    B. BF_3
    C. CH_4
    D. NH_3
    E. HCO_3

43. In the reaction below, which compound is acting like a conjugate acid?

    $H_2C_2O_4(aq) + H_2O(l) \leftrightarrow HC_2O_4^-(aq) + H_3O^+ (aq)$

    A. $H_2C_2O_4$
    B. H_2O
    C. $HC_2O_4^-$
    D. H_3O^+
    E. none of the above

44. The numbers of protons and neutrons, respectively, in $_8^{17}O^{2-}$ are
    A. 8 and 10
    B. 9 and 8
    C. 8 and 9
    D. 17 and 8
    E. 8 and 17

45. In which of the following species does phosphorus exhibit its highest oxidation number?
    A. P_2O_5
    B. PH_3
    C. H_3PO_3
    D. P_4
    E. PCL_3

46. In the nuclear reaction below, what is X?

    $X + proton \rightarrow {}^{22}Mg + neutron$

    A. ^{21}Ne
    B. ^{23}Mg
    C. ^{21}Mg
    D. ^{22}Na
    E. ^{23}Na

47. Precipitation of a solution will occur when
    A. ion product $> K_{sp}$
    B. ion product $= K_{sp}$
    C. ion product $< K_{sp}$
    D. Ion product will always cause precipitation.
    E. Ion product will never cause precipitation.

48. If ΔG has a negative value, the reaction
    A. is at equilibrium
    B. is nonspontaneous, but its reverse reaction is spontaneous
    C. is spontaneous and forward
    D. is exothermic
    E. is endothermic

49. Which of the following types of bonds is characterized by being brittle, a poor conductor of electricity, and held together by electrostatic forces.
    A. metallic
    B. ionic
    C. covalent
    D. molecular
    E. hydrogen

50. The point of a phase diagram at which the gas and liquid states are indistinguishable is known as the
    A. critical point
    B. triple point
    C. equivalence point
    D. titration point
    E. point of neutrality

51. In an experiment 25 grams of HCl (g) is dissolved in water to make 100 milliliters of an acidic solution. Assuming that the acid completely ionized, what is the pH of the solution?
    A. $-log [25/(0.1 \times 2)]$
    B. $-log [25 \times 0.1/36]$
    C. $-log [25/(0.1 \times 36)]$
    D. $-log [36/(0.1 \times 25)]$
    E. $-log [0.1/25]$

52. If a balloon is filled with gas until the pressure equals 43 atmospheres at 200 K, what temperature will have to be reached for the balloon pressure to reach 55 atmospheres?
    A. 256 K
    B. 1,200 K
    C. 131 K
    D. 2,500 K
    E. 1,813 K

53. In which two compounds does sulfur have the same oxidation state?
    A. SO_4 and Na_2SO_4
    B. SO_2 and Na_2SO_4
    C. SO_3 and H_2SO_4
    D. SO_2 and SO_3
    E. SO_4 and H_2S_2

54. What is the percent by mass of bromine in BrO_4^-?
    A. 39.5
    B. 24.8
    C. 49.3
    D. 55.5
    E. 16.3

55. What mass of styrene (molar mass = 104.1) will contain 4.5×10^{20} molecules of styrene?
    A. 0.00778 g
    B. 7.78×10^{-4} g
    C. 7.78×10^3 g
    D. 7.78×10^{-2} g
    E. 7.78×10^4 g

56. As carbon dioxide undergoes sublimation, which physical transformation occurs?
    A. gas to solid
    B. solid to gas
    C. solid to liquid
    D. solid to liquid to gas
    E. gas to liquid

57. Which of the following compounds consistently have the highest melting points?
    A. dipoles
    B. alkanes
    C. molecular crystals
    D. salts
    E. metals

58. Which of the following is NOT a correct chemical formula?
    A. $SrBr_2$
    B. CaO_2
    C. Mg_3N_2
    D. Na_2S
    E. AlI_3

59. When ammonium oxalate, $(NH_4)_2C_2O_4$, is dissolved in water, the ions formed are
    A. $2N^{3-}(aq) + 8H^+(aq) + 2C^{4+}(aq) + 4O^{2-}(aq)$
    B. $(NH_4)^{2+}(aq) + C_2O_4^{2-}(aq)$
    C. $2NH_4^+(aq) + C_2O_4^{2-}(aq)$
    D. $NH_4^{2+}(aq) + C_2O_4^{2-}(aq)$
    E. $2NH_4^+(aq) + 2CO_2^-(aq)$

60. A solution of KNO_3 is known to have a 0.564 molal concentration. To calculate the concentration of this solution in terms of molarity, which of the following must be specified?
    A. the density of the solution
    B. the volume of the solution
    C. the temperature of the solution
    D. the solubility product of KNO_3
    E. the K_a of nitric acid

61. A 10.0-gram sample of ethane, C_2H_6, is burned in an enclosed vessel with 40.0 grams of oxygen. Which of the following best describes the mixture when the reaction is complete?
    A. The mass of the system is 50.0 g.
    B. The limiting reactant is C_2H_6.
    C. The theoretical yield of CO_2 is 29.04 g.
    D. 21.52 g of oxygen is left over.
    E. All of the above statements are correct.

62. Which of the following sets of quantum numbers is IMPOSSIBLE?
    A. 4, 3, 1, +1/2
    B. 3, 2, –2, –1/2
    C. 5, 0, 0, –1/2
    D. 2, 2, –1, +1/2
    E. 3, 2, 0, +1/2

63. A compound consisting of carbon, hydrogen, and oxygen is known by quantitative analysis to have 38.71 percent carbon and 9.68 percent hydrogen. What is the empirical formula of this compound?
    A. CHO
    B. CH_2O
    C. CH_3O
    D. $C_2H_6O_2$
    E. CH_3

64. A substance that acts as both a Brönsted acid and a Brönsted base in an aqueous solution is
    A. HClO
    B. H_2SO_4
    C. PO_4^{3-}
    D. HSO_3^-
    E. ClO_4^-

65. The percent composition, by weight, of nitrogen in the compound $(NH_4)_2Cr_2O_7$ is

    A. $\left[\dfrac{14}{[14 + 4(1) + 2(52) + 7(16)]} \right] \times 100$

    B. $\left[\dfrac{(2)14}{[2(14) + 8(1) + 2(52) + 7(16)]} \right] \times 100$

    C. $\left[\dfrac{14}{(14 + 1 + 52 + 16)} \right] \times 100$

    D. $\left[\dfrac{(2)14}{[2(14) + 4(1) + 2(52) + 7(16)]} \right] \times 100$

    E. $\left[\dfrac{(2)14}{[8(1) + 2(52) + 7(16)]} \right] \times 100$

66. Which reaction has the most positive value of ΔS?
    A. $2NO_2 \text{ (g)} \rightarrow N_2O_4 \text{ (l)}$
    B. $2NO_2 \text{ (g)} \rightarrow N_2O_4 \text{ (g)}$
    C. $N_2O_4 \text{ (l)} \rightarrow 2NO_2 \text{ (g)}$
    D. $N_2O_4 \text{ (g)} \rightarrow 2NO_2 \text{ (g)}$
    E. $N_2O_4 \text{ (l)} \rightarrow 2NO_2 \text{ (l)}$

67. Which is the correct set of coefficients to balance the equation for the oxidation of ammonia?

    $$NH_3 + O_2 \rightarrow NO + H_2O$$

    A. 2, 3, 2, 3
    B. 3, 2, 3, 2
    C. 4, 5, 4, 6
    D. 2, 2, 2, 3
    E. 4, 6, 4, 6

68. A liter of solution contains 0.00001 mole of HCL. What is the pH of this solution?
    A. 1.0
    B. 4.0
    C. −4.0
    D. −5.0
    E. 5.0

69. Which trend in the halogen family occurs with increasing atomic number?
    A. decreasing ionic radius
    B. increasing first ionization potential
    C. decreasing electronegativity
    D. decreasing covalent radius
    E. decreasing melting points

70. How many liters of 5.0 molar ethyl alcohol (C_2H_5OH) can be prepared by dissolving 460 grams of ethyl alcohol in water? (Molecular weight of ethyl alcohol = 46)
    A. 1.0
    B. 1.5
    C. 2.0
    D. 2.5
    E. 5.0

71. In a double-bonded carbon atom
    A. hybridization between one *s* orbital and one *p* orbital occurs
    B. hybridization between one *s* orbital and two *p* orbitals occurs
    C. hybridization between one *s* orbital and three *p* orbitals occurs
    D. hybridization between two *s* orbitals and two *p* orbitals occurs
    E. no hybridization occurs

72. A carbon-carbon triple bond contains
    A. one sigma and two pi bonds
    B. one pi and two sigma bonds
    C. three sigma bonds
    D. three pi bonds
    E. three sigma and three pi bonds

73. What is the correct assignment of bond angles in the structure below?

    A. $a = 90°, b = 90°$
    B. $a = 180°, b = 109.5°$
    C. $a = 120°, b = 120°$
    D. $a = 180°, b = 120°$
    E. $a = 180°, b = 180°$

74. The most acidic hydrogen in the following compound is

    A. *a*
    B. *b*
    C. *c*
    D. *d*
    E. *e*

75. Which of the following is aromatic?

A. II only
B. II, III, and IV only
C. I, II, and IV only
D. II and IV only
E. all of the above

76. Which of the following compounds is (are) aromatic?

A.

B.

C.

D.

E. Both C and D

77. Which of the following molecules is most likely to be formed in abundance by a free-radical bromination reaction?
A. CH_3Br
B. $BrC(CH_3)_3$
C. $CH_3-CHBr-CH_2$
D. $CH_3-(CH_2)_8-CH_2Br$
E. None of these substances can be created by this reaction.

78. Which of the following compounds is (are) aromatic?

A.

B.

C.

D.

E. All of the above

79. How many peaks does CH_4 have in its ^1H NMR spectrograph?
A. 1
B. 4
C. 12
D. 16
E. The number of peaks depends on the phase of methane in the sample.

80. In the reaction

$$C_2H_5OH + CH_3O^- \leftrightarrow C_2H_5O^- + CH_3OH$$

the Brönstead-Lowry bases are

A. C_2H_5OH and CH_3O^-
B. $C_2H_5O^-$ and CH_3OH
C. C_2H_5OH and CH_3OH
D. $C_2H_5O^-$ and CH_3O^-
E. none of the above

81. Which reaction below is a possible initiation step in the free-radical chlorination of $CH_3CH_2CH_2CH_3$ by Cl_2?
    A. $Cl\bullet + CH_3CH_2CH_2CH_3 \rightarrow$
       $HCl + CH_3CH_2CH\bullet CH_3$
    B. $Cl_2 \rightarrow 2Cl\bullet$
    C. $Cl\bullet + CH_3CH_2CH_2CH_2\bullet \rightarrow$
       $CH_3CH_2CH_2CH_2Cl$
    D. $Cl\bullet + CH_3CH_2CH_2CH_3 \rightarrow$
       $CH_3CH_2CH_2CH_2\bullet + HCl$
    E. $Cl_2 + CH_3CH_2CH\bullet CH_3 \rightarrow$
       $CH_3CH_2CHClCH_3 + Cl\bullet$

82. Which of the following alkyl halides would you expect to be most reactive by an S_N2 mechanism?

    A.
    $$CH_3 - \underset{\underset{CH_3}{|}}{\overset{\overset{CH_3}{|}}{C}} - CH_2 - Br$$

    B. $CH_3 - \underset{\underset{Br}{|}}{CH} - CH_2 - CH_3$

    C. $CH_3 - CH_2 - CH_2 - CH_2 - Br$

    D.
    $$CH_3 - \underset{\underset{CH_3}{|}}{\overset{\overset{CH_3}{|}}{C}} - Br$$

    E. $CH_3 - \underset{\underset{CH_3}{|}}{CH} - \underset{\underset{I}{|}}{CH} - CH_3$

83. Which of the following compounds has the highest boiling point?
    A. CH_3CH_3

    B.

    C. $CH_3CH_2CH_2CH_3$
    D. $CH_3CH_2CH(CH_3)CH_3$
    E. $CH_3CH_2CH_2CH_2CH_3$

84. Which of the following molecules is the LEAST soluble in water?
    A.
    $$CH_3 - CH_2 - CH_2 - \overset{\overset{O}{\|}}{C} - H$$

    B. $CH_3 - CH_2 - CH_2 - CH_2 - NH_2$

    C. $CH_3 - CH_2 - O - CH_2 - CH_3$

    D.
    $$CH_3 - \overset{\overset{O}{\|}}{C} - CH_3$$

    E. $CH_3 - CH_2 - CH_2 - CH_3$

85. What is the principal product of the following reaction?
    $$CH_3 - CH = CH_2 + HCl \longrightarrow ?$$

    A. $CH_3 - \underset{\underset{Cl}{|}}{CH} - \underset{\underset{H}{|}}{CH_2}$

    B. $CH_3 - \underset{\underset{H}{|}}{CH} - \underset{\underset{Cl}{|}}{CH_2}$

    C. $CH_3 - CH = C\overset{\diagup H}{\diagdown Cl}$

    D. $CH_3 - C\,(Cl) = CH_2$

    E. $CH_2 = Br = CH_2$

86. Which of the following free radicals is the most stable?
    A. $CH_3\bullet$
    B. $(CH_3)_3C\bullet$
    C. $(CH_3)_2CH\bullet$
    D. $CH_3CH_2CH_2\bullet$
    E. $CH_3(CH_2)_8CH_2\bullet$

87. Which of the following carbocations is (are) the most stable?
    A. R_2HC^+
    B. R_3C^+
    C. H_3C^+
    D. RH_2C^+
    E. B and C are equally stable

88. What is the IUPAC name of the following compound?

A. 3-chloro-3-butanal
B. 2-chloro-3-butanal
C. 3-chloro-2-butanone
D. 2-chloro-3-butanone
E. none of the above

89. What is the IUPAC name of the following compound?

A. 4-chloro-2-methylpentanoic acid
B. 5-chlorohexanoic acid
C. 2-chloro-4-methylpentanoic acid
D. 4-chloro-2-methyl-1-carbonyl-1-pentanol
E. none of the above

90. Which of the following alkyl halides is most likely to have formed by an S_N1 mechanism?

A.
$$CH_3 - \underset{\underset{CH_3}{|}}{\overset{\overset{CH_3}{|}}{C}} - CH_2 - Br$$

B. $CH_3 - \underset{\underset{Br}{|}}{CH} - CH_2 - CH_3$

C. $CH_3 - CH_2 - CH_2 - CH_2 - Br$

D.
$$CH_3 - \underset{\underset{Br}{|}}{\overset{\overset{CH_3}{|}}{C}} - CH_3$$

E.
$$CH_3 - \underset{\underset{CH_3}{|}}{CH} - \overset{\overset{I}{|}}{CH} - CH_3$$

91. Which of the following compounds would be the best solvent for an S_N2 reaction?
A. H_2O
B. CH_3CH_2OH
C. CH_3SOCH_3
D. $CH_3CH_2CH_2CH_2CH_3$
E. NH_3

92. S_N1 reactions show first-order kinetics because
A. the rate-limiting step is the first step in the reaction
B. the rate-limiting step involves only one molecule
C. there is only one rate-limiting step
D. the reaction involves just one molecule
E. none of the above

93. For the S_N1 reaction shown below:

$(CH_3)_3CI + 2H_2O \rightarrow (CH_3)_3COH + H_3O^+ + CI^-$

the rate expression is
A. rate $= k[(CH_3)_3CI][H_2O]$
B. rate $= k[(CH_3)_3CI]$
C. rate $= k[(CH_3)_3CI]^2$
D. rate $= k[H_2O]$
E. The rate does not depend on the concentration of either reactant.

94. Which of the following represents the product obtained in the reaction below?

A.

B.

C.

D.

E. none of the above

95. The products of the following reaction:

are

A.

B.

C.

D.

E. none of the above

96. The products of the following reaction:

1) O_3 /CH_2Cl_2
2) Zn, H_2O → ?

are

A.

OH +

O
‖
H   H

B.

O
‖
      + CH_3OH

C.

O
‖
      + CO_2

D.

O   O
‖   ‖
H   H   +

E. A and C

97. Which of the following statements about *E2* reactions is FALSE?
   A. *E2* reactions are greatly affected by steric hinderance.
   B. The rate of reaction is dependent on the concentrations of the two species.
   C. *E2* reactions occur in one step.
   D. *E2* reactions are favored over S_N2 by weak bases.
   E. All of the above are true.

98. Complete combustion of C_3H_8 will yield
   I. CO_2
   II. H_2O
   III. CO
   IV. heat

   A. I only
   B. I and II only
   C. I, II, and III only
   D. I, II, and IV only
   E. I, II, III, and IV

99. Which of the following is most likely to be a gas at room temperature?
   A. C_2H_6
   B. C_2H_5OH
   C. C_2H_6O
   D. C_6H_6
   E. none of the above

100. Which of the following statements is (are) true about S_N2 reactions?
   A. They are favored by methyl and 1° substrates.
   B. They are favored by polar aprotic solvents.
   C. They are favored by strong nucleophiles.
   D. They are favored by a good leaving group.
   E. All of the above.

PERCEPTUAL ABILITY TEST

Time Limit: 60 Minutes

Part 1

For questions 1 through 15:

This section of the exam consists of 15 items similar to the example below. In each item, a three-dimensional object is shown on the left, followed by outlines of five apertures to its right.

The task is the same for each item. Conceptualize how the three-dimensional object looks from each possible side (in addition to the side shown). Then, pick the outline in which the three-dimensional object could pass if the proper side were inserted. Choose the letter corresponding to the correct aperture.

Here are rules for Part 1, the aperture section:

1. The irregular solid three-dimensional object on the left can be rotated in any direction prior to passing through the aperture.
2. The object may not be twisted or rotated in any way once it has started to be passed through the aperture. The correct answer is the exact representation of the external outline of the object viewed from the appropriate side.
3. The objects and the outlines are drawn to the same scale.
4. There are no irregularities in hidden portions of the objects. If the figure has symmetric indentations, it is assumed that the hidden portion is symmetric with the portion shown.
5. There is only one correct answer.

Example:

The correct answer is C.

Proceed to the questions.

1.

2.

10.

11.

12.

13.

14.

15.

Part 2

For questions 16 through 30:

The pictures that follow are representations of solid objects from three different views: top, front, and end views. The pictures are views drawn without perspective: the surface viewed is along parallel lines of vision. The projection that is labeled TOP VIEW is shown looking DOWN on its top surface and is pictured in the upper-left corner. The projection labeled FRONT VIEW is shown looking at the object from the FRONT and is pictured in the lower-left corner. The projection labeled END VIEW is shown looking at the object from the END (or side) and is pictured in the lower-right corner. These three views are always in their respective corners and labeled accordingly.

If there were a hole in the figure, it would be represented like this:

DOTTED lines indicate lines that exist but cannot be seen in the perspective shown.

In the following problems, TWO of the previous three views discussed will be shown with four alternatives to the right. Choose the correct letter that represents the correct view that completes the set.

Example:

The FRONT VIEW shows that there is a smaller block on top of a larger block and there is no hole. The TOP VIEW shows that the top block is round and is centered on a rectangular block. From this information gathered in the two views given, the correct answer must be B.

In the following problems, one of the three views will be omitted; it is not always the END VIEW as shown in the example.

Proceed to the questions.

16.   Choose the correct TOP VIEW.

17.   Choose the correct END VIEW.

18.   Choose the correct FRONT VIEW.

19.   Choose the correct FRONT VIEW.

20.   Choose the correct END VIEW.

21. Choose the correct TOP VIEW.

22. Choose the correct TOP VIEW.

23. Choose the correct END VIEW.

24. Choose the correct TOP VIEW.

25. Choose the correct FRONT VIEW.

26. Choose the correct END VIEW.

27. Choose the correct TOP VIEW.

28. Choose the correct END VIEW.

29. Choose the correct TOP VIEW.

30. Choose the correct FRONT VIEW.

Part 3

For questions 31 through 45:

Examine the INTERNAL ANGLES and rank them in terms of degrees from SMALL to LARGE. Select the alternative that represents the correct ranking.

Example:

A. 1 – 2 – 4 – 3
B. 2 – 1 – 4 – 3
C. 3 – 4 – 2 – 1
D. 3 – 4 – 1 – 2

1   2   3   4

The correct ranking is 2–1–4–3. Therefore, the correct answer is B.

Proceed to the questions.

31.

A. 3 – 4 – 1 – 2
B. 1 – 4 – 3 – 2
C. 3 – 1 – 4 – 2
D. 1 – 3 – 4 – 2

1   2   3   4

32.

A. 4 – 2 – 3 – 1
B. 4 – 1 – 2 – 3
C. 2 – 4 – 1 – 2
D. 4 – 2 – 1 – 3

1   2   3   4

33.

A. 2 – 1 – 4 – 3
B. 1 – 2 – 4 – 3
C. 2 – 4 – 1 – 3
D. 4 – 2 – 3 – 1

1   2   3   4

34.

A. 3 – 1 – 2 – 4
B. 1 – 3 – 2 – 4
C. 3 – 1 – 4 – 2
D. 1 – 3 – 4 – 2

1   2   3   4

35.

A. 3 – 2 – 1 – 4
B. 3 – 1 – 2 – 4
C. 2 – 4 – 1 – 3
D. 4 – 3 – 2 – 1

1   2   3   4

36.

A. 2 – 4 – 3 – 1
B. 2 – 4 – 1 – 3
C. 4 – 2 – 3 – 1
D. 4 – 3 – 2 – 1

1   2   3   4

37.

A. 4 – 3 – 1 – 2
B. 3 – 1 – 4 – 2
C. 3 – 4 – 2 – 1
D. 4 – 2 – 3 – 1

1   2   3   4

38.

A. 4 – 3 – 2 – 1
B. 2 – 4 – 3 – 1
C. 2 – 4 – 1 – 3
D. 4 – 2 – 3 – 1

1   2   3   4

39.

A. 1 – 3 – 2 – 4
B. 1 – 4 – 3 – 2
C. 4 – 1 – 2 – 3
D. 1 – 4 – 2 – 3

1   2   3   4

40.

A. 3 – 2 – 1 – 4
B. 2 – 3 – 1 – 4
C. 2 – 3 – 4 – 1
D. 3 – 2 – 4 – 1

1   2   3   4

41.

1   2   3   4

A. 1 – 2 – 4 – 3
B. 4 – 1 – 3 – 2
C. 1 – 4 – 3 – 2
D. 4 – 1 – 2 – 3

42.

1   2   3   4

A. 4 – 1 – 3 – 2
B. 4 – 1 – 3 – 2
C. 1 – 4 – 3 – 2
D. 4 – 1 – 2 – 3

43.

1   2   3   4

A. 1 – 2 – 3 – 4
B. 3 – 1 – 4 – 2
C. 1 – 3 – 4 – 2
D. 4 – 3 – 1 – 2

44.

1   2   3   4

A. 4 – 2 – 3 – 1
B. 2 – 4 – 1 – 3
C. 2 – 4 – 3 – 1
D. 4 – 2 – 1 – 3

45.

1   2   3   4

A. 1 – 4 – 3 – 2
B. 3 – 1 – 4 – 2
C. 4 – 3 – 1 – 2
D. 1 – 4 – 2 – 3

Part 4

For questions 46 through 60:

A flat, square piece of paper is folded one or more times starting from the left, proceeding stepwise to the illustrations to the right. The original position of the paper is represented by broken lines. The solid line indicates edges of the folded paper. The piece of paper is never twisted or turned and always remains within the outline of the original square. There may be ONE FOLD, TWO FOLDS, or THREE FOLDS in each item. After the last fold, a hole is punched in the paper. Your task is to unfold the paper in your mind and determine the placement of the holes on the original flat, square piece of paper. There is only one correct pattern of hole punches for each item. The black circles indicate hole punches. Choose the pattern that indicates the correct pattern of hole punches in the unfolded paper.

Practice Illustrations:

Figure 1   Figure 2   Figure 3   Figure 4

In this example Figure 1 shows the original flat, square piece of paper. Figure 2 shows the first fold. Figure 3 shows the location of the hole punch in the folded paper. The black circles in Figure 4 show the pattern of the hole punches on the unfolded paper. The answer has two holes since the paper was two layers thick in the position where the hole was punched.

Example:

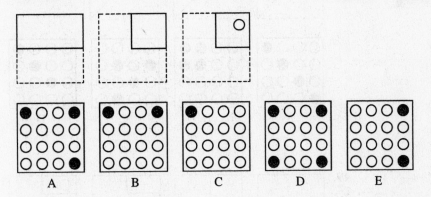

The correct answer is D. The paper was four thicknesses and therefore has four hole punches. The punch was made in the corner, so the four hole punches in the four corners are shown in black in the correct pattern.

Proceed to the questions.

58.

59.

60.

Part 5

For questions 61 through 75:

Each of the figures in this section is representative of cubes of the same size that have been cemented together. After the the cubes were cemented, the group of cubes were painted on each of the exposed sides WITH EXCEPTION TO THE BOT-TOM SIDE ON WHICH THE FIGURE IS RESTING. Some illustrations contain hidden cubes. The only hidden cubes are cubes that are necessary to support other cubes.

In each item you are to determine how many cubes have

- ONE side painted,
- TWO sides painted,
- THREE sides painted,
- FOUR sides painted, or
- FIVE sides painted.

There are no problems that will ask for the number of cubes that have none (zero) of their sides painted.

Example:
In Figure A, how many cubes have two of their sides painted?
A. 1 cube
B. 2 cubes
C. 3 cubes
D. 4 cubes
E. 5 cubes

hidden cube

FIGURE A

There are four cubes in Figure A (one is hidden supporting the top cube). The top cube has five sides painted. The hidden cube supporting it has two sides painted. The cubes in the foreground and to the left each have four sides painted. Therefore, there is only one cube that has just two sides painted and the correct answer is A.

Choose the letter that corresponds to the correct number of cubes with the given number of sides painted. Remember that THE BOTTOM OF THE CUBE IS NOT PAINTED.

Proceed to the questions.

61. In Figure A, how many cubes have one of their exposed sides painted?
A. 1 cube
B. 2 cubes
C. 3 cubes
D. 4 cubes
E. 5 cubes

FIGURE A

62. In Figure A, how many cubes have two of their exposed sides painted?
A. 1 cube
B. 2 cubes
C. 3 cubes
D. 4 cubes
E. 5 cubes

63. In Figure A, how many cubes have three of their exposed sides painted?
A. 1 cube
B. 2 cubes
C. 3 cubes
D. 4 cubes
E. 5 cubes

64. In Figure A, how many cubes have four of
their exposed sides painted?
A. 1 cube
B. 2 cubes
C. 3 cubes
D. 4 cubes
E. 5 cubes

FIGURE A

65. In Figure B, how many cubes have two of
their exposed sides painted?
A. 1 cube
B. 2 cubes
C. 3 cubes
D. 4 cubes
E. 5 cubes

FIGURE B

66. In Figure B, how many cubes have three
of their exposed sides painted?
A. 1 cube
B. 2 cubes
C. 3 cubes
D. 4 cubes
E. 5 cubes

67. In Figure C, how many cubes have one of
their exposed sides painted?
A. 1 cube
B. 2 cubes
C. 3 cubes
D. 4 cubes
E. 5 cubes

FIGURE C

68. In Figure C, how many cubes have two of
their exposed sides painted?
A. 1 cube
B. 2 cubes
C. 3 cubes
D. 4 cubes
E. 5 cubes

69. In Figure C, how many cubes have four of
their exposed sides painted?
A. 1 cube
B. 2 cubes
C. 3 cubes
D. 4 cubes
E. 5 cubes

70. In Figure D, how many cubes have two of
    their exposed sides painted?
    A. 1 cube
    B. 2 cubes
    C. 3 cubes
    D. 4 cubes
    E. 5 cubes

FIGURE D

71. In Figure D, how many cubes have four of
    their exposed sides painted?
    A. 1 cube
    B. 2 cubes
    C. 3 cubes
    D. 4 cubes
    E. 5 cubes

72. In Figure D, how many cubes have five of
    their exposed sides painted?
    A. 1 cube
    B. 2 cubes
    C. 3 cubes
    D. 4 cubes
    E. 5 cubes

73. In Figure E, how many cubes have one of
    their exposed sides painted?
    A. 1 cube
    B. 2 cubes
    C. 3 cubes
    D. 4 cubes
    E. 5 cubes

FIGURE E

74. In Figure E, how many cubes have two of
    their exposed sides painted?
    A. 1 cube
    B. 2 cubes
    C. 3 cubes
    D. 4 cubes
    E. 5 cubes

75. In Figure E, how many cubes have four of
    their exposed sides painted?
    A. 1 cube
    B. 2 cubes
    C. 3 cubes
    D. 4 cubes
    E. 5 cubes

Part 6

For questions 76 through 90:

A flat pattern will be presented in the box to the left. Your task is to mentally fold this pattern into a three-dimensional figure and choose the correct representation from the choices to the right. There is only one correct choice for each item.

Example:

Folding the pattern in the left-most box can form only one of the figures to the right. The only figure that accurately represents the shaded areas once the pattern is folded is D.

Choose the letter that represents the three-dimensional object that correctly represents the folded pattern.

Proceed to the questions.

80.

81.

82.

83.

84.

85.

86.

87.

88.

89.

90.

READING COMPREHENSION TEST

Directions: This section consists of three passages, with questions and/or incomplete statements following each passage. Read each passage; then read the questions and/or incomplete statements and answer choices carefully. For each question and/or incomplete statement, choose the best answer and blacken the corresponding space on the answer sheet. This section contains 50 items.

Time Limit: 60 minutes

Fundamentals of Tooth Movement

Clinical tooth movement requires a periodontal ligament. Forces applied to teeth are mediated through the periodontal ligament and result in remodeling of the periodontal tissues. When an appliance is attached to a tooth and the tooth is moved, the entire surface of the socket is affected. The pressure side of the tooth root compresses the periodontal ligament and alveolar bone, which results in bone resorption. On the opposite surface of the root, the movement stretches the ligament fibers, which causes tension to occur. This situation is, of course, similar in the case of a single or multirooted tooth, although it is more complex in the latter.

Sites of Remodeling

On the compression side of the ligament, collagen fiber bundles initially are disorganized and compacted. Vascular flow decreases and cell death may occur. On the tension side of the ligament, the collagen fibers are stretched. The fibroblasts become more spindle-shaped and appear oriented with their long axis in the direction of the fiber bundles. A two-rooted tooth has two or more zones of compression as well as two or more zones of tension. The bifurcation zone has a region of tension toward the left root and a region of compression toward the right root. The apical areas demonstrate transition from tension to compression and are vulnerable locations during tooth movement because too much pressure can cause death of the pulp tissue by interfering with the tooth's vascular supply.

The initial response to physical force is displacement of the tooth; permanent structural changes follow. The histological features accompanying the changes include changes in cell type and number, vascular changes, and changes in the extracellular matrix.

Transduction

The mechanism of transduction—that is, the conversion of physical force into biologic response—is not known, but numerous hypotheses have been introduced. Some of the mechanical and chemical signals proposed as initiators of metabolic changes are altered blood and lymphatic flow; pressure and volume changes within the periodontal space; distortion of matrix molecules, cell membranes, and cell cytoskeleton; stress-generated bioelectric effects from alveolar bone bending; hormonal influences; and inflammatory phenomena and other nervous and immune cellular events. The explanations propose ways for local and systemic factors to influence alveolar bone, periodontal and gingival fiber bundles, cells (mesenchymal, vascular, neural gingival epithelial), and tissue fluids. However, more investigation is needed to elucidate the cascade of changes involved in remodeling of the periodontium during tooth movement.

Force Variables

Time is an important variable in the response of alveolar bone to tooth movement. As might be expected, the histology of the compression and tension zones will change with time. Alveolar bone resorption allows for the gradual movement of the tooth into the space provided and begins on the compression front. On the tension side, bone formation compensates for tooth movement away from the bone under tension. Direct or frontal resorption is a desirable clinical goal because it is not a destructive process.

Osteoclasts appear a few hours after tooth movement begins as they are recruited from monocytes arising from blood vessels. Both osteoclasts and osteoblasts stain with oxidative enzymes. Fibroblasts proliferate, synthesize new matrix in tension sites, and participate in the degradation of necrotic periodontal ligament in areas of compression along with osteoclasts and macrophages.

Histologic Changes

The tissue response to mechanical forces in tooth movement will vary with force magnitude (light, heavy), duration (continuous, intermittent), direction, and point of application. Should the force be too great in magnitude or the movement too rapid, hyalinization of the periodontal ligament may occur. Hyalinization results in the loss of cell activity and vascularity in the pressure zone of the ligament. This zone of the ligament may appear grasslike; hence, the origin of the term. Loss of cells interrupts bone resorption, and tooth movement stops temporarily.

Another feature of hyalinization is its association with undermining resorption. Because resorption cannot occur on the compressed surface of the alveolar bone, osteoclasts are activated in the marrow spaces opposite the compressed alveolar bone surface. When the osteoclasts finish removing the intervening bone, the tooth will move again. As the osteoclasts are destroyed and resorption relieves the compression, new cells from adjacent tissues rebuild the destroyed zone. It is not yet known why compression of the ligament and alveolar bone results in undermining resorption, but lack of blood supply and cell death in the hyalinized zone may contribute. Also, changes in bioelectric potential may signal the onset of resorption.

In addition to delaying orthodontic treatment, undermining resorption of alveolar bone is potentially more damaging to the alveolar process than is direct resorption, as it may result in extensive bone loss and root resorption. What protects the root surface from damage during routine tooth movement is not known. Undermining resorption is not easily controlled, and the extent of damage is unpredictable.

Forces applied to the teeth can also produce distant changes, such as those in periosteum, endosteum, sutures, and possibly even mandibular condyles. A complete explanation of tooth movement must include mechanisms for bone remodeling in alveolar bone marrow spaces, alteration of the gingiva, and transmission of forces to distant sites. Intermittent force and continuous force cause different histological appearances. When the tissues are temporarily relieved of stress, circulation is partially restored, cell activity is restored, and repair takes place. Tooth mobility may be increased, however, which can become a problem.

A lower level of cellularity in the periodontal ligament is found in older individuals and may be related to an initial slower rate of response during tooth movement. Increased age, however, does not reduce the prospect of a successful clinical outcome.

Tipping and Bodily Movement

Tipping of a tooth results in nonuniform alteration of the sockets, whereas bodily movement affects the entire socket in a more constant fashion. When the crown tips to the left, the root apex moves to the right, producing zones of compression and tension on opposite sides of the tooth apex relative to the cervical region. Likewise, both bone resorption and bone deposition occur on the same side of a tooth as it is tipped.

In the case of a short, incompletely developed root, tipping causes resorption at two sites and tension at the opposite two sites. The root apex of a young, completely formed tooth tips in a direction opposite to the crown. In the adult, tipping is complicated by strong apical fibers that resist movement and a narrow ligament space. In this case, tipping causes less movement at the root apex, but causes resorption along most of the length of bone on the compressed side.

A micrograph of the cemental surface reveals the activity of oxidative enzymes during tooth movement in the cementoblasts adjacent to the cementum. Observe the bundles of collagen fibers projecting from the cementum. The stain indicates that the cementocytes, probably newly differentiated, have high functional activity. This is also true for the osteoblasts in the adjacent alveolar bone. New cementum will be deposited, and attachment fiber bundles will be formed in response to the tension.

Both the cementum and the alveolar bone may undergo resorption. If compression is great and occurs over a long period, both opposing surfaces will be affected.

1. If a specimen were stained with oxidative enzymes, what could be seen under a microscope?
   A. osteoclasts
   B. osteocytes
   C. periodontal ligament
   D. macrophages
   E. alveolar bone

2. How is tipping different from bodily movement?
   A. Tipping affects the entire socket.
   B. With tipping, resorption and deposition occur on opposite sides of the tooth.
   C. Bodily movement is nonuniform.
   D. Tipping does not involve osteoclasts.
   E. With tipping, resorption and deposition occur on the same side of the tooth.

3. In the bifurcation zone of a multirooted tooth there is a region of compression toward
   A. the crown
   B. the right root
   C. the root apex
   D. the left root
   E. the gingiva

4. Hyalinization may result in
   A. enamel resorption
   B. root formation
   C. excessive tooth movement
   D. extensive bone loss
   E. too much force being placed on the tooth

5. In which of the following does resorption occur?
   A. cementum
   B. alveolar bone
   C. dentin
   D. periodontal ligament
   E. A and B

6. The first visible change due to physical force on the tooth is
   A. tooth displacement
   B. a permanent structural change
   C. bone resorption
   D. pulp death
   E. bone formation

7. If a tooth is moved too quickly what may occur?
   A. Tooth movement may accelerate.
   B. Tooth movement may stop.
   C. Vascularity may increase.
   D. Cell activity may increase.
   E. Resorption may increase.

8. The conversion of a physical force into a biological force is known as
   A. a force variable
   B. a mechanical force
   C. transformation
   D. an intermittent force
   E. transduction

9. The passage suggests that in a child most resorption due to tipping occurs
   A. along the length of the root
   B. near the crown
   C. at the apex
   D. nowhere; no resorption occurs
   E. This information is not given in the passage.

10. What prevent(s) the root surface from being damaged during routine tooth movement?
    A. osteoclasts
    B. an unknown structure or mechanism
    C. osteoblasts
    D. hyalinization
    E. the periodontal ligament

11. What function(s) do fibroblasts serve?
    A. They synthesize bone.
    B. They synthesize matrix.
    C. They aid in periodontal ligament degradation.
    D. They resorb bone.
    E. B and C

12. What may result if too much pressure is placed on a tooth?
    A. death of enamel
    B. death of dentin
    C. death of cementum
    D. death of pulp
    E. all of the above

13. What may occur if pressure is applied and then temporarily removed from a tooth?
    A. Tooth mobility may increase.
    B. The tooth will return to its original position.
    C. The gingiva will be altered.
    D. Bone resorption will continue.
    E. Cell death may occur.

14. Metabolic change may be initiated by
    A. pressure changes in the periodontal space
    B. inflammation
    C. altered blood flow
    D. altered lymphatic flow
    E. all of the above

15. Direct resorption is
    A. a destructive process
    B. resorption of bone on the tension side
    C. not a destructive process
    D. not clinically desirable
    E. B and C

16. What is required for movement of a tooth to occur?
    A. cementum
    B. dentin
    C. viable pulp
    D. periodontal ligament
    E. bodily movement

Alveolar Process

The alveolar processes are those portions of the maxilla and mandible that support the roots of the teeth. They are composed of the alveolar bone proper and the supporting bone. The alveolar bone proper is the bone that lines the socket. In radiographic terms, it is referred to as the lamina dura. This process is the bony site of attachment of the periodontal ligament fibers. The supporting bone includes the remainder of the alveolar process, specifically the compact cortical plates on the outer surfaces of the alveolar processes and the spongy bone between the cortical plates and the alveolar bone proper.

The alveolar process develops as a result of tooth root elongation and tooth eruption. Alveolar bone matures as the teeth gain functional occlusion;

later, if the teeth are lost, the alveolar process disappears. Thus, the teeth are important in the development and maintenance of the alveolar bone. The alveolar bone proper is attached to the supporting cancellous and compact alveolar bone. Bone marrow containing blood vessels, nerves, and adipose tissue fills the space between the cortical plates and the alveolar bone proper. The coronal border of the alveolar process is termed the alveolar crest. It is located about 1 to 1.5 mm below the cemento-enamel junction, and is rounded in the anterior region and nearly flat in the molar area. If the teeth are in buccal or lingual position, the alveolar process will be very thin or partially missing. The area of an apical root penetrating the bone is known as a fenestration, and its occurrence at the coronal root zone is termed dehiscence.

Alveolar Bone Proper

On a histological basis, there are two types of bone: cancellous (spongy) and compact. Alveolar bone proper is a modification of compact bone, as it contains perforating fibers (Sharpey's fibers). These collagen fibers pierce the alveolar bone proper at right angles or obliquely to the surface of the long axis of the tooth. This is the means of attachment for the periodontal ligament to the tooth. The fiber bundles originating from bone are much larger than the fiber bundles inserting in cementum. Perforating fibers occur elsewhere in the skeleton, wherever ligaments and tendons insert. Purely elastic perforating fibers are also found, but not in alveolar bone proper. Because the bone of the alveolar process is regularly penetrated by collagen bundles, it has been appropriately named bundle bone or alveolar bone proper. When this bone is viewed radiographically, it is referred to as the lamina dura. The lamina dura appears more dense than does the adjacent supportive bone, but this radiographic density may be due to the mineral orientation around the fiber bundles and the apparent lack of nutrient canals. Actually, there may be no difference in mineral content between the lamina dura and the supporting bone. The lamina dura is evaluated clinically for periapical or periodontal pathology. Tension created by occlusal forces is believed to be important in the maintenance of this bone. In physiological movement of teeth, this bone is readily resorbed in zones of compression and readily formed in zones of tension. Not all alveolar bone proper appears as bundle bone. At times, there are no apparent perforating fibers in the socketlining bone. Supporting bone constantly undergoes modification in adapting to minor tooth movements, and therefore fibers may be lost or replaced from time to time in some areas of root.

Compact Supporting Bone

The compact or dense bone of the alveolar process is like that found elsewhere in the human body. Compact bone in the alveolar process extends from the alveolar crest labially or bucally to the lower border of the sockets. The cortical bone contains Haversian systems, radiating lamellae with lacunae, and canaliculi. The nutrient canals run in the direction of the long axis of the teeth and anastomose with "perforating canals" (Volkmann's canals) that pierce the bone at right or oblique angles. These canals establish a continuous system that houses the nerves and blood vessels of the bone. A sagittal view of the mandible demonstrates the vascular network in cortical bone. Compact bone comprises the bulk of the interdental alveolar process; cancellous bone is located more apically between the alveolar process proper and the cortical bone. Situated between osteons at the microscopic level are more irregular layers of bone, termed interstitial lamellae. Bone cells (osteocytes) fill the oval lacunae situated in or between the lamellae. Minute canaliculi interconnect with adjacent lacunae; they contain processes of the osteocytes that contact other cells by a system of "gap" junctions.

Cancellous Supporting Bone

The cancellous or spongy bone of the alveolar process is generally composed of heavy trabeculae. The purpose of this supporting bone is to strengthen the alveolar bone proper with struts that pass to the cortical bone. Cancellous bone contains osteocytes in the interior and osteoblasts or osteoclasts on the surface of the trabeculae. Between the bony struts that anastomose between the alveolar bone proper and the cortical bone are medullary cavities containing osteogenic cells, adipose tissue, and mature and immature blood cells. The maxillae are particularly rich in marrow tissue, such as megakaryocytes and immature white and red blood cells.

Physiological Tooth Movement

The eruptive process involves major remodeling of the alveolar processes to compensate for tooth growth and changes in position of the teeth. Repositioning of the teeth involves outward (facial and/or buccal) movement of the teeth as the face enlarges. Root growth results in growth in the height of the alveolar processes, which is compensatory for the increase in the length of the root. Although the two growth processes—tooth eruption and an increase in facial size—have different origins, both relate to positioning of the teeth and to modifications of the fine structures of Haversian and cancellous bone of the alveolar process.

There are several causative factors of alveolar bone changes. First, the increase in the height of the alveolar process associated with root lengthening is "tooth controlled." In the absence of teeth, this change does not occur. Change is especially evident in an older person whose teeth may have been lost, resulting in loss of the bone. Second, facial development involving condylar, maxillary, and mandibular growth also results in movement of the teeth. Because this process is not generated by the tooth, malformations of the face may result in tooth malalignment. Third, there will be further growth of the alveolar process unrelated to tooth eruption. This is part of the facial growth process. The teeth definitely control modifications of the alveolar process because, as a tooth moves, the alveolar bone responds with necessary compensatory changes. In this case, the resorption and deposition of bone around the teeth are a result, not the cause, of tooth movement. Thus, the alveolar process is guided in growth by tooth-related factors and extrinsic growth factors; the effects of these factors are difficult to separate as growth occurs.

Aging of Alveolar Bone

A comparison of young and old alveolar bone reveals a shift with age from alveolar processes with smoothly lined sockets, and active bone formation with numerous viable cells, to alveolar sockets that appear jagged and uneven with fewer cells. The perforating fibers are inserted in an uneven pattern. Marrow appears to have a fatty infiltration, and osteoporosis indicates loss of some bony elements.

Edentulous Jaws

The changes in the jaws resulting from tissue loading, compression, tissue conditioning, and denture retention coupled with the aging processes have not been clearly elucidated. It is apparent, however, that with age the alveolar process in edentulous jaws decreases in size; loss of maxillary bone is accompanied by an increase in the size of the maxillary sinus. The internal trabecular arrangement is more open, indicating bone loss. From a common radiographic viewpoint the locations of various structures such as glands, fatty zones, muscle masses, and blood vessels vary little in the edentulous jaws.

17. How is the periodontal ligament attached to the tooth?
    A. by perforating canals
    B. by lacunae
    C. by canaliculi
    D. by Haversian fibers
    E. by perforating fibers

18. Where is bone marrow located?
    A. in the alveolar bone proper
    B. between the cortical plates and alveolar bone proper
    C. in the cortical plates
    D. in the coronal border of the alveolar process
    E. in the compact bone

19. As the root of a tooth grows, what happens to the alveolar process?
    A. It decreases in height.
    B. It grows thicker.
    C. It grows thinner.
    D. It grows higher.
    E. It remains unchanged.

20. What is another name for bone cells?
    A. osteocytes
    B. osteoblasts
    C. lacunae
    D. lamellae
    E. canaliculi

21. Why is alveolar bone proper considered modified compact bone?
    A. It contains Sharpey's fibers.
    B. It contains Volkmann's canals.
    C. It contains fenestrations.
    D. It contains canaliculi.
    E. It contains lacunae.

22. The alveolar process develops in response to which of the following?
    A. root elongation
    B. enamel formation
    C. tooth eruption
    D. A and B
    E. A and C

23. If all teeth are lost, what, if anything, will happen to the alveolar process?
    A. It will increase in size.
    B. It will increase in density.
    C. It will decrease in density.
    D. It will decrease in size.
    E. It will remain the same.

24. What helps to maintain the lamina dura?
    A. spongy bone
    B. tension due to occlusal forces
    C. compact bone
    D. nutrient canals
    E. supporting bone

25. The bone that lines the tooth socket is called
    A. alveolar bone proper
    B. Haversian bone
    C. supporting bone
    D. cancellous bone
    E. Sharpey's bone

26. Where are osteoblasts located?
    A. inside trabeculae
    B. on the alveolar bone proper
    C. on the surface of the trabeculae
    D. in the lamina dura
    E. in "gap" junctions

27. What is the term for a coronal root penetrating the bone?
    A. fenestration
    B. perforating fiber
    C. Volkmann's canal
    D. lamina dura
    E. dehiscence

28. The nerves and blood vessels of compact bone are contained in
    A. the lamina dura
    B. cancellous bone
    C. Volkmann's canals
    D. the root
    E. the pulp

29. The growth of the alveolar process is guided by
    A. extrinsic growth factors
    B. tooth-related factors
    C. calcium intake
    D. bone density
    E. A and B

30. Where is the alveolar crest located?
    A. 1–1.5 mm above the cemento-enamel junction
    B. 2–2.5 mm below the cemento-enamel junction
    C. 1–1.5 mm below the cemento-enamel junction
    D. at the cemento-enamel junction
    E. 1–1.5 mm below the dentin-enamel junction

31. Where are immature red blood cells found in abundance?
A. bundle bone of maxillae
B. cancellous bone of maxillae
C. lamina dura of maxillae
D. compact bone of maxillae
E. cortical plates of maxillae

32. What is the function of spongy bone?
A. to strengthen the alveolar bone proper
B. to strengthen the cancellous bone
C. to provide flexibility to the alveolar bone proper
D. to carry nutrients to the alveolar bone proper
E. to strengthen the compact bone

33. What are contained in compact bone?
A. lacunae
B. lamellae
C. Haversian systems
D. canaliculi
E. all of the above

Types of Cementum

Cementum is the calcified mesenchymal tissue that forms the outer covering of the anatomic root. There are two main types of root cementum: acellular (primary) and cellular (secondary). Both consist of a calcified interfibrillar matrix and collagen fibrils.

There are two sources of collagen fibers in cementum: Sharpey's (extrinsic) fibers, which are the embedded portion of the principal fibers of the periodontal ligament and are formed by the fibroblasts; and fibers that belong to the cementum matrix per se (intrinsic) and are produced by the cementoblasts. Cementoblasts also form the noncollagenous components of the interfibrillar ground substance, such as proteoglycans, glycoproteins, and phosphoproteins.

Acellular cementum is the first to be formed and covers approximately the cervical third or half of the root; it does not contain cells. This cementum is formed before the tooth reaches the occlusal plane, and its thickness ranges from 30 to 230 µm. Sharpey's fibers make up most of the structure of acellular cementum, which has a principal role in supporting the tooth. Most of the fibers are inserted at approximately right angles into the root surface and penetrate deep into the cementum, but others enter from several different directions. Their size, number, and distribution increase with function. Sharpey's fibers are completely calcified, with the mineral crystals oriented parallel to the fibrils, as they are in dentin and bone, except in a 10- to 50-µm-wide zone near the cementodentinal junction, where they are only partially calcified. The peripheral portions of Sharpey's fibers in actively mineralizing cementum tend to be more calcified than the interior regions, according to evidence obtained by scanning electron microscopy. Acellular cementum also contains other collagen fibrils that are calcified and irregularly arranged or parallel to the surface.

Cellular cementum, formed after the tooth reaches the occlusal plane, is more irregular and contains cells (cementocytes) in individual spaces (lacunae) that communicate with each other through a system of anastomosing canaliculi. Cellular cementum is less calcified than the acellular type. Sharpey's fibers occupy a smaller portion of cellular cementum and are separated by other fibers that are arranged either parallel to the root surface or at random. Sharpey's fibers may be completely calcified or partially calcified or may have a central, uncalcified core surrounded by a calcified border.

Both acellular and cellular cementum are arranged in lamellae separated by incremental lines parallel to the long axis of the root. These lines represent rest periods in cementum formation and are more mineralized than the adjacent cementum. In addition, loss of the cervical part of the reduced enamel epithelium at the time of tooth eruption may place portions of mature enamel in contact with the connective tissue, which will then deposit over it an acellular afibrillar type of cementum.

Based on these findings, Schroeder has classified cementum as follows: Acellular afibrillar cementum (AAC) contains neither cells nor extrinsic or intrinsic collagen fibers, apart from a mineralized ground substance. It is a product of cementoblasts and in humans is found in coronal cementum.

Acellular extrinsic fiber cementum (AEFC) is composed almost entirely of densely packed bundles of Sharpey's fibers and lacks cells. It is a product of fibroblasts and cementoblasts and in humans is found in the cervical third of roots but may extend further apically.

Cellular mixed stratified cementum (CMSC) is composed of extrinsic (Sharpey's) and intrinsic fibers and contains cells. It is a coproduct of fibroblasts and cementoblasts, and in humans it appears primarily in the apical third of the roots and the apices and in furcation areas.

Cellular intrinsic fiber cementum (CIFC) contains cells but no collagen fibers. It is formed by cementoblasts, and in humans it fills resorption lacunae.

Intermediate cementum is an illdefined zone near the cementodentinal junction of certain teeth that appears to contain cellular remnants of Hertwig's sheath embedded in calcified ground substance.

The inorganic content of cementum (hydroxyapatite) is 45% to 50%, which is less than that of bone (65%), enamel (97%), or dentin (70%). Opinions differ about whether the microhardness increases or decreases with age, and no relationship has been established between aging and the mineral content of cementum.

Permeability of Cementum

In very young animals, both cellular cementum and acellular cementum are very permeable and permit the diffusion of dyes from the pulp and from the external root surface. In cellular cementum, the canaliculi in some areas are contiguous with the dentinal tubuli. With age, the permeability of cementum diminishes.

Cemento-enamel Junction

The cementum at and immediately subjacent to the cemento-enamel junction is of particular clinical importance in root scaling procedures. Three types of relationships involving the cementum may exist at the cemento-enamel junction. In about 60% to 65% of cases cementum overlaps the enamel; in about 30% there is an edge-to-edge butt joint; and in 5% to 10% the cementum and enamel fail to meet. In the last instance, gingival recession may be accompanied by an accentuated sensitivity because the dentin is exposed.

Thickness of Cementum

Cementum deposition is a continuous process that proceeds at varying rates throughout life. Cementum formation is most rapid in the apical regions, where it compensates for tooth eruption, which itself compensates for attrition. The thickness of cementum on the coronal half of the root varies from 16 to 60 µm, or about the thickness of a hair. It attains its greatest thickness (up to 150 to 200 µm) in the apical third and in the bifurcation areas; it is thicker in distal surfaces than in mesial surfaces, probably because of functional stimulation from mesial drift over time. Between the ages of 11 and 70, the average thickness of the cementum increases threefold, with the greatest increase in the apical region. Average thicknesses of 95 μm at age 20 and 215 μm at age 60 have been reported.

The term *hypercementosis* (cementum hyperplasia) refers to a prominent thickening of the cementum. It may be localized to one tooth or affect the entire dentition. Because of considerable physiologic variation in the thickness of cementum among different teeth in the same person and also among different persons, it is sometimes difficult to distinguish between hypercementosis and physiologic thickening of cementum.

Hypercementosis occurs as a generalized thickening of the cementum, with nodular enlargement of the apical third of the root. It also appears in the form of spikelike excrescences (cemental spikes) created by either the coalescence of cementicles that adhere to the root or the calcification of periodontal fibers at the sites of insertion into the cementum.

The etiology of hypercementosis varies and is not completely understood. The spikelike type of hypercementosis generally results from excessive tension from orthodontic appliances or from occlusal forces. The generalized type occurs in a variety of circumstances. In teeth without antagonists, hypercementosis is interpreted as an effort to keep pace with excessive tooth eruption. In teeth subject to lowgrade periapical irritation arising from pulp disease, it is considered to be compensation for the destroyed fibrous attachment to the tooth. The cementum is deposited adjacent to the inflamed periapical tissue. Hypercementosis of the entire dentition may occur in patients with Paget's disease.

Cementum Resorption and Repair

The cementum of erupted as well as unerupted teeth is subject to resorption. The resorptive changes may be of microscopic proportion or may be sufficiently extensive to present a radiographically detectable alteration in the root contour. Cementum resorption is extremely common. In one microscopic study, it occurred in 236 of 261 teeth (90.5%). The average number of resorption areas per tooth was 3.5. Of the 922 areas of resorption, 708 (76.8%) were located in the apical third of the root, 177 (19.2%) in the middle third, and 37 (4.0%) in the gingival third. Seventy percent of all resorption areas were confined to the cementum without involving the dentin.

Cementum resorption may be due to local or systemic causes or may occur without apparent etiology (i.e., be idiopathic). Among the local conditions in which it occurs are trauma from occlusion; orthodontic movement; pressure from malaligned erupting teeth, cysts, and tumors; teeth without functional antagonists; embedded teeth; replanted and transplanted teeth; periapical disease; and periodontal disease. Among the systemic conditions mentioned as predisposing to or inducing cemental resorption are calcium deficiency, hypothyroidism, hereditary fibrous osteodystrophy, and Paget's disease.

34. Where is intermediate dentin found?
   A. near the dentino-enamel junction
   B. near the cemento-enamel junction
   C. near the cemento-dentinal junction
   D. in Hetwig's sheath
   E. in acellular cementum

35. Most cementum resorption occurs in the
   A. middle third of the root
   B. gingival third of the root
   C. apical third of the crown
   D. middle third of the crown
   E. apical third of the root

36. Where is cementum the thickest?
    A. in the coronal third
    B. near the dentino-enamel junction
    C. near the crown
    D. in bifurcation areas
    E. near the cemento-enamel junction

37. The part of the periodontal ligament that inserts into cementum is called
    A. Sharpey's fibers
    B. cementoblasts
    C. cementoclasts
    D. fibroblasts
    E. the interfibrillar matrix

38. Some canaliculi in cellular cementum are contiguous with
    A. enamel rods
    B. acellular cementum
    C. the pulp
    D. dentinal tubuli
    E. the gingiva

39. Paget's disease may result in _____
    A. cemental spikes
    B. cementum resorption
    C. hypercementosis
    D. osteodystrophy
    E. B and C

40. A prominent thickening of the cementum is called
    A. hypocementosis
    B. acellular afibrillar cementum
    C. hypocementosis
    D. intermediate cementum
    E. interfibrillar ground substance

41. Cellular cementum generally _____ than acellular cementum.
    A. contains fewer cells
    B. is more irregular
    C. contains more Sharpey's fibers
    D. is more regular
    E. is formed earlier

42. Sensitivity may be accentuated because of
    A. failure of cementum and enamel to meet
    B. cementum and enamel forming an edge-to-edge butt joint
    C. cementum overlapping enamel
    D. enamel overlapping cementum
    E. all of the above

43. Idiopathic cementum resorption is due to
    A. systemic causes
    B. local causes
    C. orthodontic treatment
    D. trauma
    E. no apparent reason

44. In the passage hypercementosis and _____ may be used interchangeably.
    A. cementum resorption
    B. cementum hyperplasia
    C. physiologic thickening of cementum
    D. periodontal disease
    E. calcification of cementum

45. The first cementum formed
    A. is cellular
    B. is extrinsic
    C. is acellular
    D. is multinucleated
    E. B and D

46. When does cementum deposition cease?
    A. after eruption is complete
    B. when root formation is complete
    C. when enamel formation is complete
    D. when dentin formation is complete
    E. cementum deposition does not stop

47. What is the percent of hydroxyapatite in cementum?
    A. 65%
    B. 97%
    C. 70%
    D. 35%
    E. 45%

48. How are cellular and acellular cementum arranged?
    A. in lamellae
    B. in lacunae
    C. in canaliculi
    D. in a random pattern
    E. in rods

49. In which of the following are completely calcified extrinsic fibers found?
    A. cellular cementum
    B. lacunae
    C. acellular cementum
    D. canaliculi
    E. A and C

50. The calcification of periodontal fibers at the site of insertion into cementum is called
  A. physiologic thickening of cementum
  B. cemental spikes
  C. dentinal spikes
  D. hypocementosis
  E. Sharpey's fibers

QUANTITATIVE REASONING TEST

Directions: The following items are questions or incomplete statements. Read each item carefully, then choose the best answer or completion. Blacken the corresponding space on the answer sheet. This section contains 40 items.

Time Limit: 45 minutes

1. If $4^{\frac{x}{3}} = 64$, then $x = ?$
   A. −2
   B. 3
   C. 12
   D. 9
   E. 6

2. $\dfrac{\sqrt{15} \times \sqrt{3}}{\sqrt{10}} = ?$
   A. $\dfrac{3}{2}$
   B. $\dfrac{3\sqrt{2}}{2}$
   C. $2\sqrt{5}$
   D. $9\sqrt{5}$
   E. $\dfrac{\sqrt{2}}{2}$

3. What is the probability of obtaining heads in each of five tosses of a fair coin?
   A. $\dfrac{3}{5}$
   B. $\dfrac{5}{32}$
   C. $\dfrac{1}{2}$
   D. $\dfrac{5}{8}$
   E. $\dfrac{2}{5}$

4. $-8 - 6\{3 + 2[5 - (3+4) + 1] - 2\} + 7 =$
   A. 0
   B. 2
   C. 4
   D. 5
   E. −4

5. If an ordinary coin is tossed six times, what is the probability of either all heads or all tails?
   A. $\dfrac{1}{4}$
   B. $\dfrac{1}{32}$
   C. $\dfrac{1}{3}$
   D. $\dfrac{1}{8}$
   E. $\dfrac{1}{16}$

6. The value of $\dfrac{5}{6} + \dfrac{2}{3} + \dfrac{1}{4}$ is
   A. $\dfrac{9}{12}$
   B. $1\dfrac{3}{4}$
   C. $2\dfrac{1}{4}$
   D. $\dfrac{3}{4}$
   E. $1\dfrac{2}{5}$

7. The largest of five consecutive even integers is 2 less than twice the smallest. Which of the following is the largest integer?
   A. 16
   B. 18
   C. 12
   D. 20
   E. 10

8. What is the slope of a line containing points (−3,6) and (2,5)?
   A. 5
   B. $\dfrac{1}{5}$
   C. −5
   D. $-\dfrac{1}{5}$
   E. 1

9. The angles of a triangle are in the ratio 2:3:5. What is the measure of the smallest angle?
   A. 48°
   B. 36°
   C. 45°
   D. 72°
   E. 60°

10. If $3x + 2y = 8$ and $x + y = 2$, then $x - y = ?$
    A. 6
    B. 4
    C. 2
    D. −2
    E. 0

11. Which of the following is equal to $(\tan \theta)(\csc \theta)$?
    A. $\cos \theta$
    B. $\cot \theta$
    C. $\sec \theta$
    D. $\sin \theta$
    E. $\csc \theta$

12. What is the equation of the line that contains point (−3,1) and has a slope of (−2)?
    A. $y = -2x - 3$
    B. $y = 2x + 5$
    C. $y = -2x + 5$
    D. $y = -2x + 1$
    E. $y = -2x - 5$

13. Simplify: $\sqrt{\dfrac{3x^2}{12} + \dfrac{7x^2}{36}}$.
    A. $\dfrac{2}{3}x$
    B. $\dfrac{2x^2}{3}$
    C. $\dfrac{3}{4}x$
    D. $\dfrac{3x^2}{4}$
    E. $4x$

14. The sum of a number x and 6 equals 2 less than the product of 2 and the number. What is the number?
    A. $x = 6$
    B. $x = 8$
    C. $x = 10$
    D. $x = 9$
    E. $x = 5$

15. Julie has $5.50 in nickels and dimes. She has five more nickels than dimes. How many dimes does she have?
    A. 30
    B. 25
    C. 20
    D. 35
    E. 40

16. There are three consecutive even integers such that the third of the three even integers is 10 more than the sum of the first and second. What is the third integer?
    A. −8
    B. −6
    C. −4
    D. −10
    E. −2

17. Which of the following is identically equal to $\sin 2A$?
    A. $1 - \cos 2A$
    B. $2 \sin A$
    C. $1 - \cos^2 2A$
    D. $2 \sin A \cos A$
    E. $\dfrac{1}{\sec 2A}$

18. The five tires that came with Steve's new car were rotated frequently so that each tire was used exactly the same amount of time as the others. The tires were replaced when the odometer read 24,000 miles. For how many miles had each been used?
    A. 30,000 miles
    B. 24,000 miles
    C. 18,000 miles
    D. 20,000 miles
    E. 19,200 miles

19. At a convention of dentists, 1,000 dentists are from the west coast. One hundred dentists are women; 60 of the women are not from the west coast. How many male dentists are from the west coast?
    A. 850
    B. 800
    C. 900
    D. 960
    E. 940

20. Brian received a 10% increase in each of the last 2 years. His present salary is $21,780. What was his starting salary?
    A. $19,000
    B. $21,300
    C. $20,000
    D. $18,000
    E. $26,354

21. A florist bought some plants for $150.00. She sold enough at 75 cents each to meet the cost and had 100 plants left. How many plants were originally purchased by the florist?
    A. 150
    B. 250
    C. 300
    D. 350
    E. 400

22. An automobile travels at an average speed of 45 miles per hour for 1 hour and then at an average speed of 60 miles per hour for the next half hour. What is the average speed for the entire time period?
    A. 47.5 mph
    B. 50 mph
    C. 52.5 mph
    D. 55 mph
    E. 62.5 mph

23. If $\dfrac{1}{2} + \dfrac{4}{2x-1} = 6$, then $x = ?$
    A. $-\dfrac{1}{2}$
    B. $\dfrac{13}{22}$
    C. $\dfrac{19}{22}$
    D. $-\dfrac{1}{4}$
    E. $-\dfrac{15}{22}$

24. A box has the shape of a rectangular solid, with a base measuring 16 inches by 10 inches and a height of 8 inches. What is the approximate length of the sides of a cubic container having the same volume?
    A. 9.75 in.
    B. 10.85 in.
    C. 10.00 in.
    D. 12.65 in.
    E. 13.15 in.

25. If $\dfrac{1}{5}$ of 27 = 25% of x, then $x = ?$
    A. 5.4
    B. $21\dfrac{3}{5}$
    C. 1.35
    D. 21
    E. 21.5

26. An integer from 1 to 9, inclusive, is selected at random. What is the probability that the integer is a multiple of 3?
    A. $\dfrac{1}{9}$
    B. $\dfrac{2}{9}$
    C. $\dfrac{1}{3}$
    D. $\dfrac{2}{3}$
    E. 1

27. What is the rate of discount on dental equipment listing at $3,050 and selling for $2,745?
    A. 0.1%
    B. 9.0%
    C. 10.0%
    D. 10.3%
    E. 11.1%

28. If 10 cubic centimeters of 20% acid is mixed with 20 cubic centimeters of 40% acid, the percent of acid in the resulting solution is
    A. 50
    B. 30
    C. 35
    D. $33\dfrac{1}{3}$
    E. 60

29. If $x = 3 + 5h$ and $y = 3h - 5$, for what value of h will $x = 2y$?
- A. 68
- B. 34
- C. 13
- D. –4
- E. –11

30. If 85% of $\dfrac{3}{x} = 8$, then $x = ?$
- A. 2.17
- B. 0.375
- C. 0.032
- D. 0.300
- E. 0.319

31. $2\sqrt{20} + \sqrt{45} =$
- A. $5\sqrt{7}$
- B. $7\sqrt{5}$
- C. $15\sqrt{5}$
- D. $7\sqrt{10}$
- E. $3\sqrt{65}$

32. A river flows at 3 miles per hour. A man can row at 5 miles per hour in still water. If he rows 1 mile upstream and then floats back to the starting place, how many minutes will be required for the roundtrip?
- A. 30
- B. 42
- C. 50
- D. 60
- E. 65

33. When 1 is added to the numerator of the fraction $\dfrac{x}{y}$, the fraction equals $\dfrac{1}{3}$. When 3 is added to the denominator of $\dfrac{x}{y}$, the fraction equals $\dfrac{1}{6}$. What is $\dfrac{x}{y}$?
- A. $\dfrac{2}{3}$
- B. $\dfrac{2}{9}$
- C. $\dfrac{6}{17}$
- D. $\dfrac{2}{6}$
- E. $\dfrac{1}{4}$

34. If $(y + 2)x = \dfrac{1}{4}$, then $y = ?$
- A. $\dfrac{1}{4} - 2x$
- B. $\dfrac{x}{4} - 2$
- C. $\dfrac{1}{4x + 8}$
- D. $\dfrac{1}{4x} - 2$
- E. $\dfrac{1 - 8x}{4}$

35. Perform the indicated operations and simplify: $\dfrac{\dfrac{4}{3} - \dfrac{2}{5}}{2 + \dfrac{5}{3}}$
- A. $\dfrac{14}{55}$
- B. $-\dfrac{4}{7}$
- C. $-\dfrac{41}{15}$
- D. $\dfrac{14}{11}$
- E. $\dfrac{154}{45}$

36. If $x = 4$, $y = \dfrac{1}{8}$, and $z = 2\dfrac{2}{3}$, then $\dfrac{1}{x} + \dfrac{1}{4} - \dfrac{1}{z} = ?$
- A. 0
- B. $7\dfrac{7}{8}$
- C. $\dfrac{35}{24}$
- D. $\dfrac{7}{8}$
- E. $8\dfrac{5}{8}$

37. Solve the following equation: $y = \dfrac{2x + 1}{x - 3}$ for x in terms of y.
- A. $x = -\dfrac{1}{2}$
- B. $x = -4$
- C. $x = \dfrac{2y + 1}{y - 3}$
- D. $x = \dfrac{3y + 1}{y - 2}$
- E. $x = 3y + \dfrac{2y + 1}{y}$

38. What are two positive numbers whose sum is 6 and whose product is 4?
A. $2 + \sqrt{5}, 4 - \sqrt{5}$
B. $3 + \sqrt{5}, 3 - \sqrt{5}$
C. $3 + \sqrt{20}, 3 - \sqrt{20}$
D. 6, 0
E. 2, 4

39. When 2 is added to the numerator of the fraction $\frac{y}{x}$, the fraction equals $\frac{1}{4}$. When 2 is added to the denominator of $\frac{y}{x}$, the fraction equals $\frac{1}{5}$. What is $\frac{y}{x}$?
A. $\frac{10}{40}$
B. $\frac{10}{48}$
C. $\frac{12}{44}$
D. $\frac{1}{3}$
E. $\frac{1}{2}$

40. If snow is falling to the ground at a rate of 1 inch every half hour and is melting at the rate of 0.75 inch every hour, how many inches deep should the snow be after 8 hours of snowfall?
A. 10
B. 22
C. 12
D. 4
E. 2

MODEL EXAMINATION B ANSWER KEY

Survey of the Natural Sciences

1. D	11. C	21. C	31. C	41. C	51. C	61. E	71. B	81. B	91. C
2. C	12. E	22. E	32. D	42. D	52. A	62. D	72. A	82. C	92. B
3. A	13. A	23. C	33. A	43. D	53. C	63. C	73. D	83. B	93. B
4. E	14. C	24. C	34. B	44. C	54. D	64. D	74. C	84. E	94. A
5. B	15. E	25. D	35. B	45. A	55. D	65. B	75. D	85. A	95. C
6. E	16. D	26. A	36. E	46. D	56. B	66. C	76. C	86. B	96. D
7. C	17. A	27. D	37. D	47. A	57. D	67. C	77. B	87. B	97. D
8. A	18. B	28. D	38. C	48. C	58. B	68. E	78. E	88. C	98. D
9. C	19. B	29. E	39. E	49. B	59. C	69. C	79. A	89. A	99. A
10. B	20. D	30. E	40. A	50. A	60. A	70. C	80. D	90. D	100. E

Perceptual Ability Test

1. D	10. E	19. A	28. B	37. A	46. B	55. A	64. B	73. B	82. A
2. E	11. C	20. B	29. D	38. C	47. E	56. D	65. E	74. B	83. B
3. D	12. C	21. A	30. A	39. B	48. A	57. B	66. C	75. C	84. D
4. B	13. D	22. D	31. B	40. D	49. B	58. C	67. B	76. C	85. A
5. A	14. A	23. C	32. A	41. C	50. C	59. B	68. A	77. B	86. D
6. E	15. A	24. D	33. C	42. B	51. C	60. E	69. D	78. C	87. C
7. C	16. D	25. D	34. A	43. B	52. A	61. A	70. C	79. B	88. C
8. E	17. C	26. A	35. D	44. B	53. C	62. B	71. C	80. D	89. C
9. B	18. B	27. C	36. A	45. A	54. D	63. C	72. B	81. A	90. A

Reading Comprehension Test

1. A	6. A	11. E	16. D	21. A	26. C	31. B	36. D	41. B	46. E
2. E	7. B	12. D	17. E	22. E	27. E	32. A	37. A	42. A	47. E
3. B	8. E	13. A	18. B	23. D	28. C	33. E	38. D	43. E	48. A
4. D	9. C	14. E	19. D	24. B	29. E	34. C	39. E	44. B	49. E
5. E	10. B	15. C	20. A	25. A	30. C	35. E	40. C	45. C	50. B

Quantitative Reasoning Test

1. D	5. B	9. B	13. A	17. D	21. C	25. B	29. C	33. B	37. D
2. B	6. B	10. A	14. B	18. E	22. B	26. C	30. E	34. D	38. B
3. C	7. B	11. C	15. D	19. D	23. C	27. C	31. B	35. A	39. B
4. D	8. D	12. E	16. C	20. D	24. B	28. D	32. C	36. B	40. A

STANDARD SCORE TO RAW SCORE CONVERSION CHART

STANDARD SCORE	QRT	RCT	BIOLOGY	GENERAL CHEMISTRY	ORGANIC CHEMISTRY	SNS (TOTAL SCIENCE)	PAT
30	40	50	–	–	30	100	90
29	39	–	40	–	–	99	89
28	–	49	–	30	29	98	88
27	–	–	–	–	–	97	–
26	38	48	39	–	–	96	87
25	37	47	–	29	28	95	85-86
24	36	–	38	–	–	94	84
23	35	46	–	28	27	92-93	81-83
22	33-34	43-45	37	–	–	89-91	78-80
21	31-32	40-42	35-36	27	26	86-88	74-77
20	29-30	37-39	34	26	25	81-85	70-73
19	27-28	34-36	32-33	24-25	23-24	76-80	68-69
18	24-26	31-33	30-31	22-23	21-22	70-75	59-64
17	22-23	26-30	27-29	20-21	19-20	63-69	52-58
16	19-21	24-25	24-26	18-19	17-18	56-62	46-51
15	16-18	20-23	21-23	16-17	15-16	48-55	39-45
14	14-15	18-19	18-20	13-15	13-14	41-47	32-38
13	11-13	16-17	15-17	11-12	11-12	33-40	26-31
12	9-10	13-15	12-14	9-10	8-10	27-32	21-25
11	7-8	10-12	10-11	7-8	7	21-26	17-20
10	6	9	8-9	6	5-6	17-20	13-16
9	5	7-8	6-7	4-5	4	13-16	10-12
8	4	–	5	3	3	10-12	7-9
7	3	6	4	–	–	7-9	6
6	2	4-5	3	2	2	5-6	4-5
5	–	–	2	–	–	4	3
4	–	3	–	1	1	3	2
3	1	2	1	–	–	2	–
2	–	–	–	–	–	–	–
1	0	1	0	0	0	0-1	0-1

APPENDIX

ACRONYMS

You will come across more acronyms in the application process than you can possibly imagine. Some of the most frequently used acronyms are included here.

AADR	American Association for Dental Research
AADS	American Association of Dental Schools
AADSAS	American Association of Dental Schools Application Service
ADA	American Dental Association
AEGD	Advanced Education in General Dentistry
ASDA	American Student Dental Association
B.A.	Bachelor of Arts
BCP	Biology, Chemistry, Physics (AADSAS application)
B.S.	Bachelor of Science
CDA	Canadian Dental Association
DAT	Dental Admission Test (U.S.), Dental Aptitude Test (Canada)
D.D.S.	Doctor of Dental Surgery (equivalent to D.M.D.)
D.M.D.	Doctor of Dental Medicine (equivalent to D.D.S.)
DMO	Dental Maintenance Organization
EFC	Expected Family Contribution
EFN	Exceptional Financial Need Scholarship
FAF	Financial Aid Form
FAFSA	Free Application for Federal Student Aid
GPA	Grade Point Average
GPR	General Practice Residency
HEAL	Health Education Assistance Loan
HMO	Health Maintenance Organization
HPSL	Health Professions Student Loan
HPTQ	High Probability Test Question
LDS	Loans for Disadvantaged Students
M.A.	Master of Arts
M.D.	Doctor of Medicine
M.S.	Master of Science
NDA	National Dental Association
NIDCR	National Institute of Dental and Craniofacial Research (a division of NIH)
NIH	National Institutes of Health
PASS	Postdoctoral Application Support Service
PAT	Perceptual Ability Test
Ph.D.	Doctor of Philosophy
QRT	Quantitative Reasoning Test
RCT	Reading Comprehension Test
SDS	Scholarships for Disadvantaged Students
SNDA	Student National Dental Association
SNS	Survey of the Natural Sciences
TOEFL	Test of English as a Foreign Language
WHO	World Health Organization

FREQUENTLY ASKED QUESTIONS

The following list includes some of the most frequently asked questions that applicants have. The answers should clear up some of the confusion that you may feel about the exam, the application process, dental school, and the dental profession. The questions are presented in four sections:

- Questions Regarding the DAT
- Questions Regarding the Application Process
- Questions Regarding Dental School
- Questions Regarding the Profession of Dentistry

Questions Regarding the DAT

How do I get a tutorial disk to familiarize myself with the computerized format?

Try to obtain a copy from a dental school director of admissions. If unsuccessful, send $10 to:

DAT Tutorial
Department of Testing Services
211 East Chicago Avenue
Suite 1846
Chicago, Illinois 60611

You will need Microsoft Windows to run this program. The tutorial is quite simplistic and gives but one example for each section of the DAT. It is highly recommended, however, that you familiarize yourself with the computer format prior to your test date.

One unique feature is a "**MARK**" option that enables you to come back to a question that you have skipped. Also, there is an "**EXHIBIT**" option to view an attached illustration, chart, or table. If you have not familiarized yourself with the computer-based format, examination-day stress may cause you to forget about these features or to be uncertain how to use them.

You should obtain a copy of this tutorial diskette, so that you will know exactly what to expect when you sit down in front of the computer to take the DAT.

What is the scoring of the DAT?

The highest score is 30, with 18 being competitive for admittance. Refer to the *Scoring* section on page 2.

What is an average score?

About 16. This is not very competitive for admission.

What is the difference between a raw score and a standard score? Do both get sent to the dental schools that I checked on my DAT application?

A raw score is the number of correctly marked answers on a section. That number is converted to a scaled score called the standard score. The score you and the dental schools will receive is the standard score.

Is the DAT an aptitude test or an achievement test?

Webster's New World Dictionary defines an aptitude test as a test for determining the probability of a person's success in some activity for which he or she is not yet trained. The Canadian Dental Association considers its DAT to be an aptitude test. The SNS, however, is clearly an achievement test as it tests specific knowledge in the discipline of the natural sciences.

When should I begin studying for the DAT?

Three months is adequate preparation time for most test takers. Schedule your DAT accordingly.

Can I retake the DAT?

You can take the DAT as many times as you wish. The last four attempts will be reported to dental schools. You must wait at least 90 days between examinations.

What are Sylvan Learning and Technology Centers?

The Sylvan Learning Centers, Sylvan Technology Centers, and Sylvan Prometric are all divisions of Sylvan Learning Systems, Inc. Sylvan Technology Centers are under contract to the American Dental Association to administer the DAT. Sylvan also administers over 200 other types of entrance exams, board exams, and licensing exams. In short, these centers specialize in administering exams.

How are these testing centers set up?

You will take the exam on a personal computer similar to one you may have at home or one that you will find in a computer lab at your undergraduate institution. All computers have high-resolution monitors. You will take the exam in a 4-foot × 4-foot cubicle. You will be given pencil and paper to work out problems and to use for the reading comprehension test. Although the center should be quiet, you will be provided with ear plugs to prevent any distraction from another examinee's typing or mouse clicking.

Can I leave the testing center during the test battery?

You will be allowed a 15-minute break approximately halfway through the examination battery (after both the SNS and the PAT have been completed). During this break you may use the restroom, eat a snack, or leave the building. Make sure, however, that you are ready to resume the exam 15 minutes later. This break is optional.

When will I receive my scores?

When you have finished the test, your score will be printed out at the center. A report will be sent electronically to the ADA Department of Testing Services that day, and dental schools will receive your scores within 3 weeks of your test date.

What should I take to the exam?

Two forms of ID (driver's license, state ID, passport, employee ID card) are required. Both must have your signature, and one must have a current photo. (Paper and writing instruments will be provided. Be sure to arrive 30 minutes before the examination time.

Can I reschedule my exam?

Yes. However, you must call by noon two days before your test date. Call Sylvan Prometric at its National Registration Center, 800-967-1100.

I have taken the MCAT. How is the DAT different from the MCAT? How should I prepare for the DAT?

Many students taking the DAT either have already taken the MCAT or are preparing for both exams simultaneously. Here are four differences between the two exams:

1. There is no physics section on the DAT.
2. The MCAT does not have an analogous PAT section.
3. No writing sample is required on the DAT.
4. The *formats* of the questions differ.

Here are the four sections on the exam:

- *Medical College Admission Test (MCAT)*
  Verbal Reasoning: humanities-based readings
  Physical Sciences: physics, general chemistry
  Biological Sciences: biology, organic chemistry
  Writing Sample
- *Dental Admission Test (DAT)*
  Natural Sciences: biology, organic chemistry, general chemistry
  Perceptual Ability Test
  Reading Comprehension Test: science-based readings
  Quantitative Reasoning Test

The subjects common to both exams are reading analysis, general chemistry, biology, and organic chemistry. The format of the questions is quite different on the two exams. Also, many students who have taken both examinations consider the MCAT sections on biology, organic chemistry, and general chemistry to be significantly more difficult than their DAT counterparts. Therefore, in preparing for the DAT, you should briefly review the science sections and concentrate on practice for the Perceptual Ability Test, Reading Comprehension Test, and Quantitative Reasoning Test.

Questions Regarding the Application Process

What is AADSAS?

This acronym stands for American Association of Dental Schools Application Service. AADSAS is a centralized application clearinghouse; its purpose is to simplify the application process by providing one standardized application. All but a few dental schools (see next question) require that you use AADSAS to initiate the application process. The packet of application materials comes with an instruction booklet that is quite thorough and detailed in regard to filling out the application.

Which of the 54 dental schools do not participate in AADSAS?

Louisiana State University
Medical College of Georgia
University of Mississippi
University of Tennessee

How can I check the status of my AADSAS application?

Call 800-353-2237.

What can I do to maximize my chances for admission?

Send in your completed AADSAS application as soon as possible. AADSAS packets are available during June and July prior to the year of matriculation. As a wise applicant, you will have written your Personal Statement before receiving the AADSAS application. By preparing the Personal Statement in advance, you can minimize the turn-around time as this is the most time-consuming section of the application. As soon as the application is completed and double-checked for accuracy, return the packet to AADSAS, making sure all parts of the application are included.

Many schools have a rolling admissions policy; therefore, the applications received first are given the greatest consideration. When a dental school has received deposits for most of the first year seats in the spring of the year of matriculation, competition for the last few seats becomes exponentially greater. Even though AADSAS and dental schools give dates by which applications must be received for consideration, you can be sure that by March or April about 90% of the first-year class has already been chosen.

Should I send my DAT scores to AADSAS?

No. The official report will be sent from the ADA to the dental schools you indicated.

What percent of applicants actually are admitted to at least one dental school?

Approximately 53%.

How many schools should I apply to?

More than 12 schools may be excessive and fewer than 5 may not be enough. If you have above-average scores on the DAT and an above-average GPA, however, the lower number may be sufficient if you know where you want to go to school. According to recent figures, approximately 65,000 applications from 8,000 applicants were submitted to AADSAS for 4,500 available positions. These data indicate that the average student applies to 7.36 schools.

Does it matter what my undergraduate degree was in?

Provided that you have taken the prerequisites for dental school admission, your undergraduate major does not matter at all. Your life will be easier though, once you are in dental school, if you have had some biochemistry, physiology, anatomy, microbiology, or other advanced biology courses. Approximately 55% of enrolled dental students have majored in the biological sciences: 15% in chemistry/physical sciences; 13% in pre-health science; 4% in language/arts/architecture; 4% in business; and 3% in engineering.

The DAT reported score is a measure of how you performed in comparison to everyone else who took the exam. Having a background in science limited to the minimum prerequisites may put you at a disadvantage in relation to someone who has taken 60–90 credits in biology and chemistry. It is not unreasonable, however, to think that you can perform above average on the DAT with sufficient preparation. The BCP (Biology, Chemistry, Physics) GPA reported on AADSAS is representative of fewer classes; therefore, excellent grades are needed in these prerequisite courses.

Should I take classes now that I will have to take in dental school?

Doing so is not mandatory, but it will make your life a lot easier once you start your dental studies. It will be to your advantage to be familiar with the course work prior to your exposure to it in dental school. At that point, you will be expected to make clinical correlations to the basic sciences, a task that will be easier if you start with some foundation. It should be noted, however, that although a strong performance in college in advanced-level sciences will strengthen your application, it does absolutely *no* good to take these courses as an undergraduate but not perform well.

Is it advantageous to go through the Pre-Health Professions Office to obtain letters of recommendation?

Yes. See the section *Letters of Recommendation* (pages 10–12) for more information.

What is an average GPA?

Your GPA will actually be reported through AADSAS as four different numbers: the overall GPA, the science GPA, the nonscience GPA, and the BCP GPA. Because of the difficulty of most science classes, the science GPA and BCP GPA figures are typically lower than the overall GPA and nonscience GPA figures.

In general, the following GPA figures can be used to assess your competitiveness as an applicant:

3.0–3.2 → Below average
3.2–3.5 → Average
3.5–4.0 → Above average

If your science GPA or BCP GPA is below 3, you may want to consider taking additional biology and/or chemistry courses to boost this number before applying to dental schools.

My GPA is average. What can I do to make myself stand out from other applicants?

Stellar performance on the DAT. This number *can* be changed, whereas your GPA is pretty much set in stone. Remember: the two most important components of your application are your GPA and your DAT score. These are the numbers for which you will be screened in the first round of admissions. At this point, your future will hinge on a GPA and a DAT score. That's the reality of the process!

I am sure I want to go into orthodontics. Should I express my desire to become an orthodontist to the Admissions Committee?

You will learn that half of the entering class wants to go into orthodotics. The funny thing is that there are only a few spots for this specialty, and all but a few applicants will have to reevaluate their original plans. Take one step at a time. First, work on admittance to a predoctoral dental program, then concern yourself with choosing a postdoctoral specialty. Although you may have had a memorable experience with your own orthodontist, it is wise to wait until you have bent some wires in an "ortho" class to decide that orthodontics is your destined career.

I have been involved in many extracurricular activities while in college. How will this aspect of my life play into the admissions process?

Besides indicating your involvement on the AADSAS form, you will be able to include your many extracurricular activities and accomplishments in your Personal Statement, the interview, and any supplemental application requested.

I have been out of school for a few years. How will this factor into my application?

Many schools look favorably on the returning student. Returning to school after being successful in the workforce indicates two important qualities: maturity and motivation.

What should I do if I am placed on a waiting list at the school that I want to attend?

Be persistent! Let the admissions office know that this school is your first choice. Also, if you know some influential people, this would be a suitable time to get in touch with them. Waiting lists are rarely as structured as schools want you to believe.

What should I do if I am not accepted to a dental school this year?

Call the directors of admissions at the schools to which you applied and ask exactly what aspect of your application causes them to reject you. Often they will be frank and tell you outright why you were not granted admission. Take that information at face value, and do the best you can to fix obvious problems. Remember: persistence shows motivation *and* dedication.

I am coming to the United States as a foreign dental school applicant. How will this affect my application and financial aid?

See the discussion headed "A Note to Foreign Dental School Applicants" (pages 20–21) in the section *The Application Process*.

Questions Regarding Dental School

Where do I go to find out about scholarships?

When you secure a seat by remitting a deposit to a dental school, the next thing you must consider is how you are going to pay for the next 4 years of your life. Securing scholarship money takes resourcefulness and some persistence. There is a tremendous amount of money available; however, you must take the initiative to get your portion of the funds. Grants are monetary disbursements that need not be repaid, whereas loans must be repaid. About 88% of financial aid to dental students is in the form of loans, and 12% comes from scholarships or grants.

The first step is to call the financial aid office at your dental school. Perhaps a brief meeting to obtain information would be helpful as well. Then contact local and state dental societies. One way successful dentists give back to the community is through financial aid to dental students. With the tremendous cost of dental school, it is also worthwhile trying to locate private foundations that offer loans at very low interest rates (1%–5%).

Go to the library and/or a local bookstore and locate published information regarding established foundations and charitable organizations. The following two resources may be helpful:

- *ASDA Handbook: A Resource Guide for Pre-dental Students*, Call 800-621-8099, ext. 2795.
- The Financial Aid Information Home Page at *http://www.finaid.org/*

The qualifications for private grant money can be quite specific and may even appear ridiculous. To actually receive money for these sources, you will need to be persistent. Know what makes you different from the next dental student and then use these differences to your advantage.

What is the average indebtedness of the dental school graduate?

Approximately 90% of dental students utilize financial aid to some degree. Graduates of private and state-related schools, on average, owe more than graduates of public schools. Estimates of average combined living and educational expenses and average aid at the three types of schools are as follows:

- **Public Schools**
  Average cost: $87,000
  Average aid: $68,000
- **Private, State-Related Schools**
  Average cost: $122,000
  Average aid: $115,000
- **Private Schools**
  Average cost: $150,000
  Average aid: $130,000

If I choose to specialize, will it matter what dental school I went to when I apply for postdoctoral programs?

Superior performance in comparison to your peers when in dental school is much more important than the school itself. Specialty programs place heaviest emphasis on class rank, GPA, and National Board scores.

How are dental schools ranked?

There are no official rankings for dental schools; there are simply too many factors that enter into the quality of a dental education. The quality of the education offered at a dental school should be evident in the knowledge and skills of its student body. Therefore, a good measure of a dental school education is the annual scores from the first part of the National Boards. These confidential reports from the ADA are given to the deans of the 54 dental schools. It is made very clear that the intent of the board exams is not to rank schools; the boards are administered for the purpose of licensure. The scores from the boards, however, are the only method of ranking that is worth any consideration. *Proprietary rankings should be totally ignored as their evaluation criteria do not measure the education offered.*

The results on Part I of the boards will give you some idea of the didactic preparation that a school offers in the basic sciences. The ranking on Part II will give you an idea of the clinical education offered by a school. You should also realize that a school's rank on either or both parts can change from year to year. Boards are mentioned as a way to evaluate schools simply because you *will* hear admissions officers refer to their school's rankings on the board exams. The best way to obtain actual ranking information is to directly ask the dean what the school's ranks were for the past 3 or so years.

In selecting the schools to which you apply, figure out what criteria are most important to you. Then rank these schools on these bases as you obtain relevant information.

To learn the current accreditation status of any U.S. dental school, call the Commission on Dental Accreditation at 800-621-8099, ext. 2713.

What should I look for when I tour a dental school?

If you are invited for an interview, prepare a list of questions that you want answered. The interview is a time for you to get to know that school as well as a time for the school to get to know you. Here are some observations you may want to make and questions you may want to ask:

- Are the dental students mixed in with the medical students?
- When was the dental school last renovated?
- Are there a sufficient number of preclinic stations?
- How is the clinic set up? Are there individual operators?
- Are the lecture halls and audio/visual equipment adequate?
- Is there an adequate patient pool?
- What percentage of students remediate?
- What percentage graduate on time?
- Are there *buildings* dedicated to dental research, or *floors*?
- What do the students wear? Scrubs? Casual clothes?
- What is the atmosphere like? Are students and faculty friendly?

What is the average age of the first-year dental student?

The average age of first-time enrollees is approximately 24.3 years.

Questions Regarding the Profession of Dentistry

I was not granted admission to a medical school last year, and I'm now pursuing dentistry as an alternative career choice. Are these two professions really all that different?

As professions, medicine and dentistry share much in common, and therefore it is not unusual for students pursuing a career in medicine to switch to dentistry. The admission criteria are often less stringent, and dentistry is a fine alternative for those who originally intented to practice medicine. Both are highly respected members of the health care field. Nevertheless, the premedical students who use dental school as a fallback are often the first to drop out of their dental school classes. Why is this the case?

There are differences between medical school and dental school that need to be realized. In dentistry, the psychomotor skills tested through practical examinations require a high degree of manual dexterity and attention to detail. Only after detailed scrutiny of the profession of dentistry and the curricula of dental schools should a premedical student opt for a career in dentistry. An alternative for many would-be students of an allopathic medical school is osteopathy. The training and career options for the D.O. and the M.D. are becoming increasingly similar. Medical students seeking the D.O. designation undergo a thorough training in the diagnostic and therapeutic techniques of conventional medicine with an emphasis in manipulative techniques.

It is not the intention here to discourage premedical students from switching to dentistry; rather, it is to inform these students of the differences in training and practice between these professions. If you are attempting the DAT after a less than satisfactory performance on the MCAT, you should research the field of dentistry before you commit to pursuing a dental degree. Base your decision on a solid foundation of information gathered from personal observation and discussion with physicians and dentists. The most intelligent decision that you can make for yourself is one that is well thought out, is based on first-hand observation, and is most closely aligned with your interests and abilities.

I know my dental education will have to be paid for entirely by loans. Is it realistic to assume that I will earn enough money to repay these loans?

Yes. Be aware, however, that most new dentists who borrowed the maximum allowance struggle to make payments on their educational loans.

Once I'm a dentist, will it really matter what school I went to?

Maybe a handful of patients over the course of your career will care to know where you were educated. How you perform in comparison to your peers at the school that you choose is much more important.

What percentage of dentists practice general dentistry, and what percentage specializes?

Approximately 20–30% specialize in one of the ADA-recognized specialties. If you think you may want to specialize, be cautious when asking admissions officers how many students go on to residencies; the number will include students opting for GPR (General Practice Residency) and AEGD (Advanced Education in General Dentistry) programs, which do not offer specialty training.

How many recognized dental specialties are there?

See the section *The Profession of Dentistry* (pages 22–29) for an explanation of each of the eight recognized specialties.

What are the personal qualities or characteristics of an excellent dentist?
Here are some qualities that are important:

1. Compassion
2. Academic superiority and intellectual curiosity in regard to the biological sciences
3. A detail-oriented personality
4. Highly proficient manual dexterity skills
5. Ability to manage a business and personnel
6. Effective interpersonal skills

What other sources can I obtain that will provide me with information about dentistry?

See *Other Publications and Resources* on page 427 in this appendix.

WWW ADDRESSES

The best source of information regarding a particular dental school is the school itself. The following WWW addresses provide information regarding contacts, requirements, and school profiles. In most cases, the web pages are updated more frequently than are the published brochures.

It is strongly suggested that you gain access to the Internet to visit the home pages of the schools to which you are interested in submitting an application.

Organizations

- **AADS**
  http://www.aads.jhu.edu/
- **ASDA**
  http://www.asdanet.org/
- **ADA**
  http://www.ada.org/

Dental Schools in the Midwest

- **Case Western Reserve University, School of Dentistry**
  http://www.cwru.edu/dental/dent.html
- **Creighton University, School of Dentistry**
  http://cudental.creighton.edu/
- **Indiana University, School of Dentistry**
  http://www.iusd.iupui.edu/
- **Marquette University, School of Dentistry**
  http://www.dental.mu.edu/
- **Southern Illinois University, School of Dental Medicine**
  http://www.siue.edu/DMSCH/
- **The Ohio State University, College of Dentistry**
  http://www.acs.ohio-state.edu/units/dentistry/
- **University of Detroit Mercy, School of Dentistry**
  http://www.udmercy.edu/htmls/dentistry/dental.htm
- **University of Illinois at Chicago, College of Dentistry**
  http://gopher.uic.edu/11/campus/mdms
- **University of Iowa, College of Dentistry**
  http://vh.radiology.uiowa.edu/Beyond/Dentistry/DentistryHP.html
- **University of Michigan, School of Dentistry**
  http://informatics.dent.umich.edu/
- **University of Minnesota, School of Dentistry**
  http://www.umn.edu/dental/
- **University of Missouri-Kansas City, School of Dentistry**
  http://www.umkc.edu/dentistry/

- University of Nebraska Medical Center
  http://www.unmc.edu/

Dental Schools in the Northeast

- Boston University, Goldman School of Dental Medicine
  http://dentalschool.bu.edu/
- Columbia University, School of Dental and Oral Surgery
  http://cpmcnet.columbia.edu/dept/dental/
- Harvard School of Dental Medicine
  http://www.hsdm.med.harvard.edu/
- New York University, Kriser Dental Center
  http://www.nyu.edu/Dental/
- State University of New York at Buffalo, School of Dental Medicine
  http://www.sdm.buffalo.edu/
- State University of New York at Stony Brook, School of Dental Medicine
  http://www.informatics.sunysb.edu/dental/
- Temple University, School of Dentistry
  http://www.temple.edu/dentistry/
- Tufts University, School of Dental Medicine
  http://www.tufts.edu/dental/
- University of Connecticut, School of Dental Medicine
  http://www.uchc.edu
- University of Maryland at Baltimore, Dental School
  http://www.umaryland.edu/dental/
- University of Medicine and Dentistry of New Jersey, New Jersey Dental School
  http://www.umdnj.edu/
- University of Pennsylvania, School of Dental Medicine
  http://father.dental.upenn.edu/
- University of Pittsburgh, School of Dental Medicine
  http://www.pitt.edu/pittdent/

Dental Schools in the South

- Baylor College of Dentistry, A Member of the Texas A&M University System
  http://www.tambcd.edu/
- Howard University, College of Dentistry
  http://www.howard.edu/HU-HomePages/default.htm
- Louisiana State University, School of Dentistry
  http://www.lsusd.lsumc.edu/
- Medical College of Georgia, School of Dentistry
  http://www.mcg.edu/SOD/
- Medical University of South Carolina, College of Dental Medicine
  http://www.gradstudies.musc.edu/dentistry/dental.html
- Meharry Medical College, School of Dentistry
  http://www.mmc.edu/dent.htm
- Nova Southeastern University, College of Dental Medicine
  http://www.nova.edu/
- University of Alabama, School of Dentistry
  http://www.dental.uab.edu/
- University of Florida, College of Dentistry
  http://www.dental.ufl.edu/
- University of Kentucky, College of Dentistry
  http://www.uky.edu/
- University of Louisville, School of Dentistry
  http://www.dental.louisville.edu/dental/
- University of Mississippi, School of Dentistry
  http://umc.edu/dentistry/

- **University of North Carolina at Chapel Hill, School of Dentistry**
  http://www.dent.unc.edu/
- **University of Oklahoma, College of Dentistry**
  http://dent.uokhsc.edu/
- **University of Puerto Rico, School of Dentistry**
  http://w3rum.upr.clu.edu/
- **University of Tennessee, College of Dentistry**
  http://chanc.utmem.edu/catalog97/dentistry.html
- **University of Texas Health Science Center, Houston, Dental Branch**
  http://www.db.uth.tmc.edu/
- **University of Texas Health Science Center, San Antonio, Dental School**
  http://dental.uthscsa.edu/
- **Virginia Commonwealth University, School of Dentistry**
  http://views.vcu.edu/dentistry/
- **West Virginia University, School of Dentistry**
  http://www.hsc.wvu.edu/sod/

Dental Schools in the West

- **Loma Linda University, School of Dentistry**
  http://www.llu.edu/llu/dentistry/
- **Oregon Health Sciences University, School of Dentistry**
  http://www.ohsu.edu/sod/
- **University of California, Los Angeles, School of Dentistry**
  http://www.dent.ucla.edu/
- **University of California, San Francisco, School of Dentistry**
  http://itsa.ucsf.edu/dental/index.htm
- **University of Colorado, School of Dentistry**
  http://www.uchsc.edu/sd/sd/
- **University of the Pacific, School of Dentistry**
  http://www.dental.uop.edu/
- **University of Southern California, School of Dentistry**
  http://www.usc.edu/hsc/dental/
- **University of Washington, School of Dentistry**
  http://www.dental.washington.edu/

Canadian Dental Schools

- **Dalhousie University, Faculty of Dentistry**
  http://bpass.dentistry.dal.ca/
- **McGill University, Faculty of Dentistry**
  http://www.mcgill.ca/dentistry/
- **University of Alberta, Faculty of Dentistry**
  http://www.dent.ualberta.ca/
- **University of British Columbia, Faculty of Dentistry**
  http://www.dentistry.ubc.ca/
- **University Laval, Faculty of Dentistry**
  http://www.ulaval.ca/sg/annuaires/fac/mde.html
- **University of Manitoba, Faculty of Dentistry**
  http://www.umanitoba.ca/Dentistry/dental1.html
- **University of Montreal, Faculty of Dentistry**
  http://www.medent.umontreal.ca/
- **University of Saskatchewan, Faculty of Dentistry**
  http://gopher.usask.ca:70 + /11/Academic % 20Information/University % 20of % 20Saskatchewan % 20Calendar % 201993-94/College % 20of % 20Dentistry

- **University of Toronto, Faculty of Dentistry**
  http://www.utoronto.ca/dentistry/
- **University of Western Ontario, Faculty of Dentistry**
  http://dentistry.uwo.ca/

OTHER PUBLICATIONS AND RESOURCES

- *Dental Admission Testing Program: Applications and Preparation Materials,* published by the American Dental Association. This booklet contains the application form for the DAT and a sample DAT exam. It is free and can be obtained by calling 312-440-2689.

  You must obtain this booklet to apply for the DAT!

- *Admission Requirements: United States and Canadian Dental Schools,* published by the American Association of Dental Schools. This excellent guide will be invaluable in deciding to which schools you should apply. The price is about $25, and you can order it by calling the AADS at 202-667-9433.

- *Opportunities for Minority Students in United States Dental Schools,* published by the American Association of Dental Schools. This guide is about $10 and is recommended if you wish to obtain more information regarding outreach programs. Note that there is considerable overlap between this publication and *Admission Requirements: United States and Canadian Dental Schools,* also published by the AADS. Statistics regarding the ethnic breakdown of the incoming classes are included in both publications.

- *ASDA Handbook: A Resource Guide for Pre-dental Students,* published by the American Student Dental Association. The price is about $25, and it can be ordered by calling the ASDA office at 1-800-621-8099, ext. 2795.

  This publication is highly recommended!

- **The Survey Center** at the American Dental Association (ADA). The center has publications on just about anything you could think of pertaining to the DAT, dental schools, and dentistry. Unfortunately, these publications are somewhat price-prohibitive for the average applicant as the survey reports can run up to $175 for a set. For a current list of available publications and price list call the Survey Center at 312-440-2568.

- **The Internet.** For accurate and reliable information about an individual school, the very best source is that school. Contact information for individual dental schools can be obtained through the AADS *Admission Requirements: United States and Canadian Dental Schools* or via the web (see *WWW Addresses* in this appendix for individual listings).

- **Your Dentist.** Speak to your dentist about his or her experience with the profession. Remember, however, that your dentist may not be reflective of dental practitioners in general. You should also note that the overwhelming majority of dentists love nothing more than to share their experiences and opinions with an aspiring dentist; feel free, therefore, to call any practitioner, not just *your* dentist. For statistical information contact the Survey Center at the American Dental Association, which is listed above.

- **American Student Dental Association.** By joining ASDA as a predental student, you can access information and resources through this organization and the ADA. Inquire about membership by calling the ASDA office at 1-800-621-8099, ext. 2795.

PERIODIC TABLE OF THE ELEMENTS

KEY

Common oxidation states	+1, -1
Atomic number	1
Element symbol	**H**
Element name	Hydrogen
Atomic mass (or mass number of longest-lived isotope)	1.00794
Electron configuration	$1s^1$

Note: Atomic masses are based on carbon-12 = 12.000...u

s-block

GROUP

1	2
1 +1 -1 **H** Hydrogen 1.00794 $1s^1$	
3 +1 **Li** Lithium 6.941 [He]$2s^1$	4 +2 **Be** Beryllium 9.01218 [He]$2s^2$
11 +1 **Na** Sodium 22.98977 [Ne]$3s^1$	12 +2 **Mg** Magnesium 24.305 [Ne]$3s^2$
19 +1 **K** Potassium 39.0983 [Ar]$4s^1$	20 +2 **Ca** Calcium 40.078 [Ar]$4s^2$
37 +1 **Rb** Rubidium 85.4678 [Kr]$5s^1$	38 +2 **Sr** Strontium 87.62 [Kr]$5s^2$
55 +1 **Cs** Cesium 132.9054 [Xe]$6s^1$	56 +2 **Ba** Barium 137.33 [Xe]$6s^2$
87 +1 **Fr** Francium (223) [Rn]$7s^1$	88 +2 **Ra** Radium 226.0254 [Rn]$7s^2$

Transition Elements — *d-block*

GROUP

3	4	5	6	7	8	9	10	11	12
21 +3 **Sc** Scandium 44.9559 [Ar]$3d^14s^2$	22 +2 +3 +4 **Ti** Titanium 47.88 [Ar]$3d^24s^2$	23 +2 +3 +4 +5 **V** Vanadium 50.9415 [Ar]$3d^34s^2$	24 +2 +3 +6 **Cr** Chromium 51.996 [Ar]$3d^54s^1$	25 +2 +3 +4 +6 +7 **Mn** Manganese 54.9380 [Ar]$3d^54s^2$	26 +2 +3 **Fe** Iron 55.847 [Ar]$3d^64s^2$	27 +2 +3 **Co** Cobalt 58.9332 [Ar]$3d^74s^2$	28 +2 +3 **Ni** Nickel 58.69 [Ar]$3d^84s^2$	29 +1 +2 **Cu** Copper 63.546 [Ar]$3d^{10}4s^1$	30 +2 **Zn** Zinc 65.39 [Ar]$3d^{10}4s^2$
39 +3 **Y** Yttrium 88.9059 [Kr]$4d^15s^2$	40 +4 **Zr** Zirconium 91.224 [Kr]$4d^25s^2$	41 +3 +5 **Nb** Niobium 92.9064 [Kr]$4d^45s^1$	42 +6 **Mo** Molybdenum 95.94 [Kr]$4d^55s^1$	43 +4 +6 +7 **Tc** Technetium (98) [Kr]$4d^55s^2$	44 +3 **Ru** Ruthenium 101.07 [Kr]$4d^75s^1$	45 +3 **Rh** Rhodium 102.9055 [Kr]$4d^85s^1$	46 +2 +4 **Pd** Palladium 106.42 [Kr]$4d^{10}$	47 +1 **Ag** Silver 107.8682 [Kr]$4d^{10}5s^1$	48 +2 **Cd** Cadmium 112.41 [Kr]$4d^{10}5s^2$
57 +3 **La** Lanthanum 138.9055 [Xe]$5d^16s^2$	72 +4 **Hf** Hafnium 178.49 [Xe]$4f^{14}5d^26s^2$	73 +5 **Ta** Tantalum 180.9479 [Xe]$4f^{14}5d^36s^2$	74 +6 **W** Tungsten 183.85 [Xe]$4f^{14}5d^46s^2$	75 +4 +6 +7 **Re** Rhenium 186.207 [Xe]$4f^{14}5d^56s^2$	76 +3 +4 **Os** Osmium 190.2 [Xe]$4f^{14}5d^66s^2$	77 +3 +4 **Ir** Iridium 192.22 [Xe]$4f^{14}5d^76s^2$	78 +2 +4 **Pt** Platinum 195.08 [Xe]$4f^{14}5d^96s^1$	79 +1 +3 **Au** Gold 196.9665 [Xe]$4f^{14}5d^{10}6s^1$	80 +1 +2 **Hg** Mercury 200.59 [Xe]$4f^{14}5d^{10}6s^2$
89 +3 **Ac** Actinium 227.0278 [Rn]$6d^17s^2$	104 **Rf** Rutherfordium (261) [Rn]$5f^{14}6d^27s^2$	105 **Db** Dubnium (262) [Rn]$5f^{14}6d^37s^2$	106 **Sg** Seaborgium (263) [Rn]$5f^{14}6d^47s^2$	107 **Bh** Bohrium (262) [Rn]$5f^{14}6d^57s^2$	108 **Hs** Hassium (265) [Rn]$5f^{14}6d^67s^2$	109 **Mt** Meitnerium (266) [Rn]$5f^{14}6d^77s^2$	110 **Uun** Ununnilium (269) [Rn]$5f^{14}6d^87s^2$	111 **Uuu** Unununium (272) [Rn]$5f^{14}6d^97s^2$	112 **Uub** Ununbium (277) [Rn]$5f^{14}6d^{10}7s^2$

p-block

GROUP

13	14	15	16	17	18
					2 0 **He** Helium 4.00260 $1s^2$
5 +3 **B** Boron 10.81 [He]$2s^22p^1$	6 -4 +2 +4 **C** Carbon 12.011 [He]$2s^22p^2$	7 -3 +1 +2 +3 +4 +5 **N** Nitrogen 14.0067 [He]$2s^22p^3$	8 -2 **O** Oxygen 15.9994 [He]$2s^22p^4$	9 -1 **F** Fluorine 18.998403 [He]$2s^22p^5$	10 0 **Ne** Neon 20.1797 [He]$2s^22p^6$
13 +3 **Al** Aluminum 26.98154 [Ne]$3s^23p^1$	14 -4 +2 +4 **Si** Silicon 28.0855 [Ne]$3s^23p^2$	15 -3 +3 +5 **P** Phosphorus 30.97376 [Ne]$3s^23p^3$	16 -2 +4 +6 **S** Sulfur 32.066 [Ne]$3s^23p^4$	17 -1 +1 +5 +7 **Cl** Chlorine 35.453 [Ne]$3s^23p^5$	18 0 **Ar** Argon 39.948 [Ne]$3s^23p^6$
31 +3 **Ga** Gallium 69.72 [Ar]$3d^{10}4s^24p^1$	32 -4 +2 +4 **Ge** Germanium 72.61 [Ar]$3d^{10}4s^24p^2$	33 -3 +3 +5 **As** Arsenic 74.9216 [Ar]$3d^{10}4s^24p^3$	34 -2 +4 +6 **Se** Selenium 78.96 [Ar]$3d^{10}4s^24p^4$	35 -1 +1 +5 **Br** Bromine 79.904 [Ar]$3d^{10}4s^24p^5$	36 0 +2 **Kr** Krypton 83.80 [Ar]$3d^{10}4s^24p^6$
49 +3 **In** Indium 114.82 [Kr]$4d^{10}5s^25p^1$	50 +2 +4 **Sn** Tin 118.710 [Kr]$4d^{10}5s^25p^2$	51 -3 +3 +5 **Sb** Antimony 121.757 [Kr]$4d^{10}5s^25p^3$	52 -2 +4 +6 **Te** Tellurium 127.60 [Kr]$4d^{10}5s^25p^4$	53 -1 +1 +5 +7 **I** Iodine 126.9045 [Kr]$4d^{10}5s^25p^5$	54 0 +4 +6 **Xe** Xenon 131.29 [Kr]$4d^{10}5s^25p^6$
81 +1 +3 **Tl** Thallium 204.383 [Xe]$4f^{14}5d^{10}6s^26p^1$	82 +2 +4 **Pb** Lead 207.2 [Xe]$4f^{14}5d^{10}6s^26p^2$	83 +3 +5 **Bi** Bismuth 208.9804 [Xe]$4f^{14}5d^{10}6s^26p^3$	84 +2 +4 **Po** Polonium (209) [Xe]$4f^{14}5d^{10}6s^26p^4$	85 -1 **At** Astatine (210) [Xe]$4f^{14}5d^{10}6s^26p^5$	86 0 **Rn** Radon (222) [Xe]$4f^{14}5d^{10}6s^26p^6$

f-block

58 +3 +4 **Ce** Cerium 140.12 [Xe]$4f^16s^2$	59 +3 **Pr** Praseodymium 140.9077 [Xe]$4f^36s^2$	60 +3 **Nd** Neodymium 144.24 [Xe]$4f^46s^2$	61 +3 **Pm** Promethium (145) [Xe]$4f^56s^2$	62 +2 +3 **Sm** Samarium 150.36 [Xe]$4f^66s^2$	63 +2 +3 **Eu** Europium 151.96 [Xe]$4f^76s^2$	64 +3 **Gd** Gadolinium 157.25 [Xe]$4f^75d^16s^2$	65 +3 **Tb** Terbium 158.9254 [Xe]$4f^96s^2$	66 +3 **Dy** Dysprosium 162.50 [Xe]$4f^{10}6s^2$	67 +3 **Ho** Holmium 164.9304 [Xe]$4f^{11}6s^2$	68 +3 **Er** Erbium 167.26 [Xe]$4f^{12}6s^2$	69 +3 **Tm** Thulium 168.9342 [Xe]$4f^{13}6s^2$	70 +2 +3 **Yb** Ytterbium 173.04 [Xe]$4f^{14}6s^2$	71 +3 **Lu** Lutetium 174.967 [Xe]$4f^{14}5d^16s^2$
90 +4 **Th** Thorium 232.0381 [Rn]$6d^27s^2$	91 +5 **Pa** Protactinium 231.0359 [Rn]$5f^26d^17s^2$	92 +3 +4 +5 +6 **U** Uranium 238.0289 [Rn]$5f^36d^17s^2$	93 +3 +4 +5 +6 **Np** Neptunium 237.048 [Rn]$5f^46d^17s^2$	94 +3 +4 +5 +6 **Pu** Plutonium (244) [Rn]$5f^67s^2$	95 +3 +4 +5 +6 **Am** Americium (243) [Rn]$5f^77s^2$	96 +3 **Cm** Curium (247) [Rn]$5f^76d^17s^2$	97 +3 +4 **Bk** Berkelium (247) [Rn]$5f^97s^2$	98 +3 **Cf** Californium (251) [Rn]$5f^{10}7s^2$	99 +3 **Es** Einsteinium (252) [Rn]$5f^{11}7s^2$	100 +3 **Fm** Fermium (257) [Rn]$5f^{12}7s^2$	101 +2 +3 **Md** Mendelevium (258) [Rn]$5f^{13}7s^2$	102 +2 +3 **No** Nobelium (259) [Rn]$5f^{14}7s^2$	103 +3 **Lr** Lawrencium (262) [Rn]$5f^{14}6d^17s^2$

Period 1–7

LIST OF ELEMENTS WITH THEIR SYMBOLS

Element	Symbol	Element	Symbol	Element	Symbol
Actinium	Ac	Hassium	Hs	Radium	Ra
Aluminum	Al	Helium	He	Radon	Rn
Americium	Am	Holmium	Ho	Rhenium	Re
Antimony	Sb	Hydrogen	H	Rhodium	Rh
Argon	Ar	Indium	In	Rubidium	Rb
Arsenic	As	Iodine	I	Ruthenium	Ru
Astatine	At	Iridium	Ir	Rutherfordium	Rf
Barium	Ba	Iron	Fe	Samarium	Sm
Berkelium	Bk	Krypton	Kr	Scandium	Sc
Beryllium	Be	Lanthanum	La	Seaborgium	Sg
Bismuth	Bi	Lawrencium	Lr	Selenium	Se
Bohrium	Bh	Lead	Pb	Silicon	Si
Boron	B	Lithium	Li	Silver	Ag
Bromine	Br	Lutetium	Lu	Sodium	Na
Cadmium	Cd	Magnesium	Mg	Strontium	Sr
Calcium	Ca	Manganese	Mn	Sulfur	S
Californium	Cf	Meitnerium	Mt	Tantalum	Ta
Carbon	C	Mendelevium	Md	Technetium	Tc
Cerium	Ce	Mercury	Hg	Tellurium	Te
Cesium	Cs	Molybdenum	Mo	Terbium	Tb
Chlorine	Cl	Neodymium	Nd	Thallium	Tl
Chromium	Cr	Neon	Ne	Thorium	Th
Cobalt	Co	Neptunium	Np	Thulium	Tm
Copper	Cu	Nickel	Ni	Tin	Sn
Curium	Cm	Niobium	Nb	Titanium	Ti
Dubnium	Db	Nitrogen	N	Tungsten	W
Dysprosium	Dy	Nobelium	No	Ununbium	Uub
Einsteinium	Es	Osmium	Os	Ununnilium	Uun
Erbium	Er	Oxygen	O	Unununium	Uuu
Europium	Eu	Palladium	Pd	Uranium	U
Fermium	Fm	Phosphorus	P	Vanadium	V
Fluorine	F	Platinum	Pt	Xenon	Xe
Francium	Fr	Plutonium	Pu	Ytterbium	Yb
Gadolinium	Gd	Polonium	Po	Yttrium	Y
Gallium	Ga	Potassium	K	Zinc	Zn
Germanium	Ge	Praseodymium	Pr	Zirconium	Zr
Gold	Au	Promethium	Pm		
Hafnium	Hf	Protactinium	Pa		

REFERENCE TABLES FOR CHEMISTRY

PHYSICAL CONSTANTS AND CONVERSION FACTORS

NAME	SYMBOL	VALUE(S)	UNITS
Angstrom unit	Å	1×10^{-10} m	meter
Avogadro number	N_A	6.02×10^{23} per mol	
Charge of electron	e	1.60×10^{-19} C	coulomb
Electron volt	eV	1.60×10^{-19} J	joule
Speed of light	c	3.00×10^{8} m/s	meters/second
Planck's constant	h	6.63×10^{-34} J·s 1.58×10^{-37} kcal·s	joule-second kilocalorie-second
Universal gas constant	R	0.0821 L·atm/mol·K 1.98 cal/mol·K 8.31 J/mol·K	liter-atmosphere/mole-kelvin calories/mole-kelvin joules/mole-kelvin
Atomic mass unit	μ(amu)	1.66×10^{-24} g	gram
Volume standard, liter	L	1×10^{3} cm^3 = 1 dm^3	cubic centimeters cubic decimeter
Standard pressure, atmosphere	atm	101.3 kPa 760 mmHg 760 torr	kilopascals millimeters of mercury torr
Heat equivalent, kilocalorie	kcal	4.18×10^{3} J	joules

PHYSICAL CONSTANTS FOR H₂O

Molal freezing point depression . . . . 1.86°C
Molal boiling point elevation . . . . 0.52°C
Heat of fusion . . . . 79.72 cal/g
Heat of vaporization . . . . 539.4 cal/g

STANDARD UNITS

SYMBOL	NAME	QUANTITY
m	meter	length
kg	kilogram	mass
Pa	pascal	pressure
K	kelvin	thermodynamic temperature
mol	mole	amount of substance
J	joule	energy, work, quantity of heat
sec	second	time
C	coulomb	quantity of electricity
V	volt	electric potential, potential difference
L	liter	volume

SELECTED PREFIXES

FACTOR	PREFIX	SYMBOL
10^{6}	mega	M
10^{3}	kilo	k
10^{-1}	deci	d
10^{-2}	centi	c
10^{-3}	milli	m
10^{-6}	micro	μ
10^{-9}	nano	n

RELATIVE STRENGTHS OF ACIDS IN AQUEOUS SOLUTION AT 1 atm AND 298 K

CONJUGATE PAIRS			
ACID		**BASE**	K_a
HI	$= H^+ +$	I^-	very large
HBr	$= H^+ +$	Br^-	very large
HCl	$= H^+ +$	Cl^-	very large
HNO_3	$= H^+ +$	NO_3^-	very large
H_2SO_4	$= H^+ +$	HSO_4^-	large
$H_2O + SO_2$	$= H^+ +$	HSO_3^-	1.5×10^{-2}
HSO_4^-	$= H^+ +$	SO_4^{2-}	1.2×10^{-2}
H_3PO_4	$= H^+ +$	$H_2PO_4^-$	7.5×10^{-3}
$Fe(H_2O)_6^{3+}$	$= H^+ +$	$Fe(H_2O)_5(OH)^{2+}$	8.9×10^{-4}
HNO_2	$= H^+ +$	NO_2^-	4.6×10^{-4}
HF	$= H^+ +$	F^-	3.5×10^{-4}
$Cr(H_2O)_6^{3+}$	$= H^+ +$	$Cr(H_2O)_5(OH)^{2+}$	1.0×10^{-4}
CH_3COOH	$= H^+ +$	CH_3COO^-	1.8×10^{-5}
$Al(H_2O)_6^{3+}$	$= H^+ +$	$Al(H_2O)_5(OH)^{2+}$	1.1×10^{-5}
$H_2O + CO_2$	$= H^+ +$	HCO_3^-	4.3×10^{-7}
HSO_3^-	$= H^+ +$	SO_3^{2-}	1.1×10^{-7}
H_2S	$= H^+ +$	HS^-	9.5×10^{-8}
$H_2PO_4^-$	$= H^+ +$	HPO_4^{2-}	6.2×10^{-8}
NH_4^+	$= H^+ +$	NH_3	5.7×10^{-10}
HCO_3^-	$= H^+ +$	CO_3^{2-}	5.6×10^{-11}
HPO_4^{2-}	$= H^+ +$	PO_4^{3-}	2.2×10^{-13}
HS^-	$= H^+ +$	S^{2-}	1.3×10^{-14}
H_2O	$= H^+ +$	OH^-	1.0×10^{-14}

Note: $H^+(aq) = H_3O^+$

Sample equation: $HI + H_2O = H_3O^+ + I^-$

CONSTANTS FOR VARIOUS EQUILIBRIA AT 1 atm AND 298 K

$H_2O(l) = H^+(aq) + OH^-(aq)$	K_w	$= 1.0 \times 10^{-14}$
$H_2O(l) + H_2O(l) = H_3O^+(aq) + OH^-(aq)$	K_w	$= 1.0 \times 10^{-14}$
$CH_3COO^-(aq) + H_2O(l) = CH_3COOH(aq) + OH^-(aq)$	K_b	$= 5.6 \times 10^{-10}$
$Na^+F^-(aq) + H_2O(l) = Na^+(OH)^- + HF(aq)$	K_b	$= 1.5 \times 10^{-11}$
$NH_3(aq) + H_2O(l) = NH_4^+(aq) + OH^-(aq)$	K_b	$= 1.8 \times 10^{-5}$
$CO_3^{2-}(aq) + H_2O(l) = HCO_3^-(aq) + OH^-(aq)$	K_b	$= 1.8 \times 10^{-4}$
$Ag(NH_3)_2^+(aq) = Ag^+(aq) + 2NH_3(aq)$	K_{eq}	$= 8.9 \times 10^{-8}$
$N_2(g) + 3H_2(g) = 2NH_3(g)$	K_{eq}	$= 6.7 \times 10^5$
$H_2(g) + I_2(g) = 2HI(g)$	K_{eq}	$= 3.5 \times 10^{-1}$

COMPOUND	K_{SP}	COMPOUND	K_{SP}
$AgBr$	5.0×10^{-13}	Li_2CO_3	2.5×10^{-2}
$AgCl$	1.8×10^{-10}	$PbCl_2$	1.6×10^{-2}
Ag_2CrO_4	1.1×10^{-12}	$PbCO_3$	7.4×10^{-14}
AgI	8.3×10^{-17}	$PbCrO_4$	2.8×10^{-13}
$BaSO_4$	1.1×10^{-10}	PbI_2	7.1×10^{-9}
$CaSO_4$	9.1×10^{-6}	$ZnCO_3$	1.4×10^{-11}

STANDARD ENERGIES OF FORMATION OF COMPOUNDS AT 1 atm AND 298 K

COMPOUND	HEAT (ENTHALPY) OF FORMATION* KCAL/MOL ($\_H°_f$)	FREE ENERGY OF FORMATION* KCAL/MOL ($\_G_f°$)
Aluminum oxide $Al_2O_3(s)$	−400.5	−378.2
Ammonia $NH_3(g)$	−11.0	−3.9
Barium sulfate $BaSo_4(s)$	−352.1	−325.6
Calcium hydroxide $Ca(OH)_2(s)$	−235.7	−214.8
Carbon dioxide $CO_2(g)$	−94.1	−94.3
Carbon monoxide $CO(g)$	−26.4	−32.8
Copper (II) sulfate $CuSO_4(s)$	−184.4	−158.2
Ethane $C_2H_6(g)$	−20.2	−7.9
Ethene (ethylene) $C_2H_4(g)$	12.5	16.3
Ethyne (acetylene) $C_2H_2(g)$	54.2	50.0
Hydrogen fluoride $HF(g)$	−64.8	−65.3
Hydrogen iodide $HI(g)$	6.3	0.4
Iodine chloride $ICl(g)$	4.3	−1.3
Lead (II) oxide $PbO(s)$	−51.5	−45.0
Magnesium oxide $MgO(s)$	−143.8	−136.1
Nitrogen (II) oxide $NO(g)$	21.6	20.7
Nitrogen (IV) oxide $NO_2(g)$	7.9	12.3
Potassium chloride $KCl(s)$	−104.4	−97.8
Sodium chloride $NaCl(s)$	−98.3	−91.8
Sulfur dioxide $SO_2(g)$	−70.9	−71.7
Water $H_2O(g)$	−57.8	−54.6
Water $H_2O(l)$	−68.3	−56.7

*Minus sign indicates an exothermic reaction.

Sample equations:

$$2Al(s) + \frac{3}{2} O_2(g) \rightarrow Al_2O_3(s) + 400.5 \text{ kcal}$$

$$2Al(s) + \frac{3}{2} O_2(g) \rightarrow Al_2O_3(s) \ \Delta H = -400.5 \text{ kcal/mol}$$

Model Examination A

Answer Sheet

DIRECTIONS: Locate the question number to which you are responding, then fill in the circle containing the letter of the answer you have chosen.

SURVEY OF THE NATURAL SCIENCES

1. Ⓐ Ⓑ Ⓒ Ⓓ Ⓔ
2. Ⓐ Ⓑ Ⓒ Ⓓ Ⓔ
3. Ⓐ Ⓑ Ⓒ Ⓓ Ⓔ
4. Ⓐ Ⓑ Ⓒ Ⓓ Ⓔ
5. Ⓐ Ⓑ Ⓒ Ⓓ Ⓔ
6. Ⓐ Ⓑ Ⓒ Ⓓ Ⓔ
7. Ⓐ Ⓑ Ⓒ Ⓓ Ⓔ
8. Ⓐ Ⓑ Ⓒ Ⓓ Ⓔ
9. Ⓐ Ⓑ Ⓒ Ⓓ Ⓔ
10. Ⓐ Ⓑ Ⓒ Ⓓ Ⓔ
11. Ⓐ Ⓑ Ⓒ Ⓓ Ⓔ
12. Ⓐ Ⓑ Ⓒ Ⓓ Ⓔ
13. Ⓐ Ⓑ Ⓒ Ⓓ Ⓔ
14. Ⓐ Ⓑ Ⓒ Ⓓ Ⓔ
15. Ⓐ Ⓑ Ⓒ Ⓓ Ⓔ
16. Ⓐ Ⓑ Ⓒ Ⓓ Ⓔ
17. Ⓐ Ⓑ Ⓒ Ⓓ Ⓔ
18. Ⓐ Ⓑ Ⓒ Ⓓ Ⓔ
19. Ⓐ Ⓑ Ⓒ Ⓓ Ⓔ
20. Ⓐ Ⓑ Ⓒ Ⓓ Ⓔ
21. Ⓐ Ⓑ Ⓒ Ⓓ Ⓔ
22. Ⓐ Ⓑ Ⓒ Ⓓ Ⓔ
23. Ⓐ Ⓑ Ⓒ Ⓓ Ⓔ
24. Ⓐ Ⓑ Ⓒ Ⓓ Ⓔ
25. Ⓐ Ⓑ Ⓒ Ⓓ Ⓔ
26. Ⓐ Ⓑ Ⓒ Ⓓ Ⓔ
27. Ⓐ Ⓑ Ⓒ Ⓓ Ⓔ
28. Ⓐ Ⓑ Ⓒ Ⓓ Ⓔ

29. Ⓐ Ⓑ Ⓒ Ⓓ Ⓔ
30. Ⓐ Ⓑ Ⓒ Ⓓ Ⓔ
31. Ⓐ Ⓑ Ⓒ Ⓓ Ⓔ
32. Ⓐ Ⓑ Ⓒ Ⓓ Ⓔ
33. Ⓐ Ⓑ Ⓒ Ⓓ Ⓔ
34. Ⓐ Ⓑ Ⓒ Ⓓ Ⓔ
35. Ⓐ Ⓑ Ⓒ Ⓓ Ⓔ
36. Ⓐ Ⓑ Ⓒ Ⓓ Ⓔ
37. Ⓐ Ⓑ Ⓒ Ⓓ Ⓔ
38. Ⓐ Ⓑ Ⓒ Ⓓ Ⓔ
39. Ⓐ Ⓑ Ⓒ Ⓓ Ⓔ
40. Ⓐ Ⓑ Ⓒ Ⓓ Ⓔ
41. Ⓐ Ⓑ Ⓒ Ⓓ Ⓔ
42. Ⓐ Ⓑ Ⓒ Ⓓ Ⓔ
43. Ⓐ Ⓑ Ⓒ Ⓓ Ⓔ
44. Ⓐ Ⓑ Ⓒ Ⓓ Ⓔ
45. Ⓐ Ⓑ Ⓒ Ⓓ Ⓔ
46. Ⓐ Ⓑ Ⓒ Ⓓ Ⓔ
47. Ⓐ Ⓑ Ⓒ Ⓓ Ⓔ
48. Ⓐ Ⓑ Ⓒ Ⓓ Ⓔ
49. Ⓐ Ⓑ Ⓒ Ⓓ Ⓔ
50. Ⓐ Ⓑ Ⓒ Ⓓ Ⓔ
51. Ⓐ Ⓑ Ⓒ Ⓓ Ⓔ
52. Ⓐ Ⓑ Ⓒ Ⓓ Ⓔ
53. Ⓐ Ⓑ Ⓒ Ⓓ Ⓔ
54. Ⓐ Ⓑ Ⓒ Ⓓ Ⓔ
55. Ⓐ Ⓑ Ⓒ Ⓓ Ⓔ
56. Ⓐ Ⓑ Ⓒ Ⓓ Ⓔ
57. Ⓐ Ⓑ Ⓒ Ⓓ Ⓔ
58. Ⓐ Ⓑ Ⓒ Ⓓ Ⓔ
59. Ⓐ Ⓑ Ⓒ Ⓓ Ⓔ

60. Ⓐ Ⓑ Ⓒ Ⓓ Ⓔ
61. Ⓐ Ⓑ Ⓒ Ⓓ Ⓔ
62. Ⓐ Ⓑ Ⓒ Ⓓ Ⓔ
63. Ⓐ Ⓑ Ⓒ Ⓓ Ⓔ
64. Ⓐ Ⓑ Ⓒ Ⓓ Ⓔ
65. Ⓐ Ⓑ Ⓒ Ⓓ Ⓔ
66. Ⓐ Ⓑ Ⓒ Ⓓ Ⓔ
67. Ⓐ Ⓑ Ⓒ Ⓓ Ⓔ
68. Ⓐ Ⓑ Ⓒ Ⓓ Ⓔ
69. Ⓐ Ⓑ Ⓒ Ⓓ Ⓔ
70. Ⓐ Ⓑ Ⓒ Ⓓ Ⓔ
71. Ⓐ Ⓑ Ⓒ Ⓓ Ⓔ
72. Ⓐ Ⓑ Ⓒ Ⓓ Ⓔ
73. Ⓐ Ⓑ Ⓒ Ⓓ Ⓔ
74. Ⓐ Ⓑ Ⓒ Ⓓ Ⓔ
75. Ⓐ Ⓑ Ⓒ Ⓓ Ⓔ
76. Ⓐ Ⓑ Ⓒ Ⓓ Ⓔ
77. Ⓐ Ⓑ Ⓒ Ⓓ Ⓔ
78. Ⓐ Ⓑ Ⓒ Ⓓ Ⓔ
79. Ⓐ Ⓑ Ⓒ Ⓓ Ⓔ
80. Ⓐ Ⓑ Ⓒ Ⓓ Ⓔ
81. Ⓐ Ⓑ Ⓒ Ⓓ Ⓔ
82. Ⓐ Ⓑ Ⓒ Ⓓ Ⓔ
83. Ⓐ Ⓑ Ⓒ Ⓓ Ⓔ
84. Ⓐ Ⓑ Ⓒ Ⓓ Ⓔ
85. Ⓐ Ⓑ Ⓒ Ⓓ Ⓔ
86. Ⓐ Ⓑ Ⓒ Ⓓ Ⓔ
87. Ⓐ Ⓑ Ⓒ Ⓓ Ⓔ
88. Ⓐ Ⓑ Ⓒ Ⓓ Ⓔ
89. Ⓐ Ⓑ Ⓒ Ⓓ Ⓔ
90. Ⓐ Ⓑ Ⓒ Ⓓ Ⓔ

91. Ⓐ Ⓑ Ⓒ Ⓓ Ⓔ
92. Ⓐ Ⓑ Ⓒ Ⓓ Ⓔ
93. Ⓐ Ⓑ Ⓒ Ⓓ Ⓔ
94. Ⓐ Ⓑ Ⓒ Ⓓ Ⓔ
95. Ⓐ Ⓑ Ⓒ Ⓓ Ⓔ
96. Ⓐ Ⓑ Ⓒ Ⓓ Ⓔ
97. Ⓐ Ⓑ Ⓒ Ⓓ Ⓔ
98. Ⓐ Ⓑ Ⓒ Ⓓ Ⓔ
99. Ⓐ Ⓑ Ⓒ Ⓓ Ⓔ
100. Ⓐ Ⓑ Ⓒ Ⓓ Ⓔ

PERCEPTUAL ABILITY TEST

1. Ⓐ Ⓑ Ⓒ Ⓓ Ⓔ
2. Ⓐ Ⓑ Ⓒ Ⓓ Ⓔ
3. Ⓐ Ⓑ Ⓒ Ⓓ Ⓔ
4. Ⓐ Ⓑ Ⓒ Ⓓ Ⓔ
5. Ⓐ Ⓑ Ⓒ Ⓓ Ⓔ
6. Ⓐ Ⓑ Ⓒ Ⓓ Ⓔ
7. Ⓐ Ⓑ Ⓒ Ⓓ Ⓔ
8. Ⓐ Ⓑ Ⓒ Ⓓ Ⓔ
9. Ⓐ Ⓑ Ⓒ Ⓓ Ⓔ
10. Ⓐ Ⓑ Ⓒ Ⓓ Ⓔ
11. Ⓐ Ⓑ Ⓒ Ⓓ Ⓔ
12. Ⓐ Ⓑ Ⓒ Ⓓ Ⓔ
13. Ⓐ Ⓑ Ⓒ Ⓓ Ⓔ
14. Ⓐ Ⓑ Ⓒ Ⓓ Ⓔ
15. Ⓐ Ⓑ Ⓒ Ⓓ Ⓔ
16. Ⓐ Ⓑ Ⓒ Ⓓ Ⓔ
17. Ⓐ Ⓑ Ⓒ Ⓓ Ⓔ
18. Ⓐ Ⓑ Ⓒ Ⓓ Ⓔ

19. Ⓐ Ⓑ Ⓒ Ⓓ Ⓔ
20. Ⓐ Ⓑ Ⓒ Ⓓ Ⓔ
21. Ⓐ Ⓑ Ⓒ Ⓓ Ⓔ
22. Ⓐ Ⓑ Ⓒ Ⓓ Ⓔ
23. Ⓐ Ⓑ Ⓒ Ⓓ Ⓔ
24. Ⓐ Ⓑ Ⓒ Ⓓ Ⓔ
25. Ⓐ Ⓑ Ⓒ Ⓓ Ⓔ
26. Ⓐ Ⓑ Ⓒ Ⓓ Ⓔ
27. Ⓐ Ⓑ Ⓒ Ⓓ Ⓔ
28. Ⓐ Ⓑ Ⓒ Ⓓ Ⓔ
29. Ⓐ Ⓑ Ⓒ Ⓓ Ⓔ
30. Ⓐ Ⓑ Ⓒ Ⓓ Ⓔ
31. Ⓐ Ⓑ Ⓒ Ⓓ Ⓔ
32. Ⓐ Ⓑ Ⓒ Ⓓ Ⓔ
33. Ⓐ Ⓑ Ⓒ Ⓓ Ⓔ
34. Ⓐ Ⓑ Ⓒ Ⓓ Ⓔ
35. Ⓐ Ⓑ Ⓒ Ⓓ Ⓔ
36. Ⓐ Ⓑ Ⓒ Ⓓ Ⓔ
37. Ⓐ Ⓑ Ⓒ Ⓓ Ⓔ
38. Ⓐ Ⓑ Ⓒ Ⓓ Ⓔ
39. Ⓐ Ⓑ Ⓒ Ⓓ Ⓔ
40. Ⓐ Ⓑ Ⓒ Ⓓ Ⓔ
41. Ⓐ Ⓑ Ⓒ Ⓓ Ⓔ
42. Ⓐ Ⓑ Ⓒ Ⓓ Ⓔ
43. Ⓐ Ⓑ Ⓒ Ⓓ Ⓔ
44. Ⓐ Ⓑ Ⓒ Ⓓ Ⓔ
45. Ⓐ Ⓑ Ⓒ Ⓓ Ⓔ
46. Ⓐ Ⓑ Ⓒ Ⓓ Ⓔ
47. Ⓐ Ⓑ Ⓒ Ⓓ Ⓔ
48. Ⓐ Ⓑ Ⓒ Ⓓ Ⓔ
49. Ⓐ Ⓑ Ⓒ Ⓓ Ⓔ
50. Ⓐ Ⓑ Ⓒ Ⓓ Ⓔ
51. Ⓐ Ⓑ Ⓒ Ⓓ Ⓔ
52. Ⓐ Ⓑ Ⓒ Ⓓ Ⓔ
53. Ⓐ Ⓑ Ⓒ Ⓓ Ⓔ
54. Ⓐ Ⓑ Ⓒ Ⓓ Ⓔ
55. Ⓐ Ⓑ Ⓒ Ⓓ Ⓔ
56. Ⓐ Ⓑ Ⓒ Ⓓ Ⓔ
57. Ⓐ Ⓑ Ⓒ Ⓓ Ⓔ
58. Ⓐ Ⓑ Ⓒ Ⓓ Ⓔ
59. Ⓐ Ⓑ Ⓒ Ⓓ Ⓔ
60. Ⓐ Ⓑ Ⓒ Ⓓ Ⓔ
61. Ⓐ Ⓑ Ⓒ Ⓓ Ⓔ

62. Ⓐ Ⓑ Ⓒ Ⓓ Ⓔ
63. Ⓐ Ⓑ Ⓒ Ⓓ Ⓔ
64. Ⓐ Ⓑ Ⓒ Ⓓ Ⓔ
65. Ⓐ Ⓑ Ⓒ Ⓓ Ⓔ
66. Ⓐ Ⓑ Ⓒ Ⓓ Ⓔ
67. Ⓐ Ⓑ Ⓒ Ⓓ Ⓔ
68. Ⓐ Ⓑ Ⓒ Ⓓ Ⓔ
69. Ⓐ Ⓑ Ⓒ Ⓓ Ⓔ
70. Ⓐ Ⓑ Ⓒ Ⓓ Ⓔ
71. Ⓐ Ⓑ Ⓒ Ⓓ Ⓔ
72. Ⓐ Ⓑ Ⓒ Ⓓ Ⓔ
73. Ⓐ Ⓑ Ⓒ Ⓓ Ⓔ
74. Ⓐ Ⓑ Ⓒ Ⓓ Ⓔ
75. Ⓐ Ⓑ Ⓒ Ⓓ Ⓔ
76. Ⓐ Ⓑ Ⓒ Ⓓ Ⓔ
77. Ⓐ Ⓑ Ⓒ Ⓓ Ⓔ
78. Ⓐ Ⓑ Ⓒ Ⓓ Ⓔ
79. Ⓐ Ⓑ Ⓒ Ⓓ Ⓔ
80. Ⓐ Ⓑ Ⓒ Ⓓ Ⓔ
81. Ⓐ Ⓑ Ⓒ Ⓓ Ⓔ
82. Ⓐ Ⓑ Ⓒ Ⓓ Ⓔ
83. Ⓐ Ⓑ Ⓒ Ⓓ Ⓔ
84. Ⓐ Ⓑ Ⓒ Ⓓ Ⓔ
85. Ⓐ Ⓑ Ⓒ Ⓓ Ⓔ
86. Ⓐ Ⓑ Ⓒ Ⓓ Ⓔ
87. Ⓐ Ⓑ Ⓒ Ⓓ Ⓔ
88. Ⓐ Ⓑ Ⓒ Ⓓ Ⓔ
89. Ⓐ Ⓑ Ⓒ Ⓓ Ⓔ
90. Ⓐ Ⓑ Ⓒ Ⓓ Ⓔ

READING COMPREHENSION TEST

1. Ⓐ Ⓑ Ⓒ Ⓓ Ⓔ
2. Ⓐ Ⓑ Ⓒ Ⓓ Ⓔ
3. Ⓐ Ⓑ Ⓒ Ⓓ Ⓔ
4. Ⓐ Ⓑ Ⓒ Ⓓ Ⓔ
5. Ⓐ Ⓑ Ⓒ Ⓓ Ⓔ
6. Ⓐ Ⓑ Ⓒ Ⓓ Ⓔ
7. Ⓐ Ⓑ Ⓒ Ⓓ Ⓔ
8. Ⓐ Ⓑ Ⓒ Ⓓ Ⓔ
9. Ⓐ Ⓑ Ⓒ Ⓓ Ⓔ

10. Ⓐ Ⓑ Ⓒ Ⓓ Ⓔ
11. Ⓐ Ⓑ Ⓒ Ⓓ Ⓔ
12. Ⓐ Ⓑ Ⓒ Ⓓ Ⓔ
13. Ⓐ Ⓑ Ⓒ Ⓓ Ⓔ
14. Ⓐ Ⓑ Ⓒ Ⓓ Ⓔ
15. Ⓐ Ⓑ Ⓒ Ⓓ Ⓔ
16. Ⓐ Ⓑ Ⓒ Ⓓ Ⓔ
17. Ⓐ Ⓑ Ⓒ Ⓓ Ⓔ
18. Ⓐ Ⓑ Ⓒ Ⓓ Ⓔ
19. Ⓐ Ⓑ Ⓒ Ⓓ Ⓔ
20. Ⓐ Ⓑ Ⓒ Ⓓ Ⓔ
21. Ⓐ Ⓑ Ⓒ Ⓓ Ⓔ
22. Ⓐ Ⓑ Ⓒ Ⓓ Ⓔ
23. Ⓐ Ⓑ Ⓒ Ⓓ Ⓔ
24. Ⓐ Ⓑ Ⓒ Ⓓ Ⓔ
25. Ⓐ Ⓑ Ⓒ Ⓓ Ⓔ
26. Ⓐ Ⓑ Ⓒ Ⓓ Ⓔ
27. Ⓐ Ⓑ Ⓒ Ⓓ Ⓔ
28. Ⓐ Ⓑ Ⓒ Ⓓ Ⓔ
29. Ⓐ Ⓑ Ⓒ Ⓓ Ⓔ
30. Ⓐ Ⓑ Ⓒ Ⓓ Ⓔ
31. Ⓐ Ⓑ Ⓒ Ⓓ Ⓔ
32. Ⓐ Ⓑ Ⓒ Ⓓ Ⓔ
33. Ⓐ Ⓑ Ⓒ Ⓓ Ⓔ
34. Ⓐ Ⓑ Ⓒ Ⓓ Ⓔ
35. Ⓐ Ⓑ Ⓒ Ⓓ Ⓔ
36. Ⓐ Ⓑ Ⓒ Ⓓ Ⓔ
37. Ⓐ Ⓑ Ⓒ Ⓓ Ⓔ
38. Ⓐ Ⓑ Ⓒ Ⓓ Ⓔ
39. Ⓐ Ⓑ Ⓒ Ⓓ Ⓔ
40. Ⓐ Ⓑ Ⓒ Ⓓ Ⓔ
41. Ⓐ Ⓑ Ⓒ Ⓓ Ⓔ
42. Ⓐ Ⓑ Ⓒ Ⓓ Ⓔ
43. Ⓐ Ⓑ Ⓒ Ⓓ Ⓔ
44. Ⓐ Ⓑ Ⓒ Ⓓ Ⓔ
45. Ⓐ Ⓑ Ⓒ Ⓓ Ⓔ
46. Ⓐ Ⓑ Ⓒ Ⓓ Ⓔ
47. Ⓐ Ⓑ Ⓒ Ⓓ Ⓔ
48. Ⓐ Ⓑ Ⓒ Ⓓ Ⓔ
49. Ⓐ Ⓑ Ⓒ Ⓓ Ⓔ
50. Ⓐ Ⓑ Ⓒ Ⓓ Ⓔ

QUANTITATIVE REASONING TEST

1. Ⓐ Ⓑ Ⓒ Ⓓ Ⓔ
2. Ⓐ Ⓑ Ⓒ Ⓓ Ⓔ
3. Ⓐ Ⓑ Ⓒ Ⓓ Ⓔ
4. Ⓐ Ⓑ Ⓒ Ⓓ Ⓔ
5. Ⓐ Ⓑ Ⓒ Ⓓ Ⓔ
6. Ⓐ Ⓑ Ⓒ Ⓓ Ⓔ
7. Ⓐ Ⓑ Ⓒ Ⓓ Ⓔ
8. Ⓐ Ⓑ Ⓒ Ⓓ Ⓔ
9. Ⓐ Ⓑ Ⓒ Ⓓ Ⓔ
10. Ⓐ Ⓑ Ⓒ Ⓓ Ⓔ
11. Ⓐ Ⓑ Ⓒ Ⓓ Ⓔ
12. Ⓐ Ⓑ Ⓒ Ⓓ Ⓔ
13. Ⓐ Ⓑ Ⓒ Ⓓ Ⓔ
14. Ⓐ Ⓑ Ⓒ Ⓓ Ⓔ
15. Ⓐ Ⓑ Ⓒ Ⓓ Ⓔ
16. Ⓐ Ⓑ Ⓒ Ⓓ Ⓔ
17. Ⓐ Ⓑ Ⓒ Ⓓ Ⓔ
18. Ⓐ Ⓑ Ⓒ Ⓓ Ⓔ
19. Ⓐ Ⓑ Ⓒ Ⓓ Ⓔ
20. Ⓐ Ⓑ Ⓒ Ⓓ Ⓔ
21. Ⓐ Ⓑ Ⓒ Ⓓ Ⓔ
22. Ⓐ Ⓑ Ⓒ Ⓓ Ⓔ
23. Ⓐ Ⓑ Ⓒ Ⓓ Ⓔ
24. Ⓐ Ⓑ Ⓒ Ⓓ Ⓔ
25. Ⓐ Ⓑ Ⓒ Ⓓ Ⓔ
26. Ⓐ Ⓑ Ⓒ Ⓓ Ⓔ
27. Ⓐ Ⓑ Ⓒ Ⓓ Ⓔ
28. Ⓐ Ⓑ Ⓒ Ⓓ Ⓔ
29. Ⓐ Ⓑ Ⓒ Ⓓ Ⓔ
30. Ⓐ Ⓑ Ⓒ Ⓓ Ⓔ
31. Ⓐ Ⓑ Ⓒ Ⓓ Ⓔ
32. Ⓐ Ⓑ Ⓒ Ⓓ Ⓔ
33. Ⓐ Ⓑ Ⓒ Ⓓ Ⓔ
34. Ⓐ Ⓑ Ⓒ Ⓓ Ⓔ
35. Ⓐ Ⓑ Ⓒ Ⓓ Ⓔ
36. Ⓐ Ⓑ Ⓒ Ⓓ Ⓔ
37. Ⓐ Ⓑ Ⓒ Ⓓ Ⓔ
38. Ⓐ Ⓑ Ⓒ Ⓓ Ⓔ
39. Ⓐ Ⓑ Ⓒ Ⓓ Ⓔ
40. Ⓐ Ⓑ Ⓒ Ⓓ Ⓔ

Model Examination B

Answer Sheet

DIRECTIONS: Locate the question number to which you are responding, then fill in the circle containing the letter of the answer you have chosen.

SURVEY OF THE NATURAL SCIENCES

1. Ⓐ Ⓑ Ⓒ Ⓓ Ⓔ
2. Ⓐ Ⓑ Ⓒ Ⓓ Ⓔ
3. Ⓐ Ⓑ Ⓒ Ⓓ Ⓔ
4. Ⓐ Ⓑ Ⓒ Ⓓ Ⓔ
5. Ⓐ Ⓑ Ⓒ Ⓓ Ⓔ
6. Ⓐ Ⓑ Ⓒ Ⓓ Ⓔ
7. Ⓐ Ⓑ Ⓒ Ⓓ Ⓔ
8. Ⓐ Ⓑ Ⓒ Ⓓ Ⓔ
9. Ⓐ Ⓑ Ⓒ Ⓓ Ⓔ
10. Ⓐ Ⓑ Ⓒ Ⓓ Ⓔ
11. Ⓐ Ⓑ Ⓒ Ⓓ Ⓔ
12. Ⓐ Ⓑ Ⓒ Ⓓ Ⓔ
13. Ⓐ Ⓑ Ⓒ Ⓓ Ⓔ
14. Ⓐ Ⓑ Ⓒ Ⓓ Ⓔ
15. Ⓐ Ⓑ Ⓒ Ⓓ Ⓔ
16. Ⓐ Ⓑ Ⓒ Ⓓ Ⓔ
17. Ⓐ Ⓑ Ⓒ Ⓓ Ⓔ
18. Ⓐ Ⓑ Ⓒ Ⓓ Ⓔ
19. Ⓐ Ⓑ Ⓒ Ⓓ Ⓔ
20. Ⓐ Ⓑ Ⓒ Ⓓ Ⓔ
21. Ⓐ Ⓑ Ⓒ Ⓓ Ⓔ
22. Ⓐ Ⓑ Ⓒ Ⓓ Ⓔ
23. Ⓐ Ⓑ Ⓒ Ⓓ Ⓔ
24. Ⓐ Ⓑ Ⓒ Ⓓ Ⓔ
25. Ⓐ Ⓑ Ⓒ Ⓓ Ⓔ
26. Ⓐ Ⓑ Ⓒ Ⓓ Ⓔ
27. Ⓐ Ⓑ Ⓒ Ⓓ Ⓔ
28. Ⓐ Ⓑ Ⓒ Ⓓ Ⓔ

29. Ⓐ Ⓑ Ⓒ Ⓓ Ⓔ
30. Ⓐ Ⓑ Ⓒ Ⓓ Ⓔ
31. Ⓐ Ⓑ Ⓒ Ⓓ Ⓔ
32. Ⓐ Ⓑ Ⓒ Ⓓ Ⓔ
33. Ⓐ Ⓑ Ⓒ Ⓓ Ⓔ
34. Ⓐ Ⓑ Ⓒ Ⓓ Ⓔ
35. Ⓐ Ⓑ Ⓒ Ⓓ Ⓔ
36. Ⓐ Ⓑ Ⓒ Ⓓ Ⓔ
37. Ⓐ Ⓑ Ⓒ Ⓓ Ⓔ
38. Ⓐ Ⓑ Ⓒ Ⓓ Ⓔ
39. Ⓐ Ⓑ Ⓒ Ⓓ Ⓔ
40. Ⓐ Ⓑ Ⓒ Ⓓ Ⓔ
41. Ⓐ Ⓑ Ⓒ Ⓓ Ⓔ
42. Ⓐ Ⓑ Ⓒ Ⓓ Ⓔ
43. Ⓐ Ⓑ Ⓒ Ⓓ Ⓔ
44. Ⓐ Ⓑ Ⓒ Ⓓ Ⓔ
45. Ⓐ Ⓑ Ⓒ Ⓓ Ⓔ
46. Ⓐ Ⓑ Ⓒ Ⓓ Ⓔ
47. Ⓐ Ⓑ Ⓒ Ⓓ Ⓔ
48. Ⓐ Ⓑ Ⓒ Ⓓ Ⓔ
49. Ⓐ Ⓑ Ⓒ Ⓓ Ⓔ
50. Ⓐ Ⓑ Ⓒ Ⓓ Ⓔ
51. Ⓐ Ⓑ Ⓒ Ⓓ Ⓔ
52. Ⓐ Ⓑ Ⓒ Ⓓ Ⓔ
53. Ⓐ Ⓑ Ⓒ Ⓓ Ⓔ
54. Ⓐ Ⓑ Ⓒ Ⓓ Ⓔ
55. Ⓐ Ⓑ Ⓒ Ⓓ Ⓔ
56. Ⓐ Ⓑ Ⓒ Ⓓ Ⓔ
57. Ⓐ Ⓑ Ⓒ Ⓓ Ⓔ
58. Ⓐ Ⓑ Ⓒ Ⓓ Ⓔ
59. Ⓐ Ⓑ Ⓒ Ⓓ Ⓔ

60. Ⓐ Ⓑ Ⓒ Ⓓ Ⓔ
61. Ⓐ Ⓑ Ⓒ Ⓓ Ⓔ
62. Ⓐ Ⓑ Ⓒ Ⓓ Ⓔ
63. Ⓐ Ⓑ Ⓒ Ⓓ Ⓔ
64. Ⓐ Ⓑ Ⓒ Ⓓ Ⓔ
65. Ⓐ Ⓑ Ⓒ Ⓓ Ⓔ
66. Ⓐ Ⓑ Ⓒ Ⓓ Ⓔ
67. Ⓐ Ⓑ Ⓒ Ⓓ Ⓔ
68. Ⓐ Ⓑ Ⓒ Ⓓ Ⓔ
69. Ⓐ Ⓑ Ⓒ Ⓓ Ⓔ
70. Ⓐ Ⓑ Ⓒ Ⓓ Ⓔ
71. Ⓐ Ⓑ Ⓒ Ⓓ Ⓔ
72. Ⓐ Ⓑ Ⓒ Ⓓ Ⓔ
73. Ⓐ Ⓑ Ⓒ Ⓓ Ⓔ
74. Ⓐ Ⓑ Ⓒ Ⓓ Ⓔ
75. Ⓐ Ⓑ Ⓒ Ⓓ Ⓔ
76. Ⓐ Ⓑ Ⓒ Ⓓ Ⓔ
77. Ⓐ Ⓑ Ⓒ Ⓓ Ⓔ
78. Ⓐ Ⓑ Ⓒ Ⓓ Ⓔ
79. Ⓐ Ⓑ Ⓒ Ⓓ Ⓔ
80. Ⓐ Ⓑ Ⓒ Ⓓ Ⓔ
81. Ⓐ Ⓑ Ⓒ Ⓓ Ⓔ
82. Ⓐ Ⓑ Ⓒ Ⓓ Ⓔ
83. Ⓐ Ⓑ Ⓒ Ⓓ Ⓔ
84. Ⓐ Ⓑ Ⓒ Ⓓ Ⓔ
85. Ⓐ Ⓑ Ⓒ Ⓓ Ⓔ
86. Ⓐ Ⓑ Ⓒ Ⓓ Ⓔ
87. Ⓐ Ⓑ Ⓒ Ⓓ Ⓔ
88. Ⓐ Ⓑ Ⓒ Ⓓ Ⓔ
89. Ⓐ Ⓑ Ⓒ Ⓓ Ⓔ
90. Ⓐ Ⓑ Ⓒ Ⓓ Ⓔ

91. Ⓐ Ⓑ Ⓒ Ⓓ Ⓔ
92. Ⓐ Ⓑ Ⓒ Ⓓ Ⓔ
93. Ⓐ Ⓑ Ⓒ Ⓓ Ⓔ
94. Ⓐ Ⓑ Ⓒ Ⓓ Ⓔ
95. Ⓐ Ⓑ Ⓒ Ⓓ Ⓔ
96. Ⓐ Ⓑ Ⓒ Ⓓ Ⓔ
97. Ⓐ Ⓑ Ⓒ Ⓓ Ⓔ
98. Ⓐ Ⓑ Ⓒ Ⓓ Ⓔ
99. Ⓐ Ⓑ Ⓒ Ⓓ Ⓔ
100. Ⓐ Ⓑ Ⓒ Ⓓ Ⓔ

PERCEPTUAL ABILITY TEST

1. Ⓐ Ⓑ Ⓒ Ⓓ Ⓔ
2. Ⓐ Ⓑ Ⓒ Ⓓ Ⓔ
3. Ⓐ Ⓑ Ⓒ Ⓓ Ⓔ
4. Ⓐ Ⓑ Ⓒ Ⓓ Ⓔ
5. Ⓐ Ⓑ Ⓒ Ⓓ Ⓔ
6. Ⓐ Ⓑ Ⓒ Ⓓ Ⓔ
7. Ⓐ Ⓑ Ⓒ Ⓓ Ⓔ
8. Ⓐ Ⓑ Ⓒ Ⓓ Ⓔ
9. Ⓐ Ⓑ Ⓒ Ⓓ Ⓔ
10. Ⓐ Ⓑ Ⓒ Ⓓ Ⓔ
11. Ⓐ Ⓑ Ⓒ Ⓓ Ⓔ
12. Ⓐ Ⓑ Ⓒ Ⓓ Ⓔ
13. Ⓐ Ⓑ Ⓒ Ⓓ Ⓔ
14. Ⓐ Ⓑ Ⓒ Ⓓ Ⓔ
15. Ⓐ Ⓑ Ⓒ Ⓓ Ⓔ
16. Ⓐ Ⓑ Ⓒ Ⓓ Ⓔ
17. Ⓐ Ⓑ Ⓒ Ⓓ Ⓔ
18. Ⓐ Ⓑ Ⓒ Ⓓ Ⓔ

19. Ⓐ Ⓑ Ⓒ Ⓓ Ⓔ
20. Ⓐ Ⓑ Ⓒ Ⓓ Ⓔ
21. Ⓐ Ⓑ Ⓒ Ⓓ Ⓔ
22. Ⓐ Ⓑ Ⓒ Ⓓ Ⓔ
23. Ⓐ Ⓑ Ⓒ Ⓓ Ⓔ
24. Ⓐ Ⓑ Ⓒ Ⓓ Ⓔ
25. Ⓐ Ⓑ Ⓒ Ⓓ Ⓔ
26. Ⓐ Ⓑ Ⓒ Ⓓ Ⓔ
27. Ⓐ Ⓑ Ⓒ Ⓓ Ⓔ
28. Ⓐ Ⓑ Ⓒ Ⓓ Ⓔ
29. Ⓐ Ⓑ Ⓒ Ⓓ Ⓔ
30. Ⓐ Ⓑ Ⓒ Ⓓ Ⓔ
31. Ⓐ Ⓑ Ⓒ Ⓓ Ⓔ
32. Ⓐ Ⓑ Ⓒ Ⓓ Ⓔ
33. Ⓐ Ⓑ Ⓒ Ⓓ Ⓔ
34. Ⓐ Ⓑ Ⓒ Ⓓ Ⓔ
35. Ⓐ Ⓑ Ⓒ Ⓓ Ⓔ
36. Ⓐ Ⓑ Ⓒ Ⓓ Ⓔ
37. Ⓐ Ⓑ Ⓒ Ⓓ Ⓔ
38. Ⓐ Ⓑ Ⓒ Ⓓ Ⓔ
39. Ⓐ Ⓑ Ⓒ Ⓓ Ⓔ
40. Ⓐ Ⓑ Ⓒ Ⓓ Ⓔ
41. Ⓐ Ⓑ Ⓒ Ⓓ Ⓔ
42. Ⓐ Ⓑ Ⓒ Ⓓ Ⓔ
43. Ⓐ Ⓑ Ⓒ Ⓓ Ⓔ
44. Ⓐ Ⓑ Ⓒ Ⓓ Ⓔ
45. Ⓐ Ⓑ Ⓒ Ⓓ Ⓔ
46. Ⓐ Ⓑ Ⓒ Ⓓ Ⓔ
47. Ⓐ Ⓑ Ⓒ Ⓓ Ⓔ
48. Ⓐ Ⓑ Ⓒ Ⓓ Ⓔ
49. Ⓐ Ⓑ Ⓒ Ⓓ Ⓔ
50. Ⓐ Ⓑ Ⓒ Ⓓ Ⓔ
51. Ⓐ Ⓑ Ⓒ Ⓓ Ⓔ
52. Ⓐ Ⓑ Ⓒ Ⓓ Ⓔ
53. Ⓐ Ⓑ Ⓒ Ⓓ Ⓔ
54. Ⓐ Ⓑ Ⓒ Ⓓ Ⓔ
55. Ⓐ Ⓑ Ⓒ Ⓓ Ⓔ
56. Ⓐ Ⓑ Ⓒ Ⓓ Ⓔ
57. Ⓐ Ⓑ Ⓒ Ⓓ Ⓔ
58. Ⓐ Ⓑ Ⓒ Ⓓ Ⓔ
59. Ⓐ Ⓑ Ⓒ Ⓓ Ⓔ
60. Ⓐ Ⓑ Ⓒ Ⓓ Ⓔ
61. Ⓐ Ⓑ Ⓒ Ⓓ Ⓔ

62. Ⓐ Ⓑ Ⓒ Ⓓ Ⓔ
63. Ⓐ Ⓑ Ⓒ Ⓓ Ⓔ
64. Ⓐ Ⓑ Ⓒ Ⓓ Ⓔ
65. Ⓐ Ⓑ Ⓒ Ⓓ Ⓔ
66. Ⓐ Ⓑ Ⓒ Ⓓ Ⓔ
67. Ⓐ Ⓑ Ⓒ Ⓓ Ⓔ
68. Ⓐ Ⓑ Ⓒ Ⓓ Ⓔ
69. Ⓐ Ⓑ Ⓒ Ⓓ Ⓔ
70. Ⓐ Ⓑ Ⓒ Ⓓ Ⓔ
71. Ⓐ Ⓑ Ⓒ Ⓓ Ⓔ
72. Ⓐ Ⓑ Ⓒ Ⓓ Ⓔ
73. Ⓐ Ⓑ Ⓒ Ⓓ Ⓔ
74. Ⓐ Ⓑ Ⓒ Ⓓ Ⓔ
75. Ⓐ Ⓑ Ⓒ Ⓓ Ⓔ
76. Ⓐ Ⓑ Ⓒ Ⓓ Ⓔ
77. Ⓐ Ⓑ Ⓒ Ⓓ Ⓔ
78. Ⓐ Ⓑ Ⓒ Ⓓ Ⓔ
79. Ⓐ Ⓑ Ⓒ Ⓓ Ⓔ
80. Ⓐ Ⓑ Ⓒ Ⓓ Ⓔ
81. Ⓐ Ⓑ Ⓒ Ⓓ Ⓔ
82. Ⓐ Ⓑ Ⓒ Ⓓ Ⓔ
83. Ⓐ Ⓑ Ⓒ Ⓓ Ⓔ
84. Ⓐ Ⓑ Ⓒ Ⓓ Ⓔ
85. Ⓐ Ⓑ Ⓒ Ⓓ Ⓔ
86. Ⓐ Ⓑ Ⓒ Ⓓ Ⓔ
87. Ⓐ Ⓑ Ⓒ Ⓓ Ⓔ
88. Ⓐ Ⓑ Ⓒ Ⓓ Ⓔ
89. Ⓐ Ⓑ Ⓒ Ⓓ Ⓔ
90. Ⓐ Ⓑ Ⓒ Ⓓ Ⓔ

READING COMPREHENSION TEST

1. Ⓐ Ⓑ Ⓒ Ⓓ Ⓔ
2. Ⓐ Ⓑ Ⓒ Ⓓ Ⓔ
3. Ⓐ Ⓑ Ⓒ Ⓓ Ⓔ
4. Ⓐ Ⓑ Ⓒ Ⓓ Ⓔ
5. Ⓐ Ⓑ Ⓒ Ⓓ Ⓔ
6. Ⓐ Ⓑ Ⓒ Ⓓ Ⓔ
7. Ⓐ Ⓑ Ⓒ Ⓓ Ⓔ
8. Ⓐ Ⓑ Ⓒ Ⓓ Ⓔ
9. Ⓐ Ⓑ Ⓒ Ⓓ Ⓔ

10. Ⓐ Ⓑ Ⓒ Ⓓ Ⓔ
11. Ⓐ Ⓑ Ⓒ Ⓓ Ⓔ
12. Ⓐ Ⓑ Ⓒ Ⓓ Ⓔ
13. Ⓐ Ⓑ Ⓒ Ⓓ Ⓔ
14. Ⓐ Ⓑ Ⓒ Ⓓ Ⓔ
15. Ⓐ Ⓑ Ⓒ Ⓓ Ⓔ
16. Ⓐ Ⓑ Ⓒ Ⓓ Ⓔ
17. Ⓐ Ⓑ Ⓒ Ⓓ Ⓔ
18. Ⓐ Ⓑ Ⓒ Ⓓ Ⓔ
19. Ⓐ Ⓑ Ⓒ Ⓓ Ⓔ
20. Ⓐ Ⓑ Ⓒ Ⓓ Ⓔ
21. Ⓐ Ⓑ Ⓒ Ⓓ Ⓔ
22. Ⓐ Ⓑ Ⓒ Ⓓ Ⓔ
23. Ⓐ Ⓑ Ⓒ Ⓓ Ⓔ
24. Ⓐ Ⓑ Ⓒ Ⓓ Ⓔ
25. Ⓐ Ⓑ Ⓒ Ⓓ Ⓔ
26. Ⓐ Ⓑ Ⓒ Ⓓ Ⓔ
27. Ⓐ Ⓑ Ⓒ Ⓓ Ⓔ
28. Ⓐ Ⓑ Ⓒ Ⓓ Ⓔ
29. Ⓐ Ⓑ Ⓒ Ⓓ Ⓔ
30. Ⓐ Ⓑ Ⓒ Ⓓ Ⓔ
31. Ⓐ Ⓑ Ⓒ Ⓓ Ⓔ
32. Ⓐ Ⓑ Ⓒ Ⓓ Ⓔ
33. Ⓐ Ⓑ Ⓒ Ⓓ Ⓔ
34. Ⓐ Ⓑ Ⓒ Ⓓ Ⓔ
35. Ⓐ Ⓑ Ⓒ Ⓓ Ⓔ
36. Ⓐ Ⓑ Ⓒ Ⓓ Ⓔ
37. Ⓐ Ⓑ Ⓒ Ⓓ Ⓔ
38. Ⓐ Ⓑ Ⓒ Ⓓ Ⓔ
39. Ⓐ Ⓑ Ⓒ Ⓓ Ⓔ
40. Ⓐ Ⓑ Ⓒ Ⓓ Ⓔ
41. Ⓐ Ⓑ Ⓒ Ⓓ Ⓔ
42. Ⓐ Ⓑ Ⓒ Ⓓ Ⓔ
43. Ⓐ Ⓑ Ⓒ Ⓓ Ⓔ
44. Ⓐ Ⓑ Ⓒ Ⓓ Ⓔ
45. Ⓐ Ⓑ Ⓒ Ⓓ Ⓔ
46. Ⓐ Ⓑ Ⓒ Ⓓ Ⓔ
47. Ⓐ Ⓑ Ⓒ Ⓓ Ⓔ
48. Ⓐ Ⓑ Ⓒ Ⓓ Ⓔ
49. Ⓐ Ⓑ Ⓒ Ⓓ Ⓔ
50. Ⓐ Ⓑ Ⓒ Ⓓ Ⓔ

QUANTITATIVE REASONING TEST

1. Ⓐ Ⓑ Ⓒ Ⓓ Ⓔ
2. Ⓐ Ⓑ Ⓒ Ⓓ Ⓔ
3. Ⓐ Ⓑ Ⓒ Ⓓ Ⓔ
4. Ⓐ Ⓑ Ⓒ Ⓓ Ⓔ
5. Ⓐ Ⓑ Ⓒ Ⓓ Ⓔ
6. Ⓐ Ⓑ Ⓒ Ⓓ Ⓔ
7. Ⓐ Ⓑ Ⓒ Ⓓ Ⓔ
8. Ⓐ Ⓑ Ⓒ Ⓓ Ⓔ
9. Ⓐ Ⓑ Ⓒ Ⓓ Ⓔ
10. Ⓐ Ⓑ Ⓒ Ⓓ Ⓔ
11. Ⓐ Ⓑ Ⓒ Ⓓ Ⓔ
12. Ⓐ Ⓑ Ⓒ Ⓓ Ⓔ
13. Ⓐ Ⓑ Ⓒ Ⓓ Ⓔ
14. Ⓐ Ⓑ Ⓒ Ⓓ Ⓔ
15. Ⓐ Ⓑ Ⓒ Ⓓ Ⓔ
16. Ⓐ Ⓑ Ⓒ Ⓓ Ⓔ
17. Ⓐ Ⓑ Ⓒ Ⓓ Ⓔ
18. Ⓐ Ⓑ Ⓒ Ⓓ Ⓔ
19. Ⓐ Ⓑ Ⓒ Ⓓ Ⓔ
20. Ⓐ Ⓑ Ⓒ Ⓓ Ⓔ
21. Ⓐ Ⓑ Ⓒ Ⓓ Ⓔ
22. Ⓐ Ⓑ Ⓒ Ⓓ Ⓔ
23. Ⓐ Ⓑ Ⓒ Ⓓ Ⓔ
24. Ⓐ Ⓑ Ⓒ Ⓓ Ⓔ
25. Ⓐ Ⓑ Ⓒ Ⓓ Ⓔ
26. Ⓐ Ⓑ Ⓒ Ⓓ Ⓔ
27. Ⓐ Ⓑ Ⓒ Ⓓ Ⓔ
28. Ⓐ Ⓑ Ⓒ Ⓓ Ⓔ
29. Ⓐ Ⓑ Ⓒ Ⓓ Ⓔ
30. Ⓐ Ⓑ Ⓒ Ⓓ Ⓔ
31. Ⓐ Ⓑ Ⓒ Ⓓ Ⓔ
32. Ⓐ Ⓑ Ⓒ Ⓓ Ⓔ
33. Ⓐ Ⓑ Ⓒ Ⓓ Ⓔ
34. Ⓐ Ⓑ Ⓒ Ⓓ Ⓔ
35. Ⓐ Ⓑ Ⓒ Ⓓ Ⓔ
36. Ⓐ Ⓑ Ⓒ Ⓓ Ⓔ
37. Ⓐ Ⓑ Ⓒ Ⓓ Ⓔ
38. Ⓐ Ⓑ Ⓒ Ⓓ Ⓔ
39. Ⓐ Ⓑ Ⓒ Ⓓ Ⓔ
40. Ⓐ Ⓑ Ⓒ Ⓓ Ⓔ